S0-ADN-006

John DeFrain, PhD
Sylvia M. Asay, PhD
Editors

Strong Families
Around the World:
Strengths-Based Research
and Perspectives

Strong Families Around the World: Strengths-Based Research and Perspectives has been co-published simultaneously as *Marriage & Family Review*, Volume 41, Numbers 1/2 and 3/4 2007.

Pre-publication
REVIEWS,
COMMENTARIES,
EVALUATIONS . . .

"An in-depth understanding of the strengths of families from diverse cultures. . . . AN IMPORTANT ADDITION TO THE FIELD."

Linda Skogrand, PhD
Assistant and Extension Specialist
Department of Family, Consumer,
and Human Development
Utah State University

More pre-publication
REVIEWS, COMMENTARIES, EVALUATIONS . . .

"Provides an INTRIGUING INSIGHT INTO THE CONTEMPORARY CHALLENGES TO THE FAMILY as a social institution and its enduring qualities in rapidly changing cultural contexts around the world."

Mel Gray, PhD
Professor of Social Work
School of Humanities
and Social Sciences
The University of Newcastle
New South Wales, Australia

"FINALLY, A BOOK THAT PROVIDES A FAMILY STRENGTHS PERSPECTIVE THAT IS INTERNATIONAL IN SCOPE and captures the complexity of families today. . . . Provides an alternative to the focus on family problems. . . . Reveals the power of family strengths in dealing with a multitude of changes."

David H. Olson, PhD
Professor Emeritus
University of Minnesota

"Gives us a sound research based view of families from seventeen countries. . . . PROVIDES AN INVALUABLE INSIGHT into the foundations of our lives and the common strengths, which build our societies. . . . This book will provide an invaluable background to human aspirations and ways of coping with challenge. . . . I STRONGLY RECOMMEND THIS BOOK TO ALL STUDENTS AND PEOPLE WORKING TO MAKE A POSITIVE DIFFERENCE TO OUR SOCIETIES. . . . This edited book will improve our global understanding by enhancing our effectiveness at a local level."

Tina Fitchett, MEd(Hons), DipTch., DipHSc
Head of Department
Social Sciences
Manukau Institute of Technology
Auckland, New Zealand

More pre-publication
REVIEWS, COMMENTARIES, EVALUATIONS . . .

"This WONDERFULLY COM-
POSED text also explores
challenges facing the family systems and how service providers
may navigate barriers in service delivery. . . . A well structured and organized book that is HIGHLY
EFFECTIVE in providing a glimpse
into diverse family systems, and it
WILL BE A USEFUL ADDITION
AS A TEXT IN THE CLASS-
ROOM OR TO ANY LIBRARY."

**Joanne Cacciatore, PhD Can-
didate, LMSW**
Fellow in Thanatology
Arizona State University
College of Human Services
Department of Social Work
Federal IVE Program Director

MARCH 20, 2008

FOR OUR DEAR
FRIENDS EILEEN
AND MIKE —

LOVE,
JOHN

The Haworth Press, Inc.

Strong Families
Around the World:
Strengths-Based Research
and Perspectives

Strong Families Around the World: Strengths-Based Research and Perspectives has been co-published simultaneously as *Marriage & Family Review*, Volume 41, Numbers 1/2 and 3/4 2007.

Monographic Separates from *Marriage & Family Review*®

For additional information on these and other Haworth Press titles, including descriptions, tables of contents, reviews, and prices, use the QuickSearch catalog at http://www.HaworthPress.com.

Strong Families Around the World: Strengths-Based Research and Perspectives, edited by John DeFrain, PhD, and Sylvia M. Asay, PhD (Vol. 41, No. 1/2/3/4, 2007). *Insightful exploration of a conceptual framework for understanding family strengths and challenges worldwide.*

Families and Social Policy: National and International Perspectives, edited by Linda Haas and Steven K. Wisensale (Vol. 39, No. 1/2/3/4, 2006). *Examination of current research on the impact of government policy–and lack of government policy–on family life in developed and developing societies.*

The Craft of Teaching About Families: Strategies and Tools, edited by Debra L. Berke and Steven K. Wisensale (Vol. 38, No. 2/3/4, 2005). *"A superb resource for all who teach about families, this collection offers concrete examples focusing on how to teach family policy, research, and clinical techniques effectively. The breadth of coverage is impressive. . . . This book offers an exciting array of ideas and suggestions–all grounded and tested in real classrooms with real students. . . . Should be read cover-to-cover by all of us concerned with teaching the next generation of family scholars, advocates, and practitioners." (Eileen Trzcinski, PhD, Professor and Director of Social Work, Wayne State University)*

Challenges of Aging on U.S. Families: Policy and Practice Implications, edited by Richard K. Caputo, PhD (Vol. 37, No. 1/2, 2005). *Examines the policy and practical implications of the aging United States population, the changes within the family structure, caregiving by various family members, and the overall economic impact.*

Parent-Youth Relations: Cultural and Cross-Cultural Perspectives, edited by Gary W. Peterson, Suzanne K. Steinmetz, and Stephan M. Wilson (Vol. 35, No. 3/4, 2003; Vol. 36, No. 1/2/3/4, 2004). *A comprehensive examination of how culture interconnects with parent-child relationships.*

Emotions and the Family, edited by Richard A. Fabes, PhD (Vol. 34, No. 1/2/3/4 2002). *"An exciting collection. The contributors insightfully unfold the nature of emotions as relational processes in marriage and parenting, and illuminate how emotional communication, competence, and regulation color family life. Chapters on siblings, stepfamilies, economic stress, and family therapy add richness to the collective portrayal of how emotions infuse marital and parent-child relationships. Scholars of marital and family life will find this a valuable resource." (Ross A. Thompson, PhD, Carl A. Happold Distinguished Professor of Psychology, University of Nebraska)*

Gene-Environment Processes in Social Behaviors and Relationships, edited by Kirby Deater-Deckard, PhD, and Stephen A. Petrill, PhD (Vol. 33, No. 1/2/3, 2002). *"During recent years there have been somewhat fruitless battles on whether family influences or peer influences are more important in children's psychological development. This book is both innovative and helpful in seeking to bring the two sets of influences together through a range of studies using twin, adoptee, and stepfamily designs to assess how genetic and environmental influences may work together in bringing about individual differences in children's emotions, behavior and especially social relationships. The different research approaches provide some new ways of thinking about, and investigating, how interpersonal relationships develop and have their effects." (Michael Rutter, MD, FRS, Professor of Developmental Psychopathology, Institute of Psychiatry, King's College, London)*

Pioneering Paths in the Study of Families: The Lives and Careers of Family Scholars, edited by Suzanne K. Steinmetz, PhD, MSW, and Gary W. Peterson, PhD (Vol. 30, No. 3, 2000; Vol. 30, No. 4, 2001; Vol. 31, No. 1/2/3/4, 2001; Vol. 32, No. 1/2, 2001). *The fascinating autobiographies of 40 leading scholars in sociology, family studies, psychology, and child development.*

FATHERHOOD: Research, Interventions and Policies, edited by H. Elizabeth Peters, PhD, Gary W. Peterson, PhD, Suzanne K. Steinmetz, PhD, MSW, and Randal D. Day, PhD (Vol. 29, No. 2/3/4, 2000). *Brings together the latest facts to help researchers explore the father-child relationship and determine what factors lead fathers to be more or less involved in the lives of their children, including human social behavior, not living with a child, being denied visiting privileges, and social norms regarding gender differences versus work responsibilities.*

Concepts and Definitions of Family for the 21st Century, edited by Barbara H. Settles, PhD, Suzanne K. Steinmetz, PhD, MSW, Gary W. Peterson, PhD, and Marvin B. Sussman, PhD (Vol. 28, No. 3/4, 1999). *Views family from a U.S. perspective and from many different cultures and societies. The controversial question "What is family?" is thoroughly examined as it has become an increasingly important social policy concern in recent years as the traditional family has changed.*

The Role of the Hospitality Industry in the Lives of Individuals and Families, edited by Pamela R. Cummings, PhD, Francis A. Kwansa, PhD, and Marvin B. Sussman, PhD (Vol. 28, No. 1/2, 1998). *"A must for human resource directors and hospitality educators." (Dr. Lynn Huffman, Director, Restaurant, Hotel, and Institutional Management, Texas Tech University, Lubbock, Texas)*

Stepfamilies: History, Research, and Policy, edited by Irene Levin, PhD, and Marvin B. Sussman, PhD (Vol. 26, No. 1/2/3/4, 1997). *"A wide range of individually valuable and stimulating chapters that form a wonderfully rich menu from which readers of many different kinds will find exciting and satisfying selections." (Jon Bernardes, PhD, Principal Lecturer in Sociology, University of Wolverhampton, Castle View Dudley, United Kingdom)*

Families and Adoption, edited by Harriet E. Gross, PhD, and Marvin B. Sussman, PhD (Vol. 25, No. 1/2/3/4, 1997). *"Written in a lucid and easy-to-read style, this volume will make an invaluable contribution to the adoption literature." (Paul Sachdev, PhD, Professor, School of Social Work, Memorial University of Newfoundland, St. John's, Newfoundland, Canada)*

The Methods and Methodologies of Qualitative Family Research, edited by Jane F. Gilgun, PhD, LICSW, and Marvin B. Sussman, PhD (Vol 24, No. 1/2/3/4, 1997). *"An authoritative look at the usefulness of qualitative research methods to the family scholar." (Family Relations)*

Intercultural Variation in Family Research and Theory: Implications for Cross-National Studies, Volumes I and II, edited by Marvin B. Sussman, PhD, and Roma S. Hanks, PhD (Vol. 22, No. 1/2/3/4, and Vol. 23, No. 1/2/3/4, 1997). *Documents the development of family research in theory in societies around the world and inspires continued cross-national collaboration on current research topics.*

Families and Law, edited by Lisa J. McIntyre, PhD, and Marvin B. Sussman, PhD (Vol. 21, No. 3/4, 1995). *With this new volume, family practitioners and scholars can begin to increase the family's position in relation to the law and legal system.*

Exemplary Social Intervention Programs for Members and Their Families, edited by David Guttmann, DSW, and Marvin B. Sussman, PhD (Vol. 21, No. 1/2, 1995). *An eye-opening look at organizations and individuals who have created model family programs that bring desired results.*

Single Parent Families: Diversity, Myths and Realities, edited by Shirley M. H. Hanson, RN, PhD, Marsha L. Heims, RN, EdD, Doris J. Julian, RN, EdD, and Marvin B. Sussman, PhD (Vol. 20, No. 1/2/3/4, 1994). *"Remarkable! . . . A significant work and is important reading for multidisciplinary family professionals including sociologists, educators, health care professionals, and policymakers." (Maureen Leahey, RN, PhD, Director, Outpatient Mental Health Program, Director, Family Therapy Training Program, Calgary District Hospital Group)*

Families on the Move: Immigration, Migration, and Mobility, edited by Barbara H. Settles, PhD, Daniel E. Hanks III, MS, and Marvin B. Sussman, PhD (Vol 19, No 1/2/3/4, 1993). *Examines the current research on family mobility, migration, and immigration and discovers new directions for understanding the relationship between mobility and family life.*

American Families and the Future: Analyses of Possible Destinies, edited by Barbara H. Settles, PhD, Roma S. Hanks, PhD, and Marvin B. Sussman, PhD (Vol. 18, No. 3/4, 1993). *This book discusses a variety of issues that face and will continue to face families in coming years and describes various strategies families can use in their decision-making processes.*

Publishing in Journals on the Family: Essays on Publishing, edited by Roma S. Hanks, PhD, Linda Matocha, PhD, RN, and Marvin B. Sussman, PhD (Vol. 18, No. 1/2, 1993). *This helpful book contains varied perspectives from scholars at different career stages and from editors of major publication outlets, providing readers with important information necessary to help them systematically plan a productive scholarly career.*

Publishing in Journals on the Family: A Survey and Guide for Scholars, Practitioners, and Students, edited by Roma S. Hanks, PhD, Linda Matocha, PhD, RN, and Marvin B. Sussman, PhD (Vol. 17, No. 3/4, 1992). *"Comprehensive. . . . Includes listings for some 200 social science journals whose editors have expressed an interest in publishing empirical research and theoretical articles about the family." (Reference & Research Book News)*

ALL HAWORTH BOOKS AND JOURNALS
ARE PRINTED ON CERTIFIED
ACID-FREE PAPER

Strong Families Around the World: Strengths-Based Research and Perspectives

John DeFrain, PhD
Sylvia M. Asay, PhD
Editors

Strong Families Around the World: Strengths-Based Research and Perspectives has been co-published simultaneously as *Marriage & Family Review*, Volume 41, Numbers 1/2 and 3/4 2007.

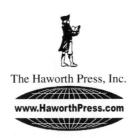

The Haworth Press, Inc.
www.HaworthPress.com

Strong Families Around the World: Strengths-Based Research and Perspectives has been co-published simultaneously as *Marriage & Family Review*, Volume 41, Numbers 1/2 and 3/4 2007.

© 2007 by The Haworth Press, Inc. All rights reserved. No part of this work may be reproduced or utilized in any form or by any means, electronic or mechanical, including photocopying, microfilm and recording, or by any information storage and retrieval system, without permission in writing from the publisher. Printed in the United States of America.

The development, preparation, and publication of this work has been undertaken with great care. However, the publisher, employees, editors, and agents of The Haworth Press and all imprints of The Haworth Press, Inc., including The Haworth Medical Press® and Pharmaceutical Products Press®, are not responsible for any errors contained herein or for consequences that may ensue from use of materials or information contained in this work. With regard to case studies, identities and circumstances of individuals discussed herein have been changed to protect confidentiality. Any resemblance to actual persons, living or dead, is entirely coincidental.

The Haworth Press is committed to the dissemination of ideas and information according to the highest standards of intellectual freedom and the free exchange of ideas. Statements made and opinions expressed in this publication do not necessarily reflect the views of the Publisher, Directors, management, or staff of The Haworth Press, Inc., or an endorsement by them.

The Haworth Press, Inc., 10 Alice Street, Binghamton, NY 13904-1580 USA

Library of Congress Cataloging-in-Publication Data

Strong families around the world : strengths-based research and perspectives / John DeFrain, Sylvia M. Asay, editors.
     p. cm.
     "Co-published simultaneously as Marriage & Family Review, Volume 41, Numbers 1/2 and 3/4 2007."
     Includes bibliographical references and index.
     ISBN 978-0-7890-3603-2 (hard cover : alk. paper)–ISBN 978-0-7890-3604-9 (soft cover : alk. paper)
     1. Family. I. DeFrain, John D. II. Asay, Sylvia M. III. Marriage & family review.
HQ734.S9739 2007
306.85–dc22

                        2007034091

The HAWORTH PRESS Inc.
Abstracting, Indexing & Outward Linking
PRINT *and* ELECTRONIC BOOKS & JOURNALS

This section provides you with a list of major indexing & abstracting services and other tools for bibliographic access. That is to say, each service began covering this periodical during the year noted in the right column. Most Websites which are listed below have indicated that they will either post, disseminate, compile, archive, cite or alert their own Website users with research-based content from this work. (This list is as current as the copyright date of this publication.)

Abstracting, Website/Indexing Coverage . . . . Year When Coverage Began

- ****Research Library Core (ProQuest CSA)****
  <http://www.proquest.com> **2006**
- *International Bibliography of Book Reviews on the Humanities and Social Sciences (IBR) (Thomson) <http://www.saur.de>* **2006**
- ****Academic ASAP (Thomson Gale)**** **1989**
- ****Academic Search Premier (EBSCO)****
  <http://search.ebscohost.com> **1993**
- ****Applied Social Sciences Index & Abstracts (ASSIA) (ProQuest CSA)**** *<http://www.csa.com>* **1993**
- ****Expanded Academic ASAP (Thomson Gale)**** **1989**
- ****Expanded Academic ASAP – International (Thomson Gale)**** . . . **1989**
- ****Expanded Academic Index (Thomson Gale)**** . . . . *
- ****InfoTrac Custom (Thomson Gale)**** **1996**
- ****InfoTrac OneFile (Thomson Gale)**** **1989**
- ****MasterFILE Premier (EBSCO)****
  <http://search.ebscohost.com> **2006**
- ****ProQuest Academic Research Library (ProQuest CSA)****
  <http://www.proquest.com> **1993**
- ****Psychological Abstracts (PsycINFO)**** *<http://www.apa.org>* . . . **1978**
- ****Research Library (ProQuest CSA)**** *<http://www.proquest.com>* . . **2006**

(continued)

(continued)

(continued)

Bibliographic Access

- *Cabell's Directory of Publishing Opportunities in Psychology <http://www.cabells.com>*
- *MedBioWorld <http://www.medbioworld.com>*
- *MediaFinder <http://www.mediafinder.com/>*
- *Ulrich's Periodicals Directory: The Global Source for Periodicals Information Since 1932 <http://www.bowkerlink.com>*

*Exact start date to come.

Special Bibliographic Notes related to special journal issues (separates) and indexing/abstracting:

- indexing/abstracting services in this list will also cover material in any "separate" that is co-published simultaneously with Haworth's special thematic journal issue or DocuSerial. Indexing/abstracting usually covers material at the article/chapter level.
- monographic co-editions are intended for either non-subscribers or libraries which intend to purchase a second copy for their circulating collections.
- monographic co-editions are reported to all jobbers/wholesalers/approval plans. The source journal is listed as the "series" to assist the prevention of duplicate purchasing in the same manner utilized for books-in-series.
- to facilitate user/access services all indexing/abstracting services are encouraged to utilize the co-indexing entry note indicated at the bottom of the first page of each article/chapter/contribution.
- this is intended to assist a library user of any reference tool (whether print, electronic, online, or CD-ROM) to locate the monographic version if the library has purchased this version but not a subscription to the source journal.
- individual articles/chapters in any Haworth publication are also available through the Haworth Document Delivery Service (HDDS).

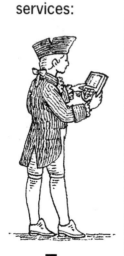

As part of
Haworth's
continuing
commitment
to better serve
our library
patrons,
we are
proud to
be working
with the
following
electronic
services:

AGGREGATOR SERVICES

EBSCOhost

Ingenta

J-Gate

Minerva

OCLC FirstSearch

Oxmill

SwetsWise

FirstSearch

Oxmill Publishing

SwetsWise

LINK RESOLVER SERVICES

1Cate (Openly Informatics)

ChemPort
(American Chemical Society)

CrossRef

Gold Rush (Coalliance)

LinkOut (PubMed)

LINKplus (Atypon)

LinkSolver (Ovid)

LinkSource with A-to-Z (EBSCO)

Resource Linker (Ulrich)

SerialsSolutions (ProQuest)

SFX (Ex Libris)

Sirsi Resolver (SirsiDynix)

Tour (TDnet)

Vlink (Extensity, formerly Geac)

WebBridge (Innovative Interfaces)

ChemPort

Gold Rush

LinkOut.
LINKING TO A WORLD OF RESOURCES

atypon

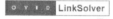
LinkSolver

ULRICH'S
RESOURCE LINKER

SerialsSolutions

S·F·X

SirsiDynix

TOUR

extensity

WebBridge

Strong Families Around the World: Strengths-Based Research and Perspectives

CONTENTS

THE MIDDLE EAST

ASIA

OCEANIA

ABOUT THE EDITORS

John DeFrain, PhD, is Extension Professor of family and community development at the University of Nebraska-Lincoln where he has been a faculty member for 32 years. His work at UNL has centered on family strengths and families in crisis. He co-founded the marital and family therapy program at UNL in 1976; was a co-founder of the National and International Building Family Strengths Symposium series that has sponsored more than 30 conferences worldwide since 1977; and currently is working to create an International Building Family Strengths Network to encourage global cooperation on behalf of families. Dr. DeFrain has coauthored and co-edited 23 books and more than 100 professional articles, including *Marriages and Families: Intimacy, Diversity, and Strengths* (5th Edition), *Building Relationships, Secrets of Strong Families, On Our Own: A Single Parent's Survival Guide, Parents in Contemporary America, Sudden Infant Death: Enduring the Loss, We Cry Out: Living with Developmental Disabilities, Stillbirth: The Invisible Death*, and *Family Treasures: Creating Strong Families*.

Sylvia M. Asay, PhD, is Associate Professor of Family Studies at the University of Nebraska at Kearney. Her research has focused on family strengths in post-communist countries and she has written several articles that describe her qualitative approach. She received a fellowship for the German and American Young Scholars' Institute from the Social Science Research Council to study post-communist transition. In addition, she has worked to develop the Cultural Transformation Model to describe the impact of students' international experiences. Dr. Asay has authored two editions of the Instructor's Manual and Test Bank for a marriage and family relationships textbook.

Comments

This collection of articles in *Strong Families Around the World* provides some insights into the challenges and strengths that are experienced by families living in 18 countries representing seven distinct geographic areas. All families in the 21st century are facing challenges, but disadvantaged populations–the indigenous natives and recent immigrants from third world countries–experience additional challenges. These are a concern, not just for citizens of the U.S., but also citizens of other countries. In the last decade or so, unprotected borders and undocumented immigration results in security issues as well as the social service, law enforcement and educational costs to borderline states (e.g., California, Arizona, New Mexico and Texas in the U.S.). These concerns, however, are not limited to the United States. Throughout Europe, South America, Africa, Asia and the Middle East, conflicts results as immigrants seeking a better life crowd the border towns of countries seen as providing a higher standard of living.

The United States has essentially been settled by those from other countries. Except for the indigenous native, all of us represent immigrants from other places in the world. In some cases this is the result of colonization which opened the borders between the colonizing nation and the nation being colonized. The large population of citizens of Indian descent in England is an example of this. In other cases, the dumping of less desirable citizens into an undeveloped country as an alternative to prison served two purposes–ridding the more developed country of undesirables, at the same time providing a workforce for newly developing country. The new colonies in the U.S., especially Georgia received immigrants from Britain (Penal Code, 2006) as did New Zealand and Australia (Synge, 2006). Capturing individuals from less developed countries and enslaving them also increased the popula-

[Haworth co-indexing entry note]: "Comments." Steinmetz, Suzanne K. Co-published simultaneously in *Marriage & Family Review* (The Haworth Press, Inc.) Vol. 41, No. 1/2, 2007, pp. xxi-xxiii; and: *Strong Families Around the World: Strengths-Based Research and Perspectives* (ed: John DeFrain, and Sylvia M. Asay) The Haworth Press, Inc., 2007, pp. xix-xxi. Single or multiple copies of this article are available for a fee from The Haworth Document Delivery Service [1-800-HAWORTH, 9:00 a.m. - 5:00 p.m. (EST). E-mail address: docdelivery@haworthpress.com].

Available online at http://mfr.haworthpress.com
© 2007 by The Haworth Press, Inc. All rights reserved. *xix*

tion of the U.S. and Mexico. Some individuals, as the result of wars and captured lands, became immigrants without ever moving when the area became part of another country. During the 18th and 19th centuries, many under-populated countries, e.g., the U.S., New Zealand or Australia, actively encouraged immigration to settle the newly opened frontiers, to till the vast farmland, or to build the railroad. However, some of these immigrants, once welcomed, have become a disadvantaged minority, in a manner similar to the indigenous population displaced by the newcomers–a phenomena seen in numerous countries across countries representing different levels of development. To survive, these families show tremendous strength in the face of adversity.

The chapters in this collection are valuable because they help us understand the social and cultural uniqueness of countries whose citizens have immigrated to the United States and many other countries that have welcomed them. While the diversity of families is clearly articulated, and there are characteristics that distinctly represent each country, their challenges, and their strengths, the similarities among all countries is also obvious.

Strong Families Around the World, a two-part collection edited by John DeFrain and Sylvia Asay is a valuable resource for those studying families in diverse cultures. Understanding the historical, cultural, geopolitical, and religious influences on families in different countries, not only provides valuable insights on families in these countries, it provides a better understanding of families from these cultures who now comprise the populations of other societies. DeFrain and Asay have assembled a rich collection written by family scholars from each country represented, arranged into seven geographic areas: Africa, the Middle East, Asia, Oceania, North America, Latin America and Europe. They have provided a wealth of information on the challenges families face, but more important the strengths that characterize these families.

The "Strength Perspective" focuses on the resilience and flexibility that enables families to adjust to the challenges in the 21st century. It is by understanding how families adjust and overcome adversity, that we can gain an understanding that will facilitate transmitting these skills to other families who are facing adversity. Ultimately, in order to adequately address the challenges that all families face, our theories, research and intervention programs will need to fully account for the multidimensional complexity of families and build on these strengths throughout the world.

NOTE

I want to acknowledge Sean Ascani for editorial assistance.

REFERENCES

Synge, M.B. The Rein of Queen Victoria. Retreived on November 9, 2006 from http://
   www.mainlesson.com/display.php?author=synge&book=victoria&story=emigrants&
   PHPSESSID=a9af92f6da162442c959ea53f7316082
Penal Colony. Retrieved on November 9, 2006 from http://en.wikipedia.org/wiki/
   Penal_colony

Suzanne K. Steinmetz
General Editor
Marriage & Family Review

Preface:
Family Strengths from a Cross-Cultural and Theoretical Perspective

I am very pleased to make some initial comments about this very important collection of original articles edited by John DeFrain and Sylvia Asay, both about its major accomplishments and briefly describe some theoretical implications of the family strengths perspective. This project should be viewed as the best collection of chapters currently in existence on an important aspect of family studies from a cross-cultural perspective.

A family strengths perspective is the central theme of this work which seeks to pursue the very worthy goal of identifying common aspects of families that serve as resources for dealing with normative and non-normative challenges during the life course. Such a perspective guides us to focus primarily on the family systemic unit of analysis rather than the individual unit of analysis–or the central theme of this edited book is that *family relationships* are the primary target of a family strengths perspective, not the psychological make-up of distinct persons. At the very least, this perspective focuses on the consequence of family systemic-level phenomena or "family strengths" on the experience and well-being of individuals who together form families.

Even more important is the idea here that family systemic phenomena, or family strengths, must be examined and understood from a cultural perspective, an approach that much of Western social science has failed to consider at the forefront of making sense of the social world (Berry, Poortinga, Segall, Dasen, 2002; Kagitcibasi, 1996). A central assumption in this edited book is that family life around the globe may

[Haworth co-indexing entry note]: "Preface: Family Strengths from a Cross-Cultural and Theoretical Perspective." Peterson, Gary W. Co-published simultaneously in *Marriage & Family Review* (The Haworth Press, Inc.) Vol. 41, No. 1/2, 2007, pp. xxv-xxix; and: *Strong Families Around the World: Strengths-Based Research and Perspectives* (ed: John DeFrain, and Sylvia M. Asay) The Haworth Press, Inc., 2007, pp. xxiii-xxvii. Single or multiple copies of this article are available for a fee from The Haworth Document Delivery Service [1-800-HAWORTH, 9:00 a.m. - 5:00 p.m. (EST). E-mail address: docdelivery@haworthpress.com].

Available online at http://mfr.haworthpress.com
© 2007 by The Haworth Press, Inc. All rights reserved.

have common dimensions of family strength but, with the important caveat, that what is specifically defined as a *strength* is shaped in formative ways by cultural diversity around the globe. Examining family strengths from a cultural or cross-cultural perspective, in my view, means that families should be scrutinized both for patterns shared across cultures that approach universality (i.e., referred to as *universalism*) and for evidence of distinctiveness provided by each culture (i.e., referred to as cultural *relativism*).

Considerable controversy exists, of course, between the perspectives of *cultural universalism* versus *cultural relativity* for studying both family life in general and family strengths in particular. Based on their work, DeFrain and Asay take the reasonable position that certain aspects of family life may be evident across cultures in similar ways that define what they believe to be "strength" within families. These basic building blocks of family strength include (1) appreciation and affection, (2) commitment, (3) positive communication, (4) spending enjoyable time together, (5) spiritual well-being, and (6) the ability to manage stress and crisis effectively (DeFrain & Stinnett, 2002). By identifying these commonalities across cultures, DeFrain and Asay lean toward an *etic* approach to cross-cultural social science, which means that family relationships can be assumed to have some invariant patterns that exist across social groups. Consequently, there is an element of the "outsider's" view here in the sense that comparative analysis is being used to identify commonalities that may be universal across cultures.

That very fact, however, that the authors of these chapters are native to the cultures they are writing about balances this edited collection with the *emic* tradition, the alternative perspective to an etic viewpoint. An emic, or relativist approach, is used to view family strengths from an "insiders" perspective, making sure that the meanings, values, and norms from a specific culture being examined are taken into account and used for making interpretations. A consistent emic view would focus on family strengths within one culture and fosters the belief that making comparisons across communities is a risky venture to avoid.

Although these strategies are often posed as being at odds, I prefer the middle ground position that studies of emic, or indigenous relationship patterns, and etic, or comparative searches for cross-cultural patterns, are not opposites but are complementary. It is very likely that many shades of gray exist between discovering cultural similarity and cultural originality in family strengths. Efforts to characterize these approaches as being fundamentally antagonistic strikes me as a process of building false dichotomies that are much more simplistic than the circumstances that exist in social life. I view such a perspective as an exercise in categorical thinking (and the creation of false categories)–when, in fact, the two strategies for viewing cultural life can be used in a complementary manner to enrich each other. Much like the idea that clear social expectations for human behavior may exist in some circumstances and transcend cultural boundaries, it is also true that many areas of social life are left ambiguous for creative interpretation by individuals and cultural creativity across communities.

An example of compatibility between the search for "universal family strengths" and recognition of cultural originality would be within the area of general family strength described as *appreciation and affection.* Certainly, it would seem to be a safe bet that most, if not all families around the globe, have ways of fostering cohesiveness in their relationships by expressing behavior and emotions that communicate appreciation, affection, warmth, nurturance or similar ideas. Consequently, it is very accurate for a family strengths model to identify this critical dimension of social life as a key feature that helps to bind together individuals who participate in the great diversity of family structures and relationships around the globe. However, *exactly how* this appreciation and affection (i.e., a general family strength) is expressed in specific detail may vary greatly, depending on specific norms that govern gender roles, authority structures, parent-child relations, marital roles, interpersonal relationships, intimacy, and sexuality in a diverse array of cultures. For example, within one culture, affection may emphasize direct, egalitarian expressions of physical affection, overt praise, and eye-to eye contact, whereas, in other cultures, affection is more commonly a covert or more indirect expression involving respect for authority, obedience to the demands of elders, spending positive time with each other, and loyalty to elders' teachings. As a result of this specific cultural variation within a generalized family strength, I am a strong advocate of constantly trying to identify similarities across cultures but also believe in using caution about asserting that common patterns at a general level have exactly the same meaning and consequence across cultures. Consequently, in my view, the best stance to take on these issues is that the *ethnocentric* perspective or the "one size fits all" view is an oversimplification of what it means to find commonality across cultures. Instead, the most accurate view of "universalism" is that substantial differences do exist across cultures, but most probably within the context of general similarities that all families tend to share regardless of culture, ethnicity, gender, class, and structure. Consequently, "universals" do exist but cultural diversity within family strengths is likely to be found in the details that are nestled within broader commonalities.

A final comment relates to my view that a family strengths perspective is a very valuable *theory of middle range* in the sense that it identifies a basic aspect of family life that explains how families function effectively and adapt (i.e., aspects of family relationships that provide "strength" or resources for meeting the challenges of development and social life). It draws our attention to a positive view of family life and provides a counter perspective to social scientists who study families primarily from a social problems viewpoint.

Given this major conceptual achievement, further conceptual thinking is now needed to link family strengths ideas to more general theory that exists about family relationships (White, 2005; White & Klein, 2002). For example, we should probably consider how family strengths can be conceptualized from a family systems perspective. Should family strengths, for example, be conceptualized as having an *equal balance* between process mechanisms in relationships emphasizing morphogenesis versus homeostasis or would different cultures lean one direction or another in terms of which of these processes is emphasized? In contrast, from a conflict theory perspective, should family strengths be defined as family relationships where conflict is managed sufficiently to foster reasonable stability, but without eliminating inevitable conflicts that foster necessary developmental change within families across the life course? Turning to exchange theory, the question arises–Would a strong family be one where there is equity in the social exchanges that occur among family members (e.g., a fair balance of rewards and costs received across family members) within relationships and a sense of distributive justice (i.e., a feeling of receiving sufficient rewards for the investments incurred) that is prevalent across family members? And finally, from a symbolic interaction-role viewpoint, would a family demonstrate strength when members define their relationships as meeting their role expectations, without experiencing high levels of role discrepancies that may foster dissatisfaction and instability in family life?

The major point here is that I strongly encourage readers of this volume to benefit from this benchmark volume by examining these excellent chapters and then think about the theoretical implications of a family strengths perspective. This volume should be used as a primary basis for further work that is, in part, a theoretical exploration aimed at gaining greater understanding of what family strengths consist across cultures. Specifically, how can we use this valuable perspective and use it to increase our understanding of families by linking it to other theoretical perspectives at an increasingly general level of analysis? I congratulate John DeFrain, Sylvia Asay, and the authors of these articles for creating such a major scholarly work that provides so much knowledge about family strengths across cultures.

REFERENCES

Berry, J.W., Poortinga, Y.H., Segall, M.H., & Dasen, P.R. (2002). *Cross-cultural psychology: Research and applications.* Cambridge, MA: Cambridge University Press.

DeFrain, J., & Stinnett, N. (2002). Family strengths. In J.J. Ponzetti et al. (Eds.), *International encyclopedia of marriage and family* (2nd Ed.). New York: Macmillan Reference. Group.

Kagitcibasi, C. (1996). *Family and human development across cultures: A view from the other side.* Mahwah, NJ: Lawrence Erlbaum Associates.

White, J. A. (2005). *Advancing family theories.* Thousand Oaks, CA: Sage.

White, J.M. & Klein, D.M. (2002). *Family theories.* Thousand Oaks, CA: Sage Publications.

Gary W. Peterson
Professor and Chair
Department of Family Studies and Social Work
Miami University
Oxford, OH

Strong Families Around the World: An Introduction to the Family Strengths Perspective

John DeFrain
Sylvia M. Asay

SUMMARY. The family is one of society's oldest and most resilient institutions. Although the structure of the family may vary around the world, the value of *family* endures. Most of the research on families, historically speaking, has focused primarily on the problems or weaknesses of families. Over the past three decades, researchers have studied families from a strengths-based perspective. Around the world researchers have found that families are amazingly similar. The similarities point to a set of qualities that describe the characteristics of strong families. These qualities are showing appreciation and affection, commitment, positive communication, enjoyable times together, spiritual well-being, and the ability to manage stress and crisis effectively. Twenty-two propositions have also been suggested that have relevance in how we look at families in general. The information has relevance and purpose and should serve to inform and expand our thinking about families. The information may have significance to some specific areas and particular fields, especially to the areas of family services, family education, marital and family therapy, and social policy. doi:10.1300/J002v41n01_01

[Haworth co-indexing entry note]: "Strong Families Around the World: An Introduction to the Family Strengths Perspective." DeFrain, John and Sylvia M. Asay. Co-published simultaneously in *Marriage & Family Review* (The Haworth Press, Inc.) Vol. 41, No. 1/2, 2007, pp. 1-10; and: *Strong Families Around the World: Strengths-Based Research and Perspectives* (ed: John DeFrain, and Sylvia M. Asay) The Haworth Press, Inc., 2007, pp. 1-10. Single or multiple copies of this article are available for a fee from The Haworth Document Delivery Service [1-800-HAWORTH, 9:00 a.m. - 5:00 p.m. (EST). E-mail address: docdelivery@haworthpress.com].

Available online at http://mfr.haworthpress.com
© 2007 by The Haworth Press, Inc. All rights reserved.
doi:10.1300/J002v41n01_01

[Article copies available for a fee from The Haworth Document Delivery Service: 1-800-HAWORTH. E-mail address: <docdelivery@haworthpress.com> Website: <http://www.HaworthPress.com> © 2007 by The Haworth Press, Inc. All rights reserved.]

KEYWORDS. Cross-cultural families, family strengths, international family strengths network, strengths-based perspective, strengths-based practice, strong families

WHY ARE STRONG FAMILIES SO IMPORTANT?

The family is perhaps society's oldest and most resilient institution. Around the world the family is valued and celebrated. From the beginning of human life on Earth, people have grouped themselves into families to find emotional, physical and collective support. Although in recent years there have been those who have predicted the failure of both marriage and the family, they not only survive but continue to change and evolve. The structure of the family may vary around the world, and yet, the value of *family* endures. People still bond into couples and seek the long-term commitment that marriage promises, even if this does not always happen. Children are born and cherished even when there is economic or political upheaval.

Families–in all their amazing diversity–are the basic, foundational social units in every society, as far as we know. Therefore, healthy individuals within healthy families are essentially at the core of a healthy society. It is the responsibility of society and in everyone's best interest to help create a positive environment for all families. This can be a labor of love for all of our social institutions: educational institutions, businesses, human and family service agencies, religious institutions, the military, health organizations, literally everyone involved in the daily life of a community.

Families are our most intimate social environment. They are the places where we begin the vital processes of socializing our children: teaching them–in partnership with countless others in the community–how to survive and thrive in the world. Life in families can bring us great joy or excruciating pain, depending upon how well family relationships are unfolding. A healthy marriage and family can be a valuable resource for helping us endure difficulties that life inevitably brings. On the other hand, unhealthy or dysfunctional relationships can create serious problems that may persist from one generation to the next.

Family Life from a Strengths-Based Perspective

Since the beginning of the 20th Century, family theorists have tried to create a theory or framework that explains the family and the place that it holds within society. According to White (2005), early family theory focused on the place of the family in American culture, creating frameworks that borrowed from other disciplines such as anthropology and economics. In the last half of the 20th century, the focus moved to the functions of the family using typologies to classify families. An interest in cross-cultural comparisons also led to a new look at previous perspectives in an effort to internationalize family theory. Since that time, researchers have largely failed to advance any new theories about the family. Is it possible that the reason that no one theory or new emerging theory has come to explain families around the world in the 21st century is that the uniqueness of families and the various ways that families function cannot be collected into one understanding?

The focus on family strengths brings into a more reasonable balance our understanding of how families succeed in the face of life's inherent difficulties. By concentrating only on a family's problems and a family's failings, we ignore the fact that it takes a positive approach in life to succeed. The family strengths perspective is a world-view or orientation toward life and families that is positive and optimistic, grounded in research conducted around the world. It does not ignore family problems but restores them to their proper place in life: as vehicles for testing our capacities as families and reaffirming our vital human connections with each other.

A HISTORICAL PERSPECTIVE ON FAMILY STRENGTHS RESEARCH

Most of the research on families, historically speaking, has focused primarily on the problems or weaknesses of families or the individuals within the family. Early research on family strengths began in the 1930s with Woodhouse's study of 250 successful families during the Great Depression, followed by Otto's work on strong families and family strengths in the early 1960s (Gabler & Otto, 1964; Otto, 1962, 1963).

Not until the 1970s did family strengths begin to gain momentum when Nick Stinnett began his work at Oklahoma State University in 1974 and subsequently at the University of Nebraska in 1977. Stinnett, DeFrain and their many colleagues then began publishing a continuous series of articles and books (Casas, et al, 1984; DeFrain, DeFrain, & Lepard, 1994; DeFrain & Stinnett, 2002; Olson & DeFrain, 2006; Stinnett & DeFrain, 1985; Stinnett & O'Donnell, 1996; Stinnett & Sauer, 1977; Xie, DeFrain, Meredith, & Combs, 1996). Family strengths conferences, beginning in 1978, proved to be a catalyst for research on strong families. Nine volumes of proceedings were published as a result of the National Symposium on Building Family Strengths series (Stinnett, Chesser, & DeFrain, 1979; Stinnett, Chesser, DeFrain, & Knaub, 1980; Stinnett, DeFrain, et al., 1981; Stinnett, DeFrain, et al., 1982; Rowe, DeFrain, et al., 1984; Williams, Lingren, et al., 1985; VanZandt, Lingren, et al, 1986; Lingren, et al., 1987). An International Family Strengths Network (IFSN) began working on a series of family strengths gatherings in the late 1990s, and to date there have been more than 30 conferences held in North America, Asia and Australia with upcoming gatherings planned for Africa, Europe, the Middle East, North America and Australia.

Over the past three decades researchers at the University of Nebraska–Lincoln led by John DeFrain, at the University of Alabama-Tuscaloosa led by Nick Stinnett, at the University of Minnesota-St. Paul led by David H. Olson, plus affiliated institutions in the United States and around the world have studied families from a strengths-based perspective. The similarities that are found among research with families globally point to a set of qualities that describe the characteristics of strong families. When people from country to country and culture to culture talk about what makes their family strong, these are some of the traits they identify:

Appreciation and Affection
Caring for each other
Friendship
Respect for Individuality
Playfulness
Humor

Commitment
Trust
Honesty
Dependability
Faithfulness
Sharing

Positive Communication
Giving compliments
Sharing feelings
Avoiding blame
Being able to compromise
Agreeing to disagree

Enjoyable Time Together
Quality time in great quantity
Good things take time
Enjoying each other's company
Simple good times
Sharing fun times

Spiritual Well-Being	**The Ability to Manage Stress and Crisis Effectively**
Hope	Adaptability
Faith	Seeing crises as challenges and opportunities
Compassion	Growing through crises together
Shared ethical values	Openness to change
Oneness with humankind	Resilience

Research on strong families has not only resulted in models for better understanding the qualities of strong families; it has also suggested a number of propositions that have relevance in how we look at families in general, and how we can successfully live in our own families.

Twenty-Two Propositions Derived from the Family Strengths Research

Understanding the family is not a static set of ideas or rigorously-testable hypotheses, but more like a family itself: a constantly growing and changing dialogue about the nature of strong marriages and strong families. Our training as skeptical social and behavioral scientists teaches us to be very cautious when talking about universals. And yet our studies of strong families in North and South America, Europe, Africa, Asia, and Oceania, lead us to the conclusion that there are remarkable similarities among families who feel good about their lives together and express satisfaction in their competence in dealing with the challenges that life brings. These similarities are much more apparent than the differences from culture to culture.

Over the past three decades, researchers looking at couples and families from a strengths perspective have developed a number of propositions derived from their work around the world that we believe merit serious consideration:

- *Families, in all their remarkable diversity, are the basic foundation of human cultures.* Strong families are critical to the development of strong communities, and strong communities promote and nurture strong families.
- *All families have strengths.* And, all families have challenges and areas of potential growth. If one looks only for problems in a family, one will see only problems. If one also looks for strengths, one will find strengths.
- *It's not about structure, it's about function.* When talking about families, it is common to make the mistake of focusing on external family structure or the type of family rather than internal family functioning. But, the fact is there are strong single-parent families,

strong stepfamilies, strong nuclear families, strong extended families, strong families with gay and lesbian members, strong two-parent families, and so forth.

- *Strong marriages are the center of many strong families.* The couple relationship is an important source of strength in many families with children who are doing well. Parents need to find ways to nurture a positive couple relationship for the good of everyone in the family.
- *Strong families tend to produce great kids*; and a good place to look for great kids is in strong families.
- *If you grew up in a strong family as a child, it will probably be easier for you to create a strong family of your own as an adult.* But, it's also quite possible to do so if you weren't so lucky and grew up in a seriously troubled family.
- *The relationship between money and family strengths is tenuous.* Once a family has adequate financial resources the relentless quest for *more* is not likely to increase the family's quality of life, happiness together, or the strength of their relationships with each other.
- *Strengths develop over time.* When couples start out in life together, they sometimes have considerable difficulty adjusting to each other, and these difficulties are quite predictable. Adjusting to each other is not an easy task. Many couples who are unstable at first end up creating a healthy, happy family.
- *Strengths are often developed in response to challenges.* A couple and family's strengths are tested by life's everyday stressors and also by the significant crises that all of us face sooner or later.
- *Strong families don't tend to think much about their strengths, they just live them.* It is, however, useful to carefully examine a family's strengths and discuss precisely how family members use them to great advantage.
- *Strong families, like people, are not perfect.* Even in the strongest of families we can sometimes be like porcupines: prickly, disagreeable, eager and ready to enjoy conflict with each other. But we also have a considerable need to cuddle up with each other for warmth and support. A strong family is a work of art continually in progress, always in the process of growing and changing.
- *When seeking to unite groups of people, communities, and even nations,* uniting around the cause of strengthening families–a cause we can all sanction–can be a powerful strategy.
- *Human beings have the right and responsibility to feel safe, comfortable, happy, and loved.*

MULTIDISCIPLINARY APPROACHES AND APPLICATIONS TO STRENGTHS-BASED PRACTICE

This two-part project will be a discussion of strong families around the world. The first part will focus on three areas of the world and the individual countries represented in each of these areas: Africa (South Africa, Botswana, Kenya, Somalia); the Middle East (Israel, Oman); and Asia (China, India, Korea). The second part will focus on the strong families of Oceania (Australia, New Zealand); North America (Canada, United States of America); Latin America (Mexico, Brazil); and Europe (Russia, Greece, Romania).

The focus is on strong families. Readers will not only notice diversity in the families that are described, but the way in which the authors have chosen to express their perspectives on families and cultures. The strengths of families from culture to culture are remarkably similar, but these strengths sometimes are expressed in creative ways imbued in the culture. For example, because of the popularity of sports in New Zealand, a sports metaphor describes New Zealand family attitudes toward solidarity and resilience quite well.

A preliminary study of strengths of New Zealand families found that a sense of being a team inspired positive responses to stressors. Similar to the notions of teamwork in the ever popular arena of sport in New Zealand, families consistently spoke in terms of being a team, being dedicated to the team, pulling together, one person's strengths making up for the weaknesses of another, each having a part to play, making sacrifices for the good of the team, working hard, and sticking together in the face of tough times.

Other authors chose to focus on the tremendous influence that history and rich cultural tradition holds within their country. In addition, the authors also represent a variety of disciplines and backgrounds that add interest to the story of the families in their country. The authors are researchers and scholars in the fields of cultural anthropology, education, family studies, modern languages, psychology, social work and sociology. This greatly contributes to the diversity in how the chapters are conceived and organized.

HOW CAN THE INFORMATION PRESENTED FROM THE VARIOUS AUTHORS BE USED AND APPLIED?

There are a variety of ways that we can learn from the experiences of families around the world. The information has relevance and purpose and should serve to inform and expand our thinking about families. The information may have significant relevance to some specific areas and particular fields. Application to the areas of family services, family education, marital and family therapy, and social policy are discussed below.

Family services. Globalization has provided opportunities for people all over the world to interact and collaborate within organizations or through employment. Migration and immigration occurs as people leave their native countries seeking better lives. Individuals, communities, and governments that provide services to displaced families require information about their cultures that are effective. Services are needed that meet the needs within the context of their cultures and must provide help that is relevant and familiar. For example, providing help to a family who is looking for adequate housing will require an understanding of their cultural living patterns and being able to point them to housing that will meet their needs for comfort, safety, and security.

Family education. Where it is being provided, educational programs for families are often culture specific and based on the majority culture. To provide education that meets the needs of all cultures will require an understanding of family life in other cultures. Parenting practices, marital traditions, and family patterns look differently around the world and have developed in a variety of ways for a specific purpose. For example, infant feeding may differ around the world because of resources, cultural practices, and issues of personal acceptance. Even though current research may point out best practices in terms of health and well-being, cultural norms need to be considered and respected.

Marital and family therapy. Individuals and couples who seek therapy will benefit from a therapist or counselor who understands their culture. It is not easy to help someone through a difficult period of life when you have no knowledge or understanding of their basic orientation to life. Different cultures have different ways of knowing and of thinking, different priorities in life, and different approaches to viewing and solving problems. For example, someone from a collectivist culture would find it difficult to think about solving a problem that would involve an individual outcome.

Developing social policy. Making decisions and setting social policy that will affect a variety of cultures requires a basic understanding of those who will be impacted. It is important that lawmakers recognize that certain decisions must take into account the cultural differences that will be represented within that decision. Setting a policy that requires someone to go against their cultural norm will mean that the policy with be met with resistance, will be ignored, or will not be utilized. For example, if a policy is put into effect that requires a particular dress code that goes against the cultural or religious dress tradition, it will be offensive and seen as a violation in the individual's eyes.

It is our responsibility as a global citizen to be aware of those around us. It is a sign of respect when we consider and value the cultural differences of others. Wherever you live it is likely that you have and will continue to encounter people from different cultures. From personal experience, we have been profoundly changed as a result of opening our hearts and minds to those from other cultures who have so much to teach us about life. It will be valuable if, as you read through the articles in this volume, you allow yourself to go beyond viewing the words through *your own* lens to begin to see it through *their* eyes. You will be changed too!

As you read through the articles, it will become evident that work is being done in countless places and countless ways around the world to strengthen and support families. You will begin to see commonalities that all families face regardless of their location, family patterns, or ethnicity. Families everywhere enjoy the benefits of healthy relationships and bravely endure the challenges that emanate from both internal and external forces. Your faith in the value and purpose of family will be strengthened as you read the accounts of the ways that families around the world band together in times of immeasurable joy and celebration as well as in times of immense sorrow and grief. That precious piece of life connects us all.

REFERENCES

Casas, C., Stinnett, N., DeFrain, J., & Lee, P. (1984). Family strengths in Latin America. *Family Perspective* (Winter).

DeFrain, J., DeFrain, N., & Lepard, J. (1994). Family strengths and challenges in the South Pacific: An exploratory study. *International Journal of the Sociology of the Family, 24*, 25-47.

DeFrain, J., & Stinnett, N. (2002). Family strengths. In J.J. Ponzetti et al. (Eds.), *International encyclopedia of marriage and family* (2nd Ed.). New York: Macmillan Reference Group.

Gabler, J., & Otto, H. (1964). Conceptualization of family strengths in the family life and other professional literature. *Journal of Marriage and the Family, 26*, 221-223.

Lingren, H. G., Kimmons, L., Lee, P., Rowe, G., Rottman, L., Schwab, L., & Williams, R. (Eds.), (1987). *Family strengths (Vol. 8-9): Pathways to well-being.* Lincoln, NE: University of Nebraska Press.

Olson, D. H., & DeFrain, J. (2006). *Marriages and families: Intimacy, strengths, and diversity* (5th Ed.). New York: McGraw-Hill.

Otto, H. A. (1962). What is a strong family? *Marriage and Family Living, 24*, 77-81.

Otto, H. A. (1963). Criteria for assessing family strength. *Family Process, 2*, 329-339.

Rowe, G., Lingren, H., Van Zandt, S., Williams, R., DeFrain, J., & Stinnett, N. (Eds.). (1984). *Family strengths (Vol. 5): Continuity and diversity.* Lincoln, NE: University of Nebraska Press.

Stinnett, N., Chesser, B., & DeFrain, J. (Eds.). (1979). *Building family strengths (Vol. 1) Blueprints for action.* Lincoln, NE: University of Nebraska Press.

Stinnett, N., Chesser, B., DeFrain, J., & Knaub, P. (Eds.). (1980). *Family strengths (Vol. 2): Positive models for family life.* Lincoln, NE: University of Nebraska Press.

Stinnett, N., & DeFrain, J. (1985). *Secrets of strong families.* Boston: Little, Brown.

Stinnett, N., DeFrain, J., King, K., Knaub, P., & Rowe, G. (Eds.). (1981). *Family strengths (Vol. 3): Roots of well-being.* Lincoln, NE: University of Nebraska Press.

Stinnett, N., DeFrain, J., King, K., Lingren, H., Van Zandt, S., & Williams, R. (Eds.). (1982). *Family strengths (Vol. 4): Positive support systems.* Lincoln, NE: University of Nebraska Press.

Stinnett, N., & O'Donnell, M. (1996). *Good kids.* New York: Doubleday.

Stinnett, N., & Sauer, K. (1977). Relationship characteristics of strong families. *Family Perspective, 11*, 3-11.

Van Zandt, S., Lingren, H., Rowe, G., Zeece, P., Kimmons, L., Lee, P., Shell, D., & Stinnett, N. (Eds.). (1986). *Family strengths (Vol. 7): Vital connections.* Lincoln, NE: University of Nebraska Press.

White, J. A. (2005). *Advancing family theories.* Thousand Oaks, CA: Sage.

Williams, R., Lingren, H., Rowe, G., Van Zandt, S., & Stinnett, N. (Eds.). (1985). *Family strengths (Vol. 6): Enhancement of interaction.* Lincoln, NE: University of Nebraska Press.

Woodhouse, C. G. (1930). A study of 250 successful families. *Social Forces, 8*, 511-532.

Xie, X., DeFrain, J., Meredith, W., & Combs, R. (1996). Family strengths in the People's Republic of China. *International Journal of the Sociology of the Family, 26*, 17-27.

doi:10.1300/J002v41n01_01

AFRICA

Family Strengths:
South Africa

Busisiwe Nkosi
Priscilla Daniels

SUMMARY. South Africa faces the formidable challenge of redressing the imbalances created by repressive apartheid policies. These policies resulted in the erosion of civil society typified by unequal and inequitable access to resources and opportunities. This condition resulted in the attrition of the asset base of families and exposed the majority of African families to physical, political and economic disasters. Yet, despite these challenges, South African families have always maintained a certain extraordinary power, which guards their systems, thereby enabling them to sustain themselves, often under the most difficult conditions. This article

Busisiwe Nkosi is Senior Researcher, Health Economics and HIV/AIDS Research Division, University of KwaZulu-Natal, 48 Patterson, Newcastle, 2940, South Africa (E-mail: nkosib@ukzn.ac.za). Priscilla Daniels is Associate Professor, Department of Human Ecology and Dietetics, University of Western Cape, Private Bag X17, Bellville, 7535, South Africa (E-mail: pdaniels@uwc.ac.za).

Address correspondence to: Busisiwe Nkosi.

[Haworth co-indexing entry note]: "Family Strengths: South Africa." Nkosi, Busisiwe, and Priscilla Daniels. Co-published simultaneously in *Marriage & Family Review* (The Haworth Press, Inc.) Vol. 41, No. 1/2, 2007, pp. 11-26; and: *Strong Families Around the World: Strengths-Based Research and Perspectives* (ed: John DeFrain, and Sylvia M. Asay) The Haworth Press, Inc., 2007, pp. 11-26. Single or multiple copies of this article are available for a fee from The Haworth Document Delivery Service [1-800-HAWORTH, 9:00 a.m. - 5:00 p.m. (EST). E-mail address: docdelivery@haworthpress.com].

Available online at http://mfr.haworthpress.com
© 2007 by The Haworth Press, Inc. All rights reserved.
doi:10.1300/J002v41n01_02

hopes to advance systematic understanding of literature pertaining to South African family strengths. doi:10.1300/J002v41n01_02 *[Article copies available for a fee from The Haworth Document Delivery Service: 1-800-HAWORTH. E-mail address: <docdelivery@haworthpress.com> Website: <http://www.HaworthPress.com> © 2007 by The Haworth Press, Inc. All rights reserved.]*

KEYWORDS. *Botho*, family strengths, family structures, humanity, indigenous knowledge systems, resilience, social capital, *ubuntu*

INTRODUCTION

To understand the practices of the African family and domestic arrangements, one has to view it from an African perspective. Too often African family systems are compared to that of Western family systems without taking cognizance of the context of this diverse continent. There is no universal family structure, and issues such as poverty, droughts, violence, and the HIV/AIDS pandemic which are synonymous with Africa have impacted upon the African family. The most serious problem facing African families in general and South African families in particular is the devastation caused by the ravages of the HIV/AIDS pandemic. Sub-Saharan Africa carries the highest burden of disease, and South Africa, particularly KwaZulu Natal, is brutally affected by HIV/AIDS (Ackerman & de Klerk 2002). Over one million people are infected, and it was estimated that nearly 400,000 people would die from AIDS in recent years. While these issues are a reality and do raise serious concerns, they have overshadowed the strengths and potentials inherent within the African Family. This article seeks to identify the strengths African families possess and the challenges which families contest within a South African context.

SOUTH AFRICA TODAY

South Africa is such a pluralistic society that it is humanly impossible to discuss the family strengths of all the ethnic groups. Like other countries, some families are so devastated that it is not clear that they have any family at all, while others are in strong, cohesive, effectively functioning family systems.

Demographics of South Africa

The population of South Africa is estimated at 44 million (Statistics South Africa, 2001). About 79% are Africans, 8.9% Colored, 9.6% White, 2.5% Indian. The population deemed as dependent, those younger than 15 and older than 64 years, is greater than the population between the 15 to 64 age category which represents the pool from which the productive part of the population is drawn (Olivier, Smit, & Kalula, 2003). The burden of supporting the dependent part of the population is greater among Africans. In respect to the population as a whole, the dependency ratio (the percent of the population younger than 15 and older than 64 as a percentage of the total population) is relatively high and typical of a developing economy. The high dependency ratio places huge obligations upon society to provide social support at the household, community, and national levels.

There is a paucity of data regarding South African families. Where the data exist, the focus is often on deficiencies and calamities. Many reasons have been provided for the breakdown of families in a South African context and Kadalie (1994) captures this succinctly when she asserts that "the migrant labor system, influx control, forced resettlement and the pass laws have been responsible for the break up of the variety of African family forms which existed previously before 1913 Land Act, Apartheid, and left us with a legacy of family arrangements . . ." (p. 39). She also emphasizes that families in the urban middle and working classes are being broken up by high incidences of divorce and that this has reshaped conventional notions of the family.

The Socio-Economic, Political Environment in South Africa

South Africa is caught up in a state of transformation and this is identified by Siqwana-Ndulo (1998) as a "powerful current of change, throwing them off-balance as it inevitably moves them in a particular direction" (p. 409). It is evident that South Africa's unique history and its current state of change has impacted on the nature of family life, and while the family forms have changed, it cannot be simplified as a progression from "primitive to modern family forms" (Siqwana-Ndulo, 1998, p. 409). The history of the native peoples of South Africa has been one of progressive impoverishment, diminishment, exploitation, and brutal treatment (Barbarin & Richter, 2001; Van Onselen, 1996). This was reflected in the migration of a black labor force that impacted on the family as males were the breadwinners leaving the families behind. The apartheid system that did so much damage ended in 1994 with South Africa's first democratic government. Van Onselen (1996) argues that "contemporary South African values evoke both hope and despair in equal measure" (p. vii). The long-awaited democratic government evokes hope for the majority of the marginalized families, yet ironically, the urgency of unfulfilled expectations turn into despair. There is an expectation that the many years of struggle would be addressed by the democratic government and many individuals who were marginalized have the hope that their impoverished state and urgent needs would be addressed almost immediately. This is an urgent desire; however, the reality is that the new government has to deal with the legacy of the past and addressing this in its full sense requires time. The aspect of time was not factored into the consciousness of the marginalized and as a result the unfulfilled expectations turn into despair.

South Africa is encumbered by a backlog of social needs and demands, as well as economic deficits which were created by the repressive apartheid policies. The troubled economic distance between blacks and whites which was intensified by political inequities is such that Africans are over-represented in the rural areas where the incidence of various characteristics of socio-economic vulnerability are disproportionately intensified. The dimensions of the social backlogs are amplified by the inability of the economy to precipitate an inclusive growth which would absorb the previously and historically excluded majority, while on the other hand, by the same token, government has been unable to muster the resources needed to address the persistent and emerging social needs (Olivier, Smith, & Kalula, 2003). It was hoped that South Africa's macro economic policy framework, the Growth, Employment and Redistribution (GEAR) strategy and its liberalization policies would catapult the South African economy to new levels of high economic growth (Africa Recovery, 2004). The results have shown, however, that this vision was not realized and that a disappointing growth in investment and the drop in the price of gold has resulted in slow growth which has worsened unemployment and contributed to poverty and job losses.

FAMILY STRUCTURES

There is a distinct difference between Western and African family structures. The foundation of Western family structures is the institution of marriage and this is based on the principle of individualism and independence. African family systems are predominantly extended families, and this term refers to a "collectivity of people who live together, whose relationship could be traced through kinship or marriage and who considered themselves family" (Siqwana-Ndulo, 1998, p. 415).

African households are more fluid and result in more complex family structures. The term *African household* therefore denotes a common unit of social organization that combines those who reside together and who contribute to the income generation, consumption, and domestic activities as well as the extended family, who could live apart due to migration but do make contributions to household resources (Young & Ansell, 2003; Siqwana-Ndulo, 1998). Families today have undergone significant changes in structure and function. The family operates in a socio-cultural and socio-political climate that differs to a large extent from that in which the traditional black family existed (Motshologane, 1987). We should therefore highlight that extended family structures are not universal and that household structures are dependent on the availability of resources, which is the ability to be able to sustain a household.

Attributes Contributing to Unique Family Structures

There are various attributes that contribute to unique family structures. These attributes could also be identified as the challenges that South African families have to tolerate within various cultural boundaries and obvious socio-political conditions. The following discussion highlights the attributes of socio-economic conditions such as poverty, disempowerment, isolation, vulnerability, poor health and isolation (Chambers, 1983).

Poverty. By and large, those in rural communities tend to live on income below the poverty line. This situation has been exacerbated by the process of urbanization and industrialization. This has resulted in a shift from subsistence to cash economies and the family has been transformed from a productive to a consumption unit often with no means to sustain themselves due to lack of support infrastructures such as employment opportunities, education and transportation. In the case where job opportunities exist, they are often seasonal and on the margin of the economy. In the sub-Saharan region of Africa, the majority of families depend on remittances sent by migrant workers. These remittances tend to be irregular and fall far below subsistence levels (Wilson & Ramphele, 1989; Nkosi, 1998). In the absence of adequate income levels, rural communities find themselves continually trapped in the cycle of poverty. According to the Minister of Social Services and Poverty Alleviation in the Western Cape, poverty has a significant impact on individuals as the level of poverty may be so severe that individuals may not have any resources. He also asserts that "the poor need institutionalized support mechanisms" (Fransman, 2003, p. 25).

Poor health. The absence of supportive infrastructures causes families, particularly rural women, to spend time and energy in arduous manual labor pursuing tenuous scraps of opportunity in order to sustain the fragile threads of their livelihood, often to the detriment of their health. The interaction of many family and community responsibilities and obligations, often under constraining conditions, takes a toll on the lives of these communities. The plight of women who have to walk long distances to collect fuel and water and perform the bulk of agricultural activities expending their energy has been widely documented (Braidotti, 1994, Moser, 1993). The situation is most desperate during the seasons of drought and famine. With men often in the cities, women and children are hardest hit and they survive on inadequate and low calorie food intake putting their health at risk. Women often experience conflicts between poor health conditions and lack of resources (Kim, Geistfeld & Seiling, 2003). In effort to fulfill their productive and reproductive roles, women often minimize sicknesses and do not consider themselves ill until the illness is so incapacitating that they cannot fulfill their roles and obligations. In these times women especially are pushed to the limits of their physical, mental, and emotional endurance.

Isolation. Rural communities are geographically located in peripheral areas. They are isolated from centers of major socio-economic activities and find it difficult to access external services. Perceived as too poor or too illiterate, rural communities are subjected to some form of social isolation. Difficulties in accessing health and educational services, as well as basic amenities such as sanitation, water, and fuel present a daily challenge. How many of us would walk a distance as far as six or even ten miles carrying a baby on our back to reach a clinic, river, or wood for fuel? Not only are these communities isolated from the rest of the world, they are expected to perform beyond what they are able to endure.

Disempowerment. The interaction of the constraints noted above make rural communities powerless when confronted by development challenges. The tendency of government and development organizations in taking the lead in "solving" communities' problems has undermined the communities' capacities and made them objects of charity. The exclusion of input from communities makes programs designed to help them seem unfamiliar and difficult for them to address. Faced with this dilemma, communities often feel powerless.

Vulnerability. Fickle and unstable economic conditions weaken the social buffer system of families and communities. Households tend to be vulnerable during economic crisis and their capacities to withstand economic shock depend on their ability to pool external resources. However, this is severely constrained by the absence of support structures and isolation. The drudgery facing the families as they struggle to construct their livelihoods, the subsequent emotions such as the dull ache of deprivation, despair, the ennui that saps their energies, apathy, and hopelessness make families vulnerable and sensitive to shocks.

Despite these constraints, South Africa's families have always maintained a certain formidable power which guards their systems, thereby maintaining some level of self-reliance. An in-depth biography of a South African sharecropper (van Onselen, 1996) provides an account of the Kas Maine household. Resilience, resourcefulness, and versatility sustained his family in the face of an oppressive, exploitative, and unjust regime which favored white farmers at the expense of black sharecroppers. His resourcefulness and versatile skills in farming surpassed the cruelty and jealousy of his landlords. In addition, extreme drought conditions and unpredictable climate conditions, compounded by a lack of technical farming equipment, pushed the Maine household to the limits of its endurance. Yet, the Maine household worked from dawn to dusk and managed to grow grain to feed the family as well as export bags of grain and wool to adjacent territories.

Gender. The significance of gender issues is often overlooked in examining family structures. Many of South Africa's families straddle between informal economic activities, which are often not sufficient to meet the families' needs. For South African women, particularly rural women, the day-to-day grind of meeting productive and reproductive responsibilities continues as they are subjected to an undisguised patriarchal dominance. It is assumed that since women are not legally the heads of households, their roles are not substantial and that they are dependent. The fact remains that they are for the majority responsible for financial as well as organizational requirements of the household in the absence of the male due to death or as a result of seeking employment elsewhere (Muthwa, 1994, p. 168). Given the history of Southern Africa with its socio-political aspects as well as the incidence of HIV/AIDS, the role of women in families has been impacted upon in a very vital way. While women have been traditionally disadvantaged in a predominantly patriarchal system, they are over-burdened with a range of activities, from providing for nutrition, survival, and well-being (Guèye, 2000). In light of these huge responsibilities, women unfortunately do not have financial freedom as there are very few programs that assist in promoting their financial independence (Guèye, 2000).

Migration of household members is now a survival strategy for the continued existence of the family. This has traditionally been accepted as the male's responsibility; however, women's migration has been quite noteworthy. This trend should also be discussed in relation to HIV/AIDS, as women are particularly vulnerable, especially if one considers the "social and sexual disruption that accompanies migration" (Young & Ansell, 2003, p. 464). Women are at extremely high-risk and the statistics have shown that many households have become dispersed with aging relatives now reforming households with HIV/AIDS orphans. Alleviating poverty among disadvantaged groups, particularly women, could be addressed through the implementation of institutional programs aimed at empowering women in various entrepreneurial areas in order for them to gain financial independence.

ATTRIBUTES THAT MAKE
SOUTH AFRICAN FAMILIES STRONG

We have argued that families take on different structures in different circumstances. The common trend of all families, though, is to accomplish tasks such as childbearing, providing for the basic needs of family members, establishing social support networks, and essentially establishing family traditions (Cole, Clark, & Gable, 1999). The way in which these tasks are realized influences the way society functions.

There is very little literature regarding South African family strengths. In light of this limitation, the livelihoods literature provides insight into the inner sanctuaries of South African families and the anguish of family members trying to cope with daily existence (Francis, 2002; Francis, 2000; Ellis, 1998; Lipton, 1996). Research recognizes that families are unique and diverse and that strong families have certain characteristics or attributes that impact on their sustainability. The following discussion will highlight the strengths of *ubuntu*, resilience, social capital and indigenous knowledge systems.

Ubuntu/Botho (Humanity)

Ubuntu (in the Zulu language) and *botho* (in the Sotho language) are ancient African words, meaning "humanity to others." *Ubuntu* also means "I am what I am because of who we all are." We say each one of us matters and we need each other in the spirit of *ubuntu*, that we can be human only in relationship, that a person is a person only through other persons *(NewAfrican,* 2005). The building block of *ubuntu/botho* is a principle of the unity of humanity and emphasizes the importance of constantly referring to the principles of empathy, sharing and coopera-tion in an effort to resolve common problems. The social reality of Africans is governed by a particular philosophical epistemology and this is succinctly described by Mbiti (1969) who states that "individuals see themselves and their roles in society only in relation to the whole community to which they belong" (p. 108-109).

> *People rely on kinship relations and other social networks for in-formation about job availability and help with accommodation in town, as well as loans that are actually gifts, or help with childcare.* (Francis, 2002, p. 549)

Despite widespread poverty and hunger, sharing continues to sustain families even when facing adversity. Individuals within family structures still think about the next person and are willing to lend a helping hand. In a study examining coping strategies when facing food shortages, it was found that participants in rural KwaZulu Natal continue to share commodities. Coping strategies adopted by poor rural families are not exclusively guided by economic needs, but by the interaction of eco-nomic exigencies and cultural values. This is confirmed by Siqwana-Ndulo (1998) who argues that the organization of African households under new conditions and the choices made as a result of these condi-tions are influenced by their cultural values. Even though the families never knew where the next meal would come from, the *African morality* in them demanded that they share the little they have.

> *You see my sister, as human beings, here in the rural areas we sur-vive by sharing. We still do it. Even when we see food shortage in many families, it's our Zulu custom to do it. It's embedded in us. When I have something I share it with my neighbor, and she'll do the same for me.* (Nkosi, 2005, p. 65)

> *When we are faced with hunger, our minds just get stuck. Some-times we go to the neighbor and ask for food, and she'll say she is also running out of food supplies, and she will feel bad that had you been here a little earlier you could have found something, be-cause she is real concerned. . . .* (Nkosi, 2005, p. 65)

For many families, the culture of sharing provides a buffer system for the many indigent rural families who are often without any form of social support or safety net.

Resilience

Resilience is defined as the capacity of systems to recover after experiencing stress or shock (Moser, 1998). Families with highly-resilient systems have the capacity to bounce back to a normal state which is contingent upon having coping strategies reserved for periods of unusual stress. Central to the concept of resilience is sensitivity, which refers to the magnitude with which the shock is experienced. This distinction is useful in understanding the intersection between families' experience of a shock and their ability to recover. Families experiencing great sensitivity often do not have a buffer system to cushion them from the shock, thus have a low resilience threshold.

The notion of focusing on the material assets often masks the magnitude of the role of the non-material assets. That the majority of African families are characterized by underdevelopment and therefore lack material resources often exposes them to economic shocks and calamities. For many of the families "the asset base is so eroded that an economic upturn cannot reverse the damage" (Moser, 1998, p. 5). Yet, these families are able to miraculously bounce back, make things work, and *make something from nothing*. This understanding is critical given the temptation to rush to believe that financial or economic growth is a panacea for socio-economic ills facing rural families and communities. This assertion by no means undermines or underestimates the role and contribution the economy plays in poverty eradication because to do so would be self-defeating.

Social Capital

For the purpose of this chapter, social capital in a community is defined as collective norms and networks of reciprocity that contribute to working together and strengthening communities (Flora, 1997; Luther & Wall, 1998). Social capital thus forms the nucleus of family and community development, particularly among under-resourced societies. Social ties tend to be strong and members devote their energies and efforts to sustaining the larger community instead of individual needs. Social control mechanisms are sometimes clearly spelled out and sometimes the rules are so fundamental that they are taken as inviolable, thus respected.

Supported by the kinship system, the political and religious systems often include means of positive and negative sanctions to induce conformity, thereby facilitating a well-balanced social system generated by collaboration for the benefit of the members. They provide support for religious, cultural, civic, recreational, as well as economic activities. A study conducted in the small town of Wakkerstroom, South Africa, aimed at examining the role of informal networks in the development of local economies, indicated that these associations play a significant role in the development of local economies, and they provide a buffer system in the event of death or a crisis in the family or community (Nkosi, 1998). For example, in the event of death, these networks provide significant emotional, economic and financial support which otherwise would not be possible because of lack of financial and economic services in remote areas. Therefore, social networks are essential in strengthening the quality of social relations and the impact on its members. For these families, poverty is not based on income levels, but by how much members contribute to the welfare of their families and the community at large.

Ladbrook (2000) argues that there is a relationship between health and being connected to the community. Social networks provide support through illness and stressful life events, and "under illness, unemployment or the many disasters of life, support from families and communities enable its members to pull through" (p. 4). In a study examining how Zulu women in South Africa grieve the loss of their husbands, the women commented on the support they received from family and kin members, neighbors, and the church (Rosenblatt & Nkosi, 2007). While the support ranged from financial to emotional, the women indicated that they would not have survived the pain and grief of their husbands' loss without social networks. The same is true for families so scourged by HIV/AIDS that the hospitals are unable to cope with the burden of disease. HIV/AIDS is prevalent among the economically active groups and pushes families to destitution, especially due to loss of income caused by losing the family breadwinner and frequent medical costs. The social costs include an increased number of orphans setting off the disintegration of the family fabric. In this situation, families largely depended on social networks and kin members for support to help raise the children, or even pay for their education. The following examples are extracts from a South African study conducted by Makosana (2001, p. 4): "I can never overestimate the role my parent, aunts, cousins and siblings played in my education as they sent me little but important presents."

Though both my undergraduate and graduate education were funded by scholarships, my parents still sent me pocket money and my paternal uncle and aunt paid for my traveling costs.

Indigenous Knowledge Systems

Indigenous knowledge systems are localized systems developed over long periods of time and whose patterns are based upon local knowledge. While these systems may refer to any society, this term is often applied to the accumulated knowledge and environmental understanding in non-Western rural societies (Asibey, 1994). In the most general sense, indigenous knowledge systems are not considered scientific and are not written down. Because they are based on localized knowledge systems, they are difficult to transmit to other societies.

Indigenous knowledge systems are instrumental in providing traditional communities with intimate knowledge of their local environs. The knowledge systems enable families to view life in a holistic manner and there is a sacred relationship and connectedness between the people, environment, ancestors and religious beliefs, and this chain is highly respected. It has been reported that evaluation of traditional family and agricultural practices based on indigenous knowledge systems demonstrates that these systems have a scientific base within and are still surviving (Asibey, 1994). Such knowledge is demonstrated by mixed cropping and the promotion of local varieties of plants which enhance the conservation of local biodiversity largely practiced in countries such as Zimbabwe, South Africa, and Mozambique. Mixed or multi-cropping techniques are now proven to be scientifically sound because of their ability to retain soil fertility, thereby preventing crop failure. Despite high illiteracy which characterizes rural women, they rely on indigenous knowledge systems to preserve food stocks in times of droughts, and they have in-depth knowledge of plant taxonomy which they apply in the utilization and sustenance of natural resources. This attribute is critical for rural families and communities whose environments have been altered by urbanization and technology, thus indigenous knowledge systems provide the inner strength to endure hardships and really make something from nothing. Table 1 summarizes the previous discussions and how challenges experienced within family structures can be overcome through the strengths inherent in the family.

Intervention programmes have been largely absent in identifying and facilitating family strengths as a means of addressing challenges faced by African families. Possible programmes could incorporate the research,

TABLE 1. Attributes of Black African Families

Challenges African families face	Strengths of African families in response to the challenges
Socio-economic conditions: • poverty • unemployment • education	Cultural values: • *Ubuntu* • Social capital • Indigenous knowledge systems
Gender	Resilience
Powerlessness	Social capital

theory and practical wisdom about the best practices in recognizing strengths of families. These could include collaborative partnerships with families. Methods of cross-cultural communication would be developed and relationships formed to facilitate the understanding of culture and diversity in families, while honoring and acknowledging these differences through interventions which could create changes in attitudes and behaviors (Louw & Avenant, 2002, p. 149).

CONCLUSION

This chapter highlights the family dynamics inherent in South African communities and the remarkable strengths that these communities possess. South African communities are characterized by a paradox of extreme material deprivation and richness in social networks and indigenous knowledge. Inspired by the family strengths model, this chapter identified attributes central to strong communities as dictated by context and place. Some parallels can be drawn from the family strengths model and communities that make something from nothing. For example, where social capital facilitates collaboration for mutual benefit, commitment, spending enjoyable time together, and a workable communication system (identified from the family strengths model) are crucial ingredients. The social support systems play a significant role in enabling individuals or groups to cope with a crisis or stressful event. It seems that families and communities function well in spite of the adversity they face. The reality that the foundation for building strong communities lies in their strengths and assets is not debatable. No governmental organization, political powers, financial or material resources can effectively solve problems facing families and communities nor can they destroy the strength and willingness of the people to succeed. The challenge is to tap into the strengths and translate this resource base into meaningful outcomes in the development process. It is amazing that such a valuable resource base should have been underutilized for so long. This would necessitate the development of partnerships between government, public service sectors and communities possibly within higher educational institutions where teaching and training initiatives are geared at addressing social inequities.

REFERENCES

Ackerman, L., & de Klerk, G. (2002). Social factors that make South African women vulnerable to HIV infection. *Health Care for Women International, 2*, 163-172.

Africa Recovery, United Nations (2004). Shifting GEAR. Retrieved on 19 January 2006 from http://www.africarecovery.org

Asibey, E. O. A. (1994, April). Indigenous knowledge systems and prudent natural resources management. A report of the Southern Africa regional workshop. Harare, Zimbabwe, pp. 3-6, 20-22.

Barbarin, O. A., & Richter, L. M. (2001). *Mandela's children*. New York: Routledge.

Braidotti, R. (1994). *Women, environment and sustainable development: Towards a theoretical synthesis*. London: Zed Books.

Chambers, R. (1983). *Rural development: Putting the last first*. New York: Longman Scientific Technical.

Cole, K. A., Clark, J. A., & Gable, S. (1999). Promoting family strengths. Columbia, Missouri, USA: University of Missouri Extension. Retrieved on 23 February 2006 from http://www.missouri.edu/~hdfswww/FOK-files/article-family-strengths.pdf#search='family%20strengths'

Ellis, F. (1998). Household strategies and rural livelihood diversification. *The Journal of Development Studies, 35*, 1-38.

Family Unity Club Worldwide. (2000). *Where problems meet solutions*. Retrieved on 19 January 2006 from http://www.famunity-worldwide.com.

Flora, C. B. (1998-1999). Quality of life versus standard of living. *Rural Development News, 22*, 1-3.

Francis, E. (2002). Rural livelihoods, institutions and vulnerability in North West Province. *Journal of Southern African Studies, 28*, 531-550.

Francis, F. (2000). *Rural livelihoods and diversity in developing countries*. Oxford: University Press.

Fransman, M. (2003). The role of higher education in poverty alleviation. *Gazette conference edition: Unity in diversity, the way forward*. South African Association of Family Ecology and Consumer Sciences (SAAFECS), 7th National Conference, University of Western Cape, September 17-20, 2003.

Guèye, E. H. F. (2000). Women and family poultry production in rural Africa. *Development in Practice, 10*, 98-102.

Kadalie, R. (1994). The changing role expectations of working women in the family. Conference proceedings, Women: The Key to Healthy Families. Bellville: South Africa: University of Western Cape Printers.

Kim, E., Geistfeld, L. V., & Seiling, S. B. (2003). The disenfranchised poor: Rural low-income women and health care decisions. *Consumer Interest Annual, 49,* 1-7.

Ladbrook, D. (2000). *Relationship quality and the future of death.* Unpublished paper presented at the International Symposium on Building Family Strengths. Lincoln, Nebraska USA: University of Nebraska.

Lipton, M. (1996) *Land, labour and livelihoods in rural South Africa.* Durban, South Africa: Indicator Press, University of Natal.

Louw, B., & Avenant, C. (2002). Culture as context for intervention: Developing a culturally congruent early intervention program. *International Pediatrics, 17,* 145-150.

Luther, V., & Wall, M. (1998). *Clues to rural community survival.* Lincoln, Nebraska, USA: Heartland Center for Leadership Development.

Makosana, N. Z. (2001). Accessing higher education in apartheid South Africa: A gender perspective. *Jenda: A Journal of Culture and African Women Studies,* ISSN, 1530-5686. Retrieved on 23 February 2006 from http://www.iiav.nl/ezines/web/ JENda/Vol1 (2000)nr1/jcndajournal/makosana.html

Mbiti, J. S. (1969). *African religions and philosophy.* Suffolk, UK: The Chaucer Press, Richard Clay Ltd.

Moser, C. O. N. (1998). The asset vulnerability framework: Reassessing urban poverty reduction strategies. *World Development, 26,* 1-19.

Moser, C. O. N. (1993). *Gender planning and development: Theory, practice and training.* Routledge: New York.

Muthwa, S. (1994). Female household headship and household survival in Soweto. *Journal of Gender Studies, 3,* 165-175.

Nkosi, B. C. (1998). *Development options for the advancement of women: The case of Esizameleni, Wakkerstroom, Mpumalanga Province.* Unpublished master's dissertation. Wakkerstroom, South Africa: University of Natal Pietermaritzburg.

Nkosi, B. C. (2005). *Household food security and health behaviors in rural communities of KwaZulu-Natal, South Africa.* Unpublished doctoral dissertation. St. Paul, Minnesota: University of Minnesota.

NewAfrican (2005). Lest we forget. January edition. London: IC Publication.

Olivier, M. P., Smit, N., & Kalula, E. R. (Eds.). (2003). Social security: A legal analysis. Butterworth: LexisNexis.

Olson, D. H., McCubbin, H. I., Barnes, H., Larsen, A., Muxen, M., &: Wilson, M. (1989). *Families: What makes them work?* (2nd ed.). Los Angeles, CA: Sage.

Rosenblatt, P. C., & Nkosi, B. C. (2007). South African Zulu widows in a time of poverty and social change. *Journal of Death Studies, 31*(1), 67-85.

Siqwana-Ndulo, N.W. (1998). Rural African family structure in the Eastern Cape Province, South Africa. *Journal of Comparative Family Studies, 29,* 407-417.

Statistics South Africa (2001). Primary tables South Africa: Census 1996 and 2001 compared. Retrieved on 18 August 2003 from: http://www.statssa.gov.za/census01/ html/RSAPrimary.pdf

van Onselen, C. (1996). *The seed is mine: The life of Kas Maine, a South African sharecropper, 1894-1985.* New York: Hill and Wang.

Wilson,W., & Ramphele, M. (1989). *Uprooting poverty.* Cape Town, South Africa: David Phillips Publishers.

Young, L., & Ansell, N. (2003). Fluid households, complex families: The impacts of children's migration as a response to HIV/AIDS in Southern Africa. *The Professional Geographer, 55,* 464-476.

doi:10.1300/J002v41n01_02

Family Strengths Perspectives
from Botswana

Lois R. Mberengwa

SUMMARY. This article discusses the challenges faced by most families in Botswana and the familial and social nets these families rely on to overcome the challenges. Both primary and secondary data were used to gather information. In-depth interviews were conducted with representatives of various tribes to get their perspective on the topic. HIV/AIDS was found to be at the centre of all social, economic, moral, spiritual, and emotional interaction among family members. Its impact is challenging traditional thinking about family structures and family life and necessitating their redefinition. doi:10.1300/J002v41n01_03 *[Article copies available for a fee from The Haworth Document Delivery Service: 1-800-HAWORTH. E-mail address: <docdelivery@haworthpress.com> Website: <http://www. HaworthPress.com> © 2007 by The Haworth Press, Inc. All rights reserved.]*

KEYWORDS. Botswanan family, family challenges, family strengths, HIV/AIDS impact traditional values

---

Lois R. Mberengwa is Senior Lecturer in the Department of Home Economics Education at the University of Botswana, P/Bag UB 0702, Gaborone, Botswana (E-mail: mberengwa@mopipi.ub.bw).

[Haworth co-indexing entry note]: "Family Strengths Perspectives from Botswana." Mberengwa, Lois R. Co-published simultaneously in *Marriage & Family Review* (The Haworth Press, Inc.) Vol. 41, No. 1/2, 2007, pp. 27-46; and: *Strong Families Around the World: Strengths-Based Research and Perspectives* (ed: John DeFrain, and Sylvia M. Asay) The Haworth Press, Inc., 2007, pp. 27-46. Single or multiple copies of this article are available for a fee from The Haworth Document Delivery Service [1-800-HAWORTH, 9:00 a.m. - 5:00 p.m. (EST). E-mail address: docdelivery@haworthpress.com].

Available online at http://mfr.haworthpress.com
© 2007 by The Haworth Press, Inc. All rights reserved.
doi:10.1300/J002v41n01_03

INTRODUCTION

Botswana is located in Sub-Saharan Africa. With a third of her population infected with HIV/AIDS, relatively high unemployment and poverty levels, a weakly diversified economy but having one of the largest Gross Domestic Product (GDP) growth rates, and a thriving multi-party democracy, families in Botswana are caught at the crossroads. They have to make critical decisions regarding their daily upkeep, their health, member roles, marriages and relationships. Often times this is a challenging task given the complex socio-environmental conditions under which they live. This chapter, therefore, first presents a profile of Botswana, and then discusses socio-environmental challenges faced by most families in Botswana and the familial and social nets these families rely on to overcome the challenges.

Both primary and secondary data sources are used. To get a clear perspective on challenges confronting today's families in Botswana and strategies they employ in an attempt to redress the challenges, in-depth interviews were conducted with four men and seven women representing the Mokgatla, Molete, Morolong, Mongwaketse, Mongwato, Mokalanga and Moyei tribes. Five had been married for more than ten years, four married between three and seven years, three were single without children, one was newly married, and one was single. They were asked for their opinions regarding issues about marriage and divorce, sex and sexual behaviors, domestic violence and abuse, politics, and economic conditions of their families in particular and those of Botswana in general. The interviews were conducted in the respondents' homes and workplaces. They were tape recorded to make it easier to capture most of their narratives and later transcribed.

BOTSWANA:
THE COUNTRY AND ITS PEOPLE

Botswana is a land-locked country whose neighbors are Zambia and Zimbabwe to the northeast, Namibia to the north and west, and South Africa to the south and southeast. Botswana's total area is equivalent to the size of France or Kenya. Most of the terrain (84%) is covered by the Kalahari Desert. The only permanent source of water is the Okavango River which flows from the north, forming the world's largest inland delta system, which is approximately the size of Israel. The capital city is Gaborone.

Only two settlements have town/city status while the rest are referred to as villages, with the big villages having achieved urban status in 1991 (Gaisie & Majelantle, 1999). Today, 54% of the population lives in these urban centers, leaving an estimated 46% who live in the rural areas (Department of Population Studies, 2005). The majority, out of a total population of 1.8 million, live along the eastern high veld which is wetter and has a more varied relief.

Various tribes are found in Botswana and these include the San (popularly known as the Bushmen), the Bangwato, Bakwena, Bakhurutshe, Bangwaketse, Bakgatla, Batlaping, Bakalanga, Barolong, Bayei, and Batawana among others (Culture and History, 2001). Botswana is, therefore, a country of so many diverse cultures, yet all are united as Batswana (agriculturalists) and speak one major language, namely Setswana. Further, the people practice diverse religions which include Christianity and traditional religious belief systems.

Mining is at the heart of Botswana's economy, making Botswana the world's largest producer of gem diamonds in the world. As such, it boasts of an impressive economic record, with growth rates averaging 13% between 1970 and 1990 (Trading and Investment, 2001). Botswana is also a relatively peaceful and politically stable country. Tourism supplements Botswana's income, contributing about 12% of its GDP. Livestock production also thrives in the rural areas and remains a social and cultural touchstone (Wikipedia, 2006). Due to the arid and poor soil conditions, Botswana remains a large importer of most of its foodstuffs, with South Africa supplying the majority of the food. As we will see later in this chapter, farming activities are under threat due to changing sociocultural conditions, including increased migration to towns.

Socio-Environmental Challenges Faced by Families

The case of Botswana presented above is special. In about 40 years, Botswana has transformed from being one of the seven poorest nations at independence in 1966 to almost achieving developed country status in the year 2004. This rapid growth has its pros and cons. While the majority of the population might be seen to be moving with the tide and enjoying the economic benefits of development, it is likely that a significant portion of the population will be left out. This then presents a challenge to the government to make sure that every citizen of Botswana benefits and enjoys the fruits of development the country is experiencing. Issues such as homelessness, when people migrate from rural areas to cities, and an increased crime rate often accompany development in many areas of the world. In the process, some people become impoverished in various ways. Some lose touch with families back home. Dialogue and exchange of views among family members is reduced, and some lack access to information that will enable them to make critical decisions as they make this transition.

Similarly, in this fast-paced economy, people experience new forms and levels of social interaction that are a blend of both the old and new life-ways. One woman reported, "Long back people tried to live a Christian life. Life now is fast. We used to help each other but now you can't even be given a cup of tea." Another added, "Life is hard, but it's not hard, it is us who are hard," implying that people had now been transformed into different kinds of human beings. The essential value of *sharing* has thus been challenged as Botswana continues to develop into a modern society. Traditional African family life thrived on the extended family. One could always count on this family for support when in need. Today's trends show preference for the nuclear family. The importance of family is highlighted by Women and Law in Southern Africa (WLSA) (1997), and clearly expressed by one man I interviewed who observed that, "If you don't have family you are just like nothing. You can't progress without family [of your own]. You can't do anything when you are alone. You need to have family. My wife acts as an advisor . . . We advise each other. It helps us a lot." This kind of companionship or comradeship between two intimately-related people is a necessary ingredient for strong families.

The Challenge of HIV/AIDS

With a prevalence rate of 37.3%, Botswana is the second highest country in the world with people living with HIV (Fredriksson-Bass & Kanabus, (2004). HIV/AIDS has reduced the life expectancy rate to a low 39 years compared to 74.4 years before its advent in the mid-1980s (Virtual Institute for Higher Education in Africa (VIHEAF), (2005). Oftentimes, local media reports present this situation as a "pandemic," as a "national crisis" and as a "disaster." One man reckoned, "There is just too much disease today." Table 1 shows the severity of the problem of HIV/AIDS in Botswana and her neighbors. The diminishing life expectancies displayed in the table are shocking, with Botswana's projected at 26.7 years in 2010. It is hard to imagine a future generation with no elderly people if the present trend were to continue. Today, increased inter-marriage between people from different countries, regional trade, and the general movement of people all challenge prevention

TABLE 1. Average life expectancy in Botswana and its neighbors (age in years).

Country	Before AIDS	2010
Angola	41.3	35.0
Botswana	74.4	26.7
Namibia	68.8	33.8
South Africa	68.5	36.5
Zambia	68.6	34.4
Zimbabwe	71.4	34.6

Source: Virtual Institute for Higher Education In Africa (VIHEAF), Harare, Zimbabwe. Retrieved on November, 2005, from http://www.viheaf.net/VIHEAF-Lesson9.htm

strategies that need to be adopted in the Southern African region as a whole. AIDS knows no boundaries as the virus can easily filter through countries' boarders. A combined strategy that equips citizens with the knowledge and skills to prevent the spread of HIV is crucial. This can be possible if people are more caring.

In discussions, interviewees linked AIDS to sex, behavior, drugs, and alcohol. When probed to explain the relationship among these elements they offered the following responses:

The real problem is that people tend to change their behavior after taking drugs and alcohol. . . . AIDS is caused by uncontrolled sexual behavior and alcoholism.

Drinking patterns have changed such that even the youth (15 year olds) are drinking too much.

Everyone in Botswana is drinking, even the women.

People are just involved in sex in and outside marriage. People no longer reserve sex to marriage; they just have it anytime with anyone they feel like.

Sex used to be reserved for only married people. But now everyone is involved in sex irrespective of status. . . . Some even marry at this young age.

Sex, behavior and HIV go hand in hand.

Sex contributes to breaking up of families. If one's partner does not want to have sex, then the other one starts looking elsewhere.

Youth drop out in school and they have children when they are young.

Behavior contributes to sexual problems and this depends on the individual.

HIV and AIDS is out of control, even the elders are being affected.

It appears a sexual revolution (Ericksen, 2003) has happened in Botswana. An early sexual debut is common among both boys and girls and they do so without much thought. They want to experiment with sex for the fun of it. One of the women remarked that, "Girls start having sex from as early as 15 years of age, when they are still babies themselves and they do not know what they are doing." The question then to ask is: Do these young people know what they are doing? Are they not scared of contracting AIDS? Where are the parents when such things happen? Do they allow such behavior among their children? This chapter attempts to answer some of these questions.

The president of the Republic of Botswana, Mr. Festus Mogae, in his foreword to the Botswana 2003 Second Generation HIV/AIDS Surveillance (2003) observes that, "For Botswana, factors that drive the epidemic are multiple, intertwined and complex and these have social-cultural and economic antecedents" (p. 1). In other words, HIV/AIDS knows no boundaries. It cuts across the social, economic, moral or spiritual, political and emotional spheres of life.

It was encouraging to note that all interviewees recognized that HIV/AIDS is a deadly disease and that action is needed to contain its spread. The Botswana National Policy on HIV/AIDS (1998) confirms this increase in knowledge among the populace by stating that, "In 1993, more than 90% of interviewed youths had correct knowledge about HIV transmission; between 80% and 50% correctly stated two methods of prevention and 50% to 60% used condoms consistently with 90% casual sexual partners" (p. 2). Such increase is attributed to government's "political and economic commitment to [HIV/AIDS] control by declaring war against it." One man offered the strategy for action by saying, "It's all about self behavior, if you don't change your lifestyle we are going to perish . . . There is a thing like self-respect; most don't respect themselves; so you have to first give yourself respect and then give other people respect." This man's response mirrors prevention strategies that have been adopted by both the government, non-governmental organizations (NGOs), and other private organizations, that focus on people either as individuals or as family units taking action to combat the disease mostly through behavior change. Mogae

(2003) recognizes partnerships between the private sector and civil societies, including people living with HIV/AIDS (PLWA) organizations, joining together in fighting the pandemic. Current trends, however, show that despite the increase in knowledge about the disease, the disease continues to spread and its impact continues to be felt among families and communities.

Prevention strategies are now encouraging people to take personal responsibility for HIV/AIDS. Everyone should now ask the critical question: "What should I do to stop AIDS?" The 15-to- 40 age group that is most sexually active and thus affected, often adopts a carefree attitude–not caring whether they get the disease or not, and not caring about the possibility that they can pass it on to the next person. This attitude needs to stop and they should think more critically about the consequences of AIDS to future generations and the country. HIV/AIDS activists should move beyond mere calls for awareness to the implementation of more dynamic strategies. For example, according to the BBC World (November, 2005) the Ugandan government now offers scholarships to girls who are still virgins on completion of high school to go to university and other tertiary education systems. This is an incentive to stop girls from indulging in sex prematurely. The issue of abstinence as a cultural strength in bringing behavior change will be explored further in the chapter.

The Challenge of Marriage

Next to HIV and AIDS, keeping the family intact (together) is increasingly becoming a big social concern in Botswana. One man described the issue of marriage as a "big challenge in itself. . . . There are so many problems with marriages, they do not last."

The Botswana Gazette (2005), a local weekly newspaper, notes that, "the rising number of divorce cases threaten the institution of marriage in the country" (p. 5). A total of 279 divorce cases were recorded in the first five months of the year 2005 in the country's two high courts. Most of these were attributed to domestic violence. Interviewees revealed the following reasons why "families are falling apart" in Botswana:

- The youth tend to marry early and most of these marriages end up in divorce.
- Divorce is caused by competition, human rights, and gender equality.

- Families are breaking up because of material things we are running after.
- A lot of people are not married hence they do not respect our marriage.
- Some marriages are not genuine; some women consider other things like money and leisure.
- People are no longer interested in marriage, even those that are in it are struggling to sustain it.
- In-laws also interfere in marriages and contribute to divorce.
- Adultery.
- Poor communication among couples.
- Women being exposed to alternative means of help and empowerment strategies.
- Behavior contributes to divorce.
- People are no longer valuing marriage, hence they can easily divorce.

If the above causes of divorce are analyzed, it would be found that they touch across economic and social relationships, familial obligations, values, and empowerment concerns. The issue of couples divorcing does not just affect the couple concerned, but its consequences also extend to those other members who live in close proximity to them, often shaking the social fabric that bound the couple together in the first place. In a divorce, relationships become strained. Children, if any, become perplexed as they do not know whether to side with the father or mother.

Traditionally, marriage is the social institution that permitted procreation to take place. Children born out of wedlock were often labeled social outcasts and mocked. In Botswana, however, it appears that single parenting is becoming more and more common. It has been observed that most Batswana do not marry during their life span, particularly females. Gaisie and Majelantle's (1999) study revealed that the tendency to remain single throughout one's life is much more pronounced among females than males. In their study, almost 29% (28.7%) of females aged 35-44 and 21.32% of those aged 45-54 had never married, compared to 25.21% and 13.74% among men, respectively. In addition, *Botswana Television* (2005) reports that 80% of those who went for the Prevention of Mother to Child Transmission Treatment (PMTCT) program (a program for pregnant mothers who have tested positive), were not married and that 40% of children under 14 did not know their father's identity. While these statistics might initially be quite shocking, one does not help but ask the reasons for such an increase in single parenting and female-headed households. Is single parenting now the "preferred" family type in Botswana–whether it is by choice or otherwise?

Other equally interesting evolving trends related to marriage that impact family life in Botswana include the facts that: cohabitation and/or visiting unions are becoming increasingly significant; and the tendency to remain married during one's lifetime is greater among males than females, particularly after 45 years (Gaisie & Majelantle, 1999). Such trends impact family forms and interactions, family cohesion, and the nature of relationships. In studying family strengths, there is a need to reflect on these evolving family forms and try to establish how societal attitudes toward them have been affected. It is a fact that single-parenting has already made its impact in Botswana's demographics and people are caught up in a complex web between accepting the new and hanging on to the past.

The Challenge of Domestic Violence, Spousal and Child Abuse

Person-to-person violence is increasingly growing into a cancer in Botswana society. Reports of child abuse and "passion killings" (a phenomenon where one person first kills his lover and then kills himself) are frequently reported in the media. For example, front page news in *The Midweek Sun* (October 12, 2005) read: "Love crisis: Beware the man you sleep with may be your killer" (p. 1). In this report, 62 people were reported to have died in passion killings since January, 2005. Fifty-six murders had been recorded the previous year in 2004. Trying to understand the causes of passion killings (or "craze" as it is referred in the paper) is equally puzzling. One man observed that, "People are led into relationships that are not genuine by sexual behavior and other sources of entertainment and they end up being frustrated and start to fight and abuse one another." When the relationship goes wrong, the couple starts fighting because they do not know how to handle the situation. Other views expressed were that:

- Men don't want to accept that they are guilty (wrong) and it is often the man who attacks the woman and then kills himself.
- Sometimes these are caused by people having too many rights which was not the case in the past.
- Child abuse is now common. The existence of stepchildren is fueling child abuse.
- Sometimes children are being abused because they are now staying with relatives rather than their own biological parents.

- Over consumption of this beverage [alcohol] is common, not only among men but also women. Men, when distressed, often take solace in the bottle and when they return home, take it out on the wives and children.
- Some men can't control themselves when intoxicated.
- Long back husband and wife respected each other and there were fewer misunderstandings.

According to *The Midweek Sun* (October 12, 2004) "the unprecedented social changes that have occurred in the last 40 years which have complicated life, especially for men" are the causes of passion killings. In addition, "Due to the culture of patriarchal upbringing some men who still believe that they can determine the initiation and termination of a relationship may end up killing when they feel used and jilted." Unfortunately, the situation of passion killings was "reaching psycho-contagic proportions where people are now idolizing and copying what other killers are doing" (p. 3), and this signaled societal moral decay. Headlines such as, "Man (42) rapes four-year-old" (*Echo*, 2005, p. 7) surely challenge people's thinking about such trends. One is bound to ask what is happening to our society. What has gone wrong? What has happened to those social safety nets that would protect our children? It seems people no longer value the sanctity of life. Traditionally, the care and socialization of a child was entrusted to the whole village and no one would harm a child because their welfare was everybody's concern. Today it is different. Neighbors, uncles, or even fathers are reported to be sexually abusing children. The issue of passion killings and other forms of violence in Botswana requires individual, familial, communal, and national commitment to those values that made our forefathers teach us to say, "It takes a village to raise a child."

Challenges of Family Roles

Botswana's economy is traditionally built on subsistence farming and a communal way of life. The people interviewed kept referring to the "good old times" when they used to plough. "My mother would be here with us. Husband used to go and look for a job and send us money. Everything was for the family. Today it is more of "I want to have my own things. He wants to have his own. I will sell my own cattle [cows]...." Women used to not work [outside the family]. "Today he goes his way and I go my own way," said one woman referring to elements of individualism that have taken control of families. This woman's words also reflect the typical stereotypical tradition that takes "man" as the provider for the family, while the woman plays her role as *basadi* (a Setswana word for "the one who stays at home"), looking after the children and household. Another added, "People have forgotten about ploughing. They no longer want to stay in the villages. We are consuming all the time, not producing any more. We do not want to do anything for ourselves, not doing anything to sustain ourselves . . . we should vary the means of getting money. Encourage gardening. . . ."

The challenge of these trends as we study family strengths is: how can we maintain stability in the family and at the same time continue to satisfy family functions? It is a fact that there has been a shift in the expected roles of men and women. One area where significant change can be seen is in raising children. One man observed,

> Raising children is a challenge but it's one of the most interesting things in the family. It's a challenge because you have to provide them with everything they want and it's interesting because you see yourself as someone [important] among other people and it's challenging when it comes to education. You have to teach your children from A-Z, how they should behave, work with other people, and how to cooperate.

A woman argued that, "Women should still raise children, men do not take the responsibility. If they don't, who will take care of the children?" Another woman responded, "Raising children used to not be a big problem. Children did not go to school but now they [parents] need to raise money to take children to school. The young people no longer look after their children. They give them to their mothers." This is especially true as more and more Batswana women leave their homes for paid employment or to further their education.

Evidently, if role expectations are not fulfilled, relationships are likely to be strained. While in some countries such as Sweden and the United Kingdom some men can willingly trade roles as "housedads" or "housefathers," most men in Botswana would find this embarrassing. To change these societal attitudes and role expectations requires that we start doing something about it in our homes, including capitalizing on the strength of our children. Children are excellent at mimicking. They can mimic adults and their siblings from a very early age. For example, those who grow up seeing their fathers changing diapers are more likely to practice that same behavior when they grow into adults. As a man evolves into this "new man," some old practices need to be discarded in order to make way for new ones and this is a big challenge. If not carefully managed, role distribution among family members has the potential to destroy relationships and families.

The Challenge of Politics

Although Botswana legislation recognizes the role of women in politics, the public seems not to appreciate the role played by women who are in politics. Except for three of the eleven people I interviewed, the rest were of the opinion that women should leave politics alone. Experience has shown that the women do not handle politics well, they claimed. "Politics is not good for women. [We must recognize that] man is the head of family but women want to take that role." When women join politics they are still regarded as inferior. "The women chiefs are undermined," remarked one man. "There is use of bad words/language in politics and women should not partake in this." While the role of *Kgosi* (chief) was appreciated, most of the people were cognizant of the fact that the chief's role was being modernized.

"The *Kgosi* is not as traditional as they used to be. Again, people do not value the *Kgotla* system anymore; they no longer go for meetings," one man said. "Traditionally, it was better, the *Kgosi* used to be innocent. With diamonds everywhere you can't trust them now," another man argued. One woman reported, "After elections [politicians] stop their promises." Through many of the interviews, they kept referring to "corrupt politicians." It was clear that the older generation would want to maintain the traditional *Kgotla*, while the young want to modernize it. We will explore some of the strengths derived from this system of governance later in this chapter.

Economic Challenges

Botswana as a nation is doing quite well on the economic front. However, unemployment is one of the major challenges with which the country is battling. In the year 2004, it was reported that 17% of students who had graduated from the University of Botswana in 2003 were without jobs (Department of Institutional Planning, 2004). At the same time, the official national unemployment figure was almost 24% (*The World Factbook*, 2006). Effects of unemployment are mostly felt at the grassroots where basic survival becomes a big challenge. One man put it simply, "If not working you can't feed your family. You cannot take your children to school. Sometimes I have no money; it's not enough. The government is not helping." Another, though he is employed, remarked that, "We are dying. You cannot buy what you can eat the whole day. Things have gone up and we buy one item at a time because we are buying everything from A-Z. . . . People no longer plough. We used to have enough to eat. Now you need to look inside your pocket for everything." Other statements:

- Raising children has become very expensive because we only rely on income from salaries.
- Prices have gone up and most people are jobless.
- We end up supporting other members of the extended family in addition to our own family commitments.
- Because of money, not enough jobs, prostitution is increasing.

These statements indicate the hardships generally felt by the common man as a result of the absence or gradual loss of buying power. This has been made more complicated by additional factors including the devaluation of the local currency (the *Pula*), and HIV/AIDS. As discussed above, Botswana is a society in mourning. Everyone has been affected or is infected with HIV (Mogae, 2003) and this has caused people to question and redefine some of their traditional practices. For example, one woman remarked, "The time we take before burying our loved ones is too long. . . . Sometimes it takes more than a week, and meanwhile you have to feed the people three meals a day, and it becomes very expensive. Where does the money come from?" Another commented, "Long back, people used to chip in during funerals with anything they have. They came to the funeral carrying something on their heads. Some would bring firewood. Now you have to buy [even the firewood]. Multitudes come and you have to feed them."

The advent of HIV/AIDS has had serious social and economic consequences for Botswana. The process of mourning and burying the deceased is becoming more stressful than the death itself due to financial costs associated with the funerals. In the process, culturally appropriate knowledge and practices are being reconstructed.

From what we have seen so far, it is clear that as the Botswana society transforms into modernity, some of the traditional practices and values that might seem outdated are being challenged by youths and adults alike. For example, while the concept of extended family might be seen as a strong African principle (Mberengwa & Johnson, 2004), young people view this as deprivation of personal space, as was noted by one young man during an interview. The unwritten African law of "what's yours is mine, leads to the weight of going through life with the extended family leaving little personal space." In addition, important decisions are made on a person's behalf because they are either children or not in the right family position (Ministry of Local Government, 2001). Courtship practices which tend to be done in secrecy away from parents, the issues of *lobola* (dowry), and inheritance are cultural practices that need to be re-examined as new forms of families and new ways of family interaction evolve in Botswana.

Family Strengths

Given the above scenarios, one might ask: What is left of families in Botswana? Is the family as an institution becoming more and more irrelevant in people's lives? What strengths persist in the Botswana culture that can help rescue the family from collapsing? It appears that most of the challenges cited above revolve around the issues of marriage and HIV/AIDS, so our discussion in this section will anchor on these two adversities and see how families negotiate the otherwise disastrous consequences. Strengthening marriage is the pivot of family survival. If the family is strong, a marriage is successful.

Setswana is the culture of the people of Botswana. When asked to identify aspects of this culture that might have a positive influence on families, one woman quickly remarked, "Bring back the initiation days," referring to the old practice where young people were taught about the process of marriage and *proper* behavior as a man or woman. One of the specific issues they were taught and encouraged to do was to refrain from sexual intercourse before marriage. Dating and socialization between the opposite sexes was discouraged. Girls were expected to be virgins at the time of marriage and this would bring pride to the parents, aunts, and all. Failure to observe this practice would shame the family, let alone the whole tribe.

A harsh side of abstinence existed. One young man who had gone through the process remarked: "Abstinence is painful. It is like walking in a desert carrying a bottle of water and not being able to drink from it" (Latitude, 2005). However, he added, "The pain and waiting were worth it." Today, some sectors of the society capitalize on the practice of abstinence from sex as one of the ways that can be used to combat the spread of HIV/AIDS among the youth. The strength of this strategy comes out in the separation of the sexes. In typical Botswana culture, boys lived at the cattle post looking after the livestock while the women and girls lived at the villages. Boys and girls, men and women, even married couples could be further separated during other ceremonies, church services, and some holy days. Separation was also a way of controlling knowledge about sex. The challenge, when we compare with life today, was to discover ways of connecting and bonding without sex. Thus, marriage would be a union of "two pure people." It is unlike today where knowledge is impossible to control with the advent of the television, the internet, novels, and magazines.

All interviewees acknowledged that today's marriages do not survive. The big question then is: what can be done to the marriages to strengthen them so that they can last? The key mechanism that needs to be invigorated is that of guidance. The problem is that there is no more preparation for marriage. Marriage was a milestone that one had to strive to achieve, unlike today, when some individuals just find themselves in different forms of unions. "People need to be informed of how to take care of your husband or wife. What are your expectations as a man or woman? All those things are important," reported one woman. Along the same line of thought, another woman remarked, "How to be a woman, how to be a man–if brought back can help change behavior . . . Although you may say girls married early, *they were guided*, and they knew what they were going into." This guidance was provided through well-established mechanisms within the extended family structure. With the gradually-diminishing role being played by the extended family in Botswana today, the gap continues to widen about who is there to provide the counseling that is so much needed to harness some of these social problems. A significant proportion of households are without adults due to HIV/AIDS, hence, the advent of child-headed families. Who is there to counsel these adult-children? What is society doing to make their lives easier? Again, at the community level, we find missing the strength that was once embedded in the functioning of the extended family system. A child belonged to all so the child would continue to get guidance in case the biological parents were not available. In contrast today, these children are stigmatized.

In some religious sectors of the community, prayers form an important part of the process of marriage. "Prayers bring spiritual discipline. Special prayers for a marriage commence within the church well before the two people are united," reported one church elder. He added, "Marriage is a commitment made before God and the family and should be respected." One man also remarked that people need "respect for marriages. That way we will have fewer divorce cases, if it can be done. It will also reduce HIV and AIDS."

Other suggested strategies that could save marriages:

Couples also need to know that when faced with a problem they should speak about it.

There must be love in the family and it is important to feel loved.

If people can stick to their culture it will avoid a lot of clashes.

On a more general note one woman observed, "Go back to our culture, for example of ploughing, helping each other. We have lost the helping hand. For me to help, you have to pay. Bring back that love, work together. We have lost our love for each other. . . ." Another added, "The traditional way of providing for the family through ploughing and livestock keeping is good." Once again, the strength derived from being self-reliant and doing things together, either as a family or community is being brought up as a mechanism that made it possible to solve challenges confronting communities. Ploughing was a communal event that brought people together by sharing resources–both human and material, and this made communities strong.

As stated in a previous section of this chapter, the frequency of deaths happening in a particular family are making people feel the economic strains, because responsibilities for funerals are quickly becoming a family's affair, rather than a communal event that they used to be. Traditional communal values and ways of interaction, if resuscitated, have potential to strengthen families and communities so that they are better equipped to confront whatever challenges they face. Surely, it needs an army rather than a general to fight some of these social battles facing Botswana today.

After listening to many people and reading, I constructed Table 2, which compares traditional values in Botswana society to emerging trends. It was the opinion of some interviewees that if practiced, the traditional values seem to have potential to rescue the family from collapsing. These values seemed to bind families together in the past and rid them of challenges which are causing havoc among families today.

An additional strength of the Botswana culture is embedded in its system of governance which is founded in the traditional *Kgotla* system. The *Kgotla* is the centre for the traditional political system where tribal elders hear complaints, disputes and debate village affairs. Today, the *Kgotla* has become the forum where government policies are explained to the populace and where major decisions take place. It is led by the traditional leader called the Chief who acts as the central figure around whom tribal life revolves (University of Botswana, 2005). Public consultation is an important feature of Botswana's democratic tradi-

TABLE 2. Comparison of traditional values versus emerging trends.

Traditional Values	Emerging Trends
Honesty	Corruption and deceit
Compassionate and sharing	Greed, selfishness
Discipline, self-discipline	Hooliganism
Faithfulness, commitment	Fornication (adultery)
Dignity	Immorality
Togetherness, solidarity, interdependence	Individualism
Humility	Pride
Self-reliance	Dependency

tions and the *kgotla* is meant to provide a unique forum for open discussion and a free and proper exchange of ideas and views–ideals which the present government tries to uphold. Thus, the *Kgotla*, provides a model on how to deal with disputes. At the grassroots level, people should learn about the importance of communication and arriving at shared decisions from the way issues are deliberated at the *Kgotla*. These two values seem to be lacking and are also being attributed to the breakdown of moral aspects in the nation.

My interviewees held mixed opinions about the importance of the *Kgotla* as it exists today. Many were aware that they are there to inform them about developments happening in their villages and in the country. One man remarked, "I really don't understand it. They help settle issues. People should learn to settle [their] issues at home and not run to the *Kgotla* every time." Generally, they were of the opinion that the *Kgotla* had been modernized. "The young do not want to go there for meetings anymore," one interviewee said. Another added, "Ministers don't care about people. Devaluation [of the standard of currency] is done without consulting people," thus challenging the extent to which the essential value of public consultation is practiced. Efforts must not be spared to redress the people's concerns about how the *Kgotla* is functioning now so as to harness its strength before this important structure is destroyed. What is needed is to re-inject the import values they have upheld for so many years.

Botho is a concept describing a person who has a well-rounded character, who is well mannered, courteous and disciplined. This is reflected in the Setswana saying whose English translation is, "Let not our children be without soul." This saying implies nurturing total development of children including moral aspects of life that are equally important; they should not be neglected and parents should aim for the total growth of the children.

Respect is an important aspect of the spirit of *botho*. The process for earning respect is defined by giving it, and the process for gaining empowerment is by empowering others. Most of our interviewees agreed that there was little respect left in the Botswana society. "People no longer respect especially the adults. In the past, we used even to kneel for adults, but its no longer the case these days," reported one woman. "It is difficult to control kids now. They no longer live with parents," added another. "From primary school kids are out of hand because of the issue of equal rights; they know they are not supposed to be beaten. People are now influenced by human rights," observed one man.

The pain and concern of these interviewees is felt as they describe how some of the cultural values that used to bind their society were being eroded. What can be done to bring back the respect that seemed to cushion societies? It appears that, just like in the issue of marriage discussed above, the solution lies in education and modeling appropriate behavior to our children. It is respect that binds relationships, siblings, couples, family members, and societies together.

Botswana should capitalize on its economic strength and rescue the family. Unlike most African countries, Botswana is politically stable with no wars. Marked technological advancements and improved infrastructure that facilitate easier communication and transportation continue to be made. These make it possible for the government to embark on progressive and comprehensive programs for dealing with HIV/AIDS and other national development programs, such as the provision of improved infrastructure including schools and clinics, so that they can benefit all people countrywide. These have already started bearing fruit as reported above, regarding knowledge about HIV/AIDS. Other progressive national policies also exist. For example, Botswana is the only African country with women chiefs (currently three), who provide a vital link between the grassroots and government.

CONCLUSIONS

Significant social changes have taken place in the 40 years since Botswana's independence in 1966, transforming social life from a predominantly agricultural rural society to a fast-paced modern society. Some people are slow to accept the changes while others flow with the tide. Bottlenecks to development efforts are to be expected and these are evident in the passion killings, teenage pregnancies, suicidal tendencies among youth, lack of discipline, dependency syndrome, and unemployment. Today, Botswana is going through a period in which HIV/AIDS is reshaping society. Social programs for both men and women, boys and girls of all ages should be put in place to cushion those in need. To date, it has been observed that these have favored women more than men, hence, the increase in social evils like passion killings (*The Botswana Gazette*, 2005).

It appears the general public is crying for a "return to the past" as a solution to the many social challenges confronting Botswana. This is a past where extended families reigned, and where communal values were upheld. This means resuscitating and redefining values and functioning systems which are quickly being eroded with modernization–values of respect, tolerance, togetherness, sharing, compassion (caring), honesty, discipline, dignity, solidarity, and many others. Let us remember and acknowledge that it is the observance of these core values that seems to have bound families and sustained the older generations that are becoming a rare species in Botswana. It is extremely dangerous to have a nation full of people with no morals. No matter how developed we become, it is a societal obligation to know what is right and wrong. Permissiveness should be controlled among the youth by upholding the do's and don'ts that seem to have held the moral fiber of the African culture including Botswana society.

REFERENCES

BBC World Live from New York. (2005, November 8). Uganda AIDS: New campaign preaches abstinence, 06:20 hrs.

Culture and History. (2001). Government of Botswana, Retrieved October 21, 2004: http://www.gov.bw/tourism/culture_and_his/culture_and_his.html

Department of Institutional Planning. (2004). 2003 Graduate destination survey report. Gaborone: University of Botswana.

Department of Population Studies. (2004). Research on migration in Botswana: Proposal. Paper presented at a Departmental Seminar (no full date). Gaborone: University of Botswana.

Echo. (2005, October 6). Man (42) rapes four-year old, p. 7.

Ericksen, J., & Steffen, S. A. (2003). Premarital sex before the "Sexual Revolution." In A. S. Skolnick, & J. H. Skolnick, (Eds.). *Family in transition* (12th Ed.), New York: Pearson Education, pp.134-142.

Fredriksson-Bass, J., & Kanabus, A. (2005). HIV and AIDS in Botswana. Retrieved February 18, 2006 from http://www.avert.org/aidsbotswana.htm Gaisie, S. K., &

Majelantle, R. G. (Eds.). (1999). *Demography of Botswana: Change in population size and structure.* Gaborone, Botswana: Mmegi Publishing House.

Latitude, SABC3. (2005). Documentary on Shambe Community: Nazareth Church. Tuesday, 1st November, 2005.

Mberengwa, L. R., & Johnson, J. M. (2004). Strengths of Southern African families and their cultural context. *Journal of Family and Consumer Sciences, 95,* 20-25.

Ministry of Local Government, Division of Social Welfare. (2001). Initial Report to the United Nations Committee for the Convention on the Rights of the Child. Gaborone: Botswana Government Printers.

Ministry of State President: The National AIDS Coordinating Agency (NACA). (2003). *Botswana 2003 Second Generation HIV/AIDS Surveillance: A Technical Report.* Gaborone: Botswana Government Printers

The Botswana Gazette. (2005, November 2). Passion killings must help us re-look at our societal values, p. 11.

The Botswana Television. (2005, November 5). Talk Back and Break the Silence. 11:30-12:30 a.m.

The Midweek Sun. (2004, October 12). Hell hath no fury than an affair gone sour, p. 3.

The World Factbook. (2006). Botswana. Retrieved February 18, 2006, from http://www.odci.gov/cia/publications/factbook/print/bc.html

Trading and Investment. (2001). Retrieved October 21, 2004, from Government of Botswana web site: http://www.gov.bw/tourism/trading/trading.html

University of Botswana (2005). The *Kgotla.* Retrieved March 25, 2005 from http://www.ub.bw/kgotla/kgotla.cfm

Virtual Institute for Higher Education in Africa (VIHEAF). (2005). The impact of HIV/AIDS in Africa. Retrieved November 16, 2005, from http://www.viheaf.net/VIHEAF-Lesson9.htm

Wikipedia. (2005). Economy of Botswana. Retrieved March 25, 2005, from http://en.wikipedia.org/wiki/Economy_of_Botswana

Women and Law in Southern Africa Research Trust WLSA). (1997). *Botswana families and women's rights in a changing environment.*Gaborone, Botswana: Printing and Publishing Botswana.

doi:10.1300/J002v41n01_03

Family Strengths
and Challenges in Kenya

Jane Rose M. Njue
Dorothy O. Rombo
Lucy W. Ngige

SUMMARY. There are myriad challenges facing Kenyan families today that include: poverty; HIV/AIDS; illiteracy; unemployment and gender inequality; infant, childhood and maternal mortality; and obsolete traditional marriage and family laws. However, the Kenyan family as an institution has survived and stood the test of time. Strong families exist and respond positively and effectively to contemporary challenges. They are cohesive, adaptive, and use communication within the social spheres which provide the context for positive interaction. Strategies that support strong families in Kenya include: promotion of family values; communitarianism in form of familism and collectivism; extended kin and family social system; communal child rearing; care of

---

Jane Rose M. Njue is Assistant Professor of Family and Child Studies, School of Family Consumer and Nutrition Science, Northern Illinois University, DeKalb, IL 60115 (E-mail: jnjue@niu.edu). Dorothy O. Rombo is a doctoral student in the Department of Family Social Science, 1985 McNeal Hall, University of Minnesota, St. Paul, MN 55108 (E-mail: romb0003@umn.edu). Lucy W. Ngige is Senior Lecturer and Chair, Department of Family and Consumer Science, Kenyatta University, P.O. BOX 43844, Nairobi, 00100 Kenya (E-mail: lwngige@yahoo.com).

Address correspondence to: Jane Rose M. Njue.

[Haworth co-indexing entry note]: "Family Strengths and Challenges in Kenya." Njue, Jane Rose M., Dorothy O. Rombo, and Lucy W. Ngige. Co-published simultaneously in *Marriage & Family Review* (The Haworth Press, Inc.) Vol. 41, No. 1/2, 2007, pp. 47-70; and: *Strong Families Around the World: Strengths-Based Research and Perspectives* (ed: John DeFrain, and Sylvia M. Asay) The Haworth Press, Inc., 2007, pp. 47-70. Single or multiple copies of this article are available for a fee from The Haworth Document Delivery Service [1-800-HAWORTH, 9:00 a.m. - 5:00 p.m. (EST). E-mail address: docdelivery@haworthpress.com].

Available online at http://mfr.haworthpress.com
© 2007 by The Haworth Press, Inc. All rights reserved.
doi:10.1300/J002v41n01_04

the elderly, sick, and members with disability; contemporary child and family-friendly legislation; women as sources of family strengths; combating and adapting to HIV/AIDS; poverty eradication; and religion. doi:10.1300/J002v41n01_04 *[Article copies available for a fee from The Haworth Document Delivery Service: 1-800-HAWORTH. E-mail address: <docdelivery@haworthpress.com> Website: <http://www.HaworthPress.com> © 2007 by The Haworth Press, Inc. All rights reserved.]*

KEYWORDS. Collectivism, communitarianism, familism, family challenges, family strengths, family values

INTRODUCTION

This chapter presents contemporary challenges facing Kenyan families and family strengths that contribute to their adaptation, survival and sustainability.

Kenyan Demographics

Kenya is located in East Africa and has a population of over 30 million people and 42 different ethnic groupings with distinct languages and culture. Life expectancy is 42 for males and 49 for females. More than half of the population is below 15 years of age and 4% are over 65 years (Kenya, 2002 Vol. III). The majority of Kenyans live in rural areas (82%) and 18% reside in urban areas. Kenyans adhere to a variety of religious affiliations such as Christianity (82%), Islam (6%), Hinduism (1%) and 11% are associated with traditional African religions (Kenya, 2002 Vol. I). In terms of human development, Kenya is ranked in the medium human development category with a Human Development Index value of 0.514 (United Nations Development Program, 2003). Kenya is a developing country and mainly non-industrialized, where agriculture is the mainstay of the economy accounting for 26% of GDP, while manufacturing makes up only 14%. The main foreign exchange earners are tea, coffee, tourism and horticulture (Kenya, 2002 Vol. II). The majority of Kenyans live below the absolute poverty line (52.3%), and the unemployment rate is above 35% (Kenya, 2002 Vol. IX). Kenya gained independence from the British Government in 1963 and therefore has undergone social transformations due to Western culture and influence.

Family Strengths and Sociocultural Context

Olson and DeFrain (2006) have outlined three broad family strengths and three sociocultural characteristics that help us to better understand family dynamics in the context of their culture. The three broad strengths, cohesion, flexibility, and communication focus on dynamics in the family as a system. The three sociocultural characteristics are the extended family, social systems, and belief systems.

Family cohesion refers to the emotional bond that family members feel toward other family members. This is expressed through commitment and spending time together, especially during family events such as weddings, births and deaths which are not only highly important to the nuclear family but to the extended family as well.

Family flexibility is the ability to change and to adapt to both normative family processes such as growth and development of members, and aging of older family members. Flexibility is also exercised to cope with non-normative events such as illness or death of a family member that cause stress to the family. Resources both material and psychological are important for flexibility. Spirituality plays a major role in coping with crisis as families acknowledge power greater than themselves when they are faced with crisis and challenges.

Family communication is important as it allows the sharing of information and feelings both negative and positive that family members have toward each other. Through communication family members are able to express mutual caring and the interdependence they have among members of the family.

Sociocultural characteristics of families are important because they place the family in a context. This context is useful in describing and understanding diversity of families from different ethnic and racial backgrounds groups. According to Olson and DeFrain (2006), these characteristics include the extended family system that comprises relatives, kin and other members connected to the family. The social system includes the economic, educational, and other related resources available to the families within a given culture. The belief system refers to families' spiritual beliefs and values that provide them with a sense of moral foci for guiding their actions and behavior. Since Kenyan families are evolving and adapting, their strengths can be seen as both inherent and indigenous and acquired. For example, traditional African spirituality and modern religions such as Christianity, Islam and Hinduism have a great influence on moral judgment and behavior in and outside the family setting.

Following are examples of challenges that Kenyan families face with examples of consequential emerging strengths.

FAMILY CHALLENGES

Kenyan families are confronted by myriad challenges, including poverty (52.3%), malnutrition and household food insecurity (48.7%), illiteracy (30%), unemployment (35%), gender inequality (Gender Development Index or GDI of 0.519), infant mortality (77 deaths per 1,000 live births), childhood mortality (116 deaths per 100,000 live births), maternal mortality (650 deaths per 100,000 live births), HIV/AIDS infection (14%), orphaned children (1.8 million), rural-urban migration (ratio, 80:20), an increase in female-headed households (37%) and child-headed households (15%), lack of environmental sanitation, access to clean and safe water supply (69%), inter-ethnic civil strife, domestic violence, and obsolete traditional marriage and family laws, among others (Kenya, 2002a; Kenya, 2000a). Each specific challenge would lead to certain outcomes in family processes and functions. However, challenges are seldom experienced singularly. Often a multitude of challenges prevail, causing a domino effect on the same family processes and functions.

Poverty, Household Food Insecurity and Malnutrition

Kenya is ranked among the 30 poorest countries in the world, holding the 146th position out of 177 countries studied by the United Nations Development Program (2003). Poverty is the inability of families and households to afford basic necessities, such as food, clothing, housing, health, and education. At the national level, 52.3% of Kenyans live below the poverty line (Kenya, 2000b). The population whose expenditure on food is insufficient to meet the recommended daily allowances of 2,250 calories per adult is 48.7%. About 30% of children under age 5 suffer from moderate malnutrition and 12% experience severe malnutrition (Kenya, 2000a). Chronic malnutrition among children is associated with prolonged periods of consuming inadequate food, intake of poor quality foodstuffs, and poor health. Food security at the household level has been compromised by unpredictable climatic conditions such as droughts and floods.

The Kenya Welfare Monitoring Surveys between 1992 and 2000 indicated an increasing trend in the proportion of the population living below the poverty line from 47% to 52.9% in rural areas and ranging from 40% to 49% in urban areas (Kenya, 2002b). Wide disparities exist when we examine poverty by gender, education, marital status, age of household head, household size, and location of residence. In general, prevalence and intensity of poverty is higher among women (63%) than men (45.9%) in urban areas, and slightly higher in rural females (54%) compared to rural males (53%). Lack of formal education increases vulnerability to poverty as indicated by the 64% of the poor population with no school attendance compared to 6.8% with tertiary education (i.e., post secondary) living in rural areas. In urban areas, the figures are 66% and 14.3% respectively. Poverty levels among single women are higher in both rural (56.1%) and urban (64.9%) areas, compared to single men where the data are 48.4% and 42.4% respectively (Kenya, 2000b, Kenya 2002 Vol. XI). Data indicates that younger heads of households with smaller household size fair better (36%) than do older household heads with larger family sizes (64%).

According to the UNDP (2003) Human Development Report on the Millennium Development Goals, poverty remains the greatest challenge of the 21st Century for developing countries. The report predicted that it will take Sub-Saharan Africa until 2147 to halve extreme poverty, until 2129 to achieve universal primary education, and until 2165 to cut child mortality by two-thirds. No date was set for hunger because the situation continues to worsen (UNDP, 2003). Difficult economic situations challenge family processes and functioning when provisions of basic needs such as food, shelter, education, and health are constrained. The outcomes lead to multigenerational effects of poor health, morbidity and mortality, conflicts over scarce resources, and poverty within households. The gap between the rich and the poor is great, for a child born in poverty has a low chance of alleviating it. Those whose parents have the resources have a guaranteed springboard for upward socio-economic mobility.

In the face of poverty, girls fare poorly compared with boys in terms of access to resources to improve their lives. They are more likely to engage in child labor, marry early, and drop out of school when funds are limited or if care is required at home. Patriarchy and poverty combine to the detriment of girls. Later in life a similar pattern is seen with rampant poverty among the female-headed households, increased morbidity and mortality, low school enrollment and declining school completion rates.

Childhood Mortality and Morbidity

The infant mortality rate is 77 per 1,000 live births, while the child mortality rate for the first 5 years of life is 116 per 1,000 live births (Kenya, 2002 Vol. V). This high mortality rate could be explained by the poor economic conditions, the rising rate of HIV/AIDS, and the rapid population growth rate. In order to address the situation of children and reduce mortality, the government has established and strengthened health programs, such as primary health care, maternal and child health services, family planning, and immunization programs (Kenya, 2002 Vol. V). There have been significant efforts to control diarrhea diseases through a national control of diarrhea diseases program and use of oral rehydration therapy with the aim of reducing childhood mortality and morbidity (UNICEF, 2004).

The Kenya expanded program on immunization has had a positive impact on immunization of children against six common childhood immunizable diseases with over 85% coverage (UNICEF, 2004). The integrated management of childhood illnesses focuses on the major causes of death in children aged below five years. Sick children are provided with appropriate treatment and checked for malnutrition, immunization and micronutrient deficiency. In addition, there is a community and household component that ensures children are given appropriate home-based care in order to reduce the number of children dying at home. Child survival has had an impact on reducing the high fertility rate from 8 in 1989 to 5 in 1999 (Kenya, 2002 Vol. IV).

HIV/AIDS

Trends indicate that the annual number of HIV/AIDS deaths is still rising steeply and has doubled over the past 6 years to about 150,000 deaths per year. New infections, however, may be dropping to around 80,000 each year. The majority of new infections occur among youth; especially young women aged 15 to 24 and young men under the age of 30. HIV/AIDS infection among adults in urban areas (10%) is almost twice as high as in rural areas (6%) (Kenya Demographic & Health Survey, 2003). Although the prevalence of HIV/AIDS in Kenya has been reduced from 13.6% in 1997 to 7% in 2003, the impact of HIV/AIDS at individual, household and community levels is felt firsthand and with the most impact, but it is also at these levels that it is hardest to measure.

Demographic indicators of HIV/AIDS in morbidity, mortality, and life expectancy rates are one thing, but their meaning for individuals and their families is another. The lasting impact in human suffering is a reality for the individuals affected as well as their families and communities for many generations (Barnett & Whiteside, 2002). The negative social impact of HIV/AIDS on families is enormous, ranging from the loss of lives to an increasing population of orphaned children estimated at 1.8 million in 2005 ("State sets up," 2005). Some of the impacts of HIV/AIDS on families include a decline in life expectancy from 65 years to 42 years, poor health and reduced capacity to work, lower productivity, and reduced incomes, savings and investments. The health-care costs are high in the face of the poor economic situation prevailing in the country. The control and management of HIV/AIDS is very expensive and puts a strain on family budgets. AIDS-related morbidity and mortality is high. It robs children of their parents and increases infant and childhood mortality.

When a family member is infected with HIV/AIDS, family functions and processes change. It becomes increasingly difficult to be a spouse, parent, provider, or continue any community role held before the infection. Family relationships change to care-giver/care-receiver, and it is usually women and girls who care for the sick person. Some families that are not resilient disintegrate with the onset of infection if relations are overly strained. Often young girls must drop out of school to assist their mothers when a father is infected, and in cases where both parents are infected and ailing, daughters may be called upon to assume the role of the household head and take up the duties of providing and caring for parents and siblings. The result is that families become poorer, children drop out of school, the standard of living declines, child survival decreases, and ultimately children are orphaned. (Kenya, 1999; State sets up scheme for orphans'upkeep, 2005).

Gender Roles and Issues

The division of roles is characteristic within any society. Within the Kenyan context, men and women control different and sometimes competing economic, social and political spheres. East African family structure is charged with duties which have far-reaching implications for the well-being of individuals, families, and the community at large (Wilson & Ngige, 2005). These features include the structuring of the African family in a patrilineal kinship system, extended family network, the role of the family in initiating the young into adulthood, the collective and institutional nature of marriage, the prevalence of polygamous marriages in the African setting, payment of bride wealth, the practice of widow inheritance, and childrearing responsibilities.

The changing roles of the members of the African family, brought about by the change in the nature of marriage, occupational and educational trends, and from novel developments in medical and reproductive health care, have posed challenges to the family that continue to confront its existence (Keller, 1980). The division of duties and the allocation of gender roles have traditionally favored men in Kenyan communities. In patrilineal communities, decision making concerning the economic and political well-being of the family has been the domain of men, while the social responsibilities, especially concerning the care and rearing of children and the day-to-day running of the family and the homestead are the responsibility of women.

The extended family, composed of filial and consanguine relatives, was the prevalent type of family pattern in traditional Kenyan society. Today, the move toward modernization and urbanization has steadily reduced family size. Smaller family units made up of a variation of the nuclear family composed of parents and children and selected dependant relatives are quickly becoming the norm (Ngige, Ondigi, & Wilson, 2005).

Women provide the larger share of labor, especially domestic, in most Kenyan communities. In the patrilineal family system, women are regarded as *outsiders* and as such have to prove their worth to the family by procreation upon marriage. Women's labor includes the duties of childbearing and rearing, family resource management (land, water), and participating in economically-viable activities to supplement the agricultural/agrarian resources. As Kenya strives to become more industrialized, the need for both skilled and unskilled labor in the urban areas has greatly increased, drawing a large percentage of young and able-bodied people from the rural areas. With men participating in migratory labor, the women are left with the responsibility of not only taking care of the family, but are also burdened with traditional men's roles of decision-making regarding the family and providing for security, safety and maintenance.

Gender Disparity

Gender is defined as a socio-cultural construct of the society that determines the identity, roles or functions, entitlement, and deprivation of men and women in society. Gender disparities occur as a result of unequal power relations and unequal access to resources by men and women. During the 1999 population and housing census, an in-depth analysis of gender dimensions was conducted in Kenya (Kenya, 2002 Vol. XI). Results indicate wide disparities between men and women in terms of access to education, employment, clean water, and sanitation.

Sex ratios. According to the 1999 population and housing census, females accounted for 50.5% of the total population. At the national level, the sex ratio was 98 males for every 100 females.

Education and gender. More females (62%) than males (38%) had not attended school. This means that there were 162 women for every 100 men who had not attended school. Of the entire population working for pay in 1999, about 71% were males and 29% were females. The implication is that wage employment is still dominated by males in both urban and rural areas.

Marital status and gender. There are more females (53%) than males (46%) who are married. The fertility level for those married is almost double (6.1) than that for the single women (3.4). In general, females are poorer than males, regardless of their marital status. During the 1999 population and housing census, it was reported that 37% of all households were headed by females, an increase from 35% in 1989. Gender disparity was also found for owner-occupied households where female heads of household accounted for 72% and male heads, 61%. This gives an indication that female-headed households gave greater priority to house ownership than their male counterparts who are more likely to rent their houses (Kenya, 2002 Vol. XI).

Access to water and sanitation. Access to piped, safe drinking water sources was low, accounting for 25% of the female-headed and 43% of the male-headed households (Kenya, 2002 Vol. X). Scarcity of clean and safe water at the household level presents a hygiene problem. Women's self help organizations have successfully managed to mobilize resources and buy water tanks for harvesting rain water from the roof of their houses in many rural areas.

Cooking fuel and gender. A higher proportion of female-headed households (75%) than male-headed households (64%) used firewood (Kenya, 2002 Vol. X). The results have an effect on women's time for collecting firewood and the management of the environment because firewood depletes forests and contributes to the expansion of arid lands. The Ministry of Environment and Natural Resources encourages every Kenyan to plant two trees for every tree that is cut down. The Green Belt movement led by women's organizations has planted over 30 million trees in Kenya in an attempt to create a balance in the ecosystem.

Levels of gender development. The Gender Development Index (GDI) for Kenya showed a medium level of development ranging from 0.501 in 1999 to 0.519 in 2001 (Kenya, 2002a). Although the increase was minimal, the indication was that there was some improvement in the situation for women due to increased literacy levels, higher participation in paid employment, and participation in key decision-making areas in the country, such as government, public, and private sectors. Sustainable development cannot be attained without gender equity (Kenya, 2002a).

Traditional marriage and family law. Polygamy–the practice of one man having multiple wives–is widespread among Kenyan communities. The 1999 national population census indicated that 13% of women were in a polygamous marriage (Kenya, 2002, Vol. IV). Marriage law and family patterns have an impact on birth rates, parental investment in offspring, and parental practices.

According to Draper (1989), parents in a polygamous marriage do not expect to be the major providers for each offspring throughout a child's life. The responsibility for the offspring is divided among kin, which reduces the parenting effort required from each parent to raise a child. As expected, women make a greater investment in the well-being of their children, partly due to the role society has delegated to them and partly to ensure the loyalty and indebtedness of their children, and in particular sons, who inherit property and power from their forebears.

Payment of bride wealth. The practice of paying bride wealth has been an important part of the marriage process. Marriage is a fundamental institution in the development of the African family, because it is not only the promise of a new generation to continue the lineage, but it is also the joining together of whole families and clans. Bride wealth, or more recently, bride price, among Kenyan communities, is a form of compensation made by the husband-to-be and his family to the future bride's family. Traditionally, the payment of bride wealth was the basis upon which the marriage was solidified and the union was legitimized.

Early marriage. The age of marriage varies from one community to the other. This mostly depends upon which marriage law to which a family subscribes. Under Kenyan Customary Law, children are ready for marriage after having reached puberty and undergoing the necessary rites of passage to elevate them to the status of adulthood (Kabeberi-Macharia Kameri-Mbote, & Mucai-Katambo, 1995). Although traditional law provides for very young children to marry (9-11 years being the average age of onset of puberty), human rights activists have been vocal in denouncing this law, citing such early marriages to be human rights violations against the child. To curb this practice, chiefs and other community leaders can veto or reverse marriages through provisions in the Chief Authority Act (Chapter 128, Laws of Kenya), restoring children to their schools and family lives. In addition, the Children's Act (2002) prohibits child marriages, provides for the annulment of such a marriage, and allows for prosecution of the adult partner and parents of the minor who give such consent.

Early marriage is a challenge for several reasons. While the law is contradictory and does not offer proper and concrete guidance in the matter of marriage under customary law, society has proven to be its own biggest barrier (Kabeberi-Macharia et al., 1995). Among several Kenyan communities, male children were the preferred choice since they would "continue the family line." However, female children were preferred for their childbearing capabilities and wealth generation, by bringing in bride-wealth payments. Some have viewed girls as an investment, much like a stock or bond that will pay for itself when it reaches maturity. In many cases, girls are forced into early marriage mostly to much older men who can afford to pay to quickly enrich greedy fathers or in an opposite case, to pay off family debts incurred by his prospective father-in-law. However, times are changing. The 1999 census report has shown an increasing age at first marriage for girls from 14 years (traditional age at marriage) to 20 years and for boys from 18 to 25 years respectively (Kenya, 2002,Vol. IV).

Widowhood and wife inheritance. Death of one's spouse is one of the most stressful and destabilizing life crises one can go through. The immediate emotional and psychological effects of bereavement can lead to physical and pathological problems (Hiltz, 1978). In patrilineal communities, the death of one's husband is especially difficult for the widow and children. Widowhood is associated with the loss of identity, financial support, and social relationships (Hiltz, 1978). With the death of the husband, the woman's social standing in the family is in question. Having lost her connection to her in-laws, many women suffer at the mercy of the cruel relatives who aspire to claim her dead husband's property and children. In communities such as the Luhyia, children belong to the man, and will remain with the deceased husband's family after the funeral, depriving the woman not only of her children, but also of her livelihood and security in old age.

Among the Luo community, the practice of wife inheritance was intended to be a solution to the critical state that a widow found herself, and to give children a sense of belonging. However, present-day practices surrounding wife inheritance have become the bane of the community, and campaigns have recently targeted banning the practice. The practice of wife inheritance has been one of the primary avenues for the spread of STDs, most notably HIV/AIDS. Inherited wives are required not only to take on the name of one of their brothers-in-law; they are also required to perform *marital duties* with the new *husband*, greatly increasing the risk of transmitting STDs and more recently the dreaded HIV/AIDS.

The Kenyan traditional marriage and family *law* on polygamy, bride-wealth expectations, arranged and early marriages, and wife inheritance are challenges that contemporary families are faced with and grappling to overcome.

Maternal mortality. Maternal mortality was estimated at 650 per 100,000 live births (Kenya Demographic and Health Survey, 2003). The causes of maternal mortality include pregnancy at an early age, poor nutrition during pregnancy, lack of antenatal care during pregnancy, and complications during home delivery managed by traditional birth attendants without assistance by trained health professionals. Rural mothers are more disadvantaged than their urban counterparts in terms of access to reproductive health care.

CASE STUDIES ON FAMILY STRENGTHS

A case study of strong and durable marriages and families in Kenya indicated that the most-valued qualities were love and mutual respect, valuing children, providing for the family, communication, and time together (Ngige, Njue, & Rombo, 2005). Founding a family is of paramount importance to Kenyan families. A single adult is considered incomplete until he or she establishes a family through marriage and childbearing. According to a couple that had been married for 45 years, companionship was the most important thing that they valued in their marriage:

> The most important thing that we value in our marriage is companionship. Without each other, none of us would have survived since all our children are married and have left us to establish their own families. (Mr. & Mrs. Kimani, personal communication, April, 2005)

Love and mutual respect between husband and wife, which are then extended to children, is the foundation of strong families. Children who are loved and cared for adequately develop strong bonds with their parents and siblings. These strong relationships continued over the life-course where children in turn take care of their aging parents gracefully and grandparents provide childcare freely and not as a result of obligation. This was demonstrated by a couple who had been married for 60 years and was still enjoying a satisfying marital relationship.

> The thing that keeps our marriage strong is mutual love and respect. When you love and respect your spouse, he or she experiences fulfillment in marriage. What else is out there to yearn for? (Mr. & Mrs. Kariuki, personal communication, April, 2005)

Children are highly valued in Kenyan families and they are considered to be the fulfillment of marriage. Children are regarded as heirs and the continuation of family lineages across generations. Children are also considered as the linkages between clans where marriage alliances have been contracted. This has led to increasing family size where the total fertility rate for married women is 6.1, but for single women it is 3.4 at the national level (Kenya, 2002 Vol. IV). In traditional society, large families were highly regarded as a status symbol as well as for economic purposes. Where child survival was very low, bearing many children ensured that some children survived. In the contemporary society, the shift has moved to smaller families and couples plan the number of children they wish to have and are able to care for adequately. Parents as the primary duty bearers have the responsibility of providing for their children in order to meet their physical and social-emotional needs. Where parents are incapacitated and cannot provide for the needs of their children, the extended family is obligated to fill the gap as indicated by grandparents who took the responsibility of raising their grandchildren upon the death of the children's father:

> The greatest blessing in our old age is to be able to enjoy the companionship of our grandchildren and to make an investment in their future. When our son-in-law died, we assured our daughter that her children would not lack any provision in their upbringing. Today all her children are either in college or working. (Mr. & Mrs. Kariuki, personal communication, April 2005)

In a predominantly extended family setting, communication is a strong bonding factor where couples and children are free with one another and with their immediate relatives in matters pertaining to family life:

Communication is the key ingredient in our marriage that we value most. Through communication, we are able to plan together and to sort out our differences without having to call upon a third party to our family affairs. (Mr. & Mrs. Wamugunda, personal communication, April 2005)

Kenyan families promote time together in all stages of family and child development. Mate selection and bride-wealth negotiations, wedding ceremonies, childbirth rituals, initiation of youths into adulthood, commissioning of older adults into the council of elders, and funerals are all marked with ceremonies as important family events. In contemporary society, birthdays and graduation ceremonies are also considered family events where members congregate to celebrate together:

During Christmas season, we have an annual family event where our children and grandchildren visit us and we have time together as a family to renew our sense of belonging and common heritage. (Mr. & Mrs. Kimani, personal communication, April 2005)

FAMILY PRACTICES

Communitarianism, Familism and Collectivism

Communitarianism is the practice of familism and collectivism over individualism in resource generation and distribution. It is a family strength in the face of adverse economic situations prevailing in the community. Familism ensures that the wealthy members of the family allocate resources to the less-endowed members in exchange for their labor, and in the end this creates a balance in resource distribution. The more educated family members contribute to meeting the education costs of younger siblings and relatives as a means of reciprocating with their parents for their own upbringing. The gains made in collectivism are greater than those made by practicing individualism in the sense that it raises the standard of living of the extended family, rather than the nuclear family alone. Familism encourages a high sense of community where the common good outweighs individual interests. At the national level, the *harambee* philosophy, which means pulling together, has provided communities with an opportunity to network together to develop schools, hospitals, churches, and social welfare funds to meet their collective needs.

Transitional changes in family life, such as additions and deletions due to birth, marriage, death, and graduation, and adulthood/rites of passage are communally arranged because they are culturally considered to be beyond a single family's capacity to cope. At the community level, the *harambee* spirit has provided individuals with financial, emotional, and participatory support when the need arises. Benevolent funds and welfare organizations have evolved out of the concept of *harambee*.

Cultural belief and collective problem solving has also contributed to sustaining families. The chief's *baraza* are local administrative offices that solve family issues of any magnitude, ranging from land ownership wrangles to sibling rivalry. Although the chief is a government employee, he or she is also recognized as an individual who operates within an extended kinship network and is therefore familiar with cultural norms that guide morals in a given community.

Extended Family and Kin

The benefits of the extended family system include intra-familial childcare arrangements and shared monitoring and supervision of young children and youths by adult relatives. Extended family networks are useful for resource generation and distribution among needy relatives. Many transitions in life are supported and celebrated within the extended family system. For example: extended family care-giving for vulnerable family members, such as the sick, the elderly, and members with a disability. Care of widows, widowers, and orphaned children is done collectively, and families uphold the concepts of "blood is thicker than water" and "marriage alliances cement lasting family friendships." Therefore, one should not neglect a person related to her or him by blood, marriage or adoption. The extended family also takes care of single parents, child-headed households, and grandparent-headed households. The kin system promotes multi-generational families living in close proximity and building strong family bonds across generations. Kenyan families have cultivated resiliency through adaptation, cohesiveness and strong kinship ties that enable them to pool together for survival.

Communal Childrearing Practices:
"It Takes a Village to Raise a Child"

Each community has its own age-old regimen for caring for the young. Several practices are carried out to ensure that the new members of the family are not only healthy and strong, but will survive to young-adulthood and establish families of their own. Maternal bonding with the newborn through carrying and holding the baby, bathing and cleaning, and breastfeeding are important measures in the psychological and emotional well-being of the child (UNICEF, 2001).

According to Draper (1989), maternal investment in the well-being of the child is significantly higher than male investment in African communities. A low level of paternal obligation in the raising of his young is translated into the prominent absence of the African man in the day-to-day childrearing practices. This pattern of childrearing practices may be the reason behind the need for communal investment in the well-being of children. Among several African families, care for children is shared amongst kin, especially among female consanguine kin. Parents do not expect to be the primary providers and care-givers throughout a child's life, especially in cases where spouses do not rely too heavily on each other as primary long-term sources of support, either for themselves or their children (Oppong & Bleek, 1982).

Care for the Elderly and the Sick

Caring for the elderly and the sick is one of the most daunting tasks that anyone can face. In these days of great advances in the medical and health sciences, curative and preventive medicine for several diseases have been discovered and applied to improve the health of the community. Despite these advancements, however, modern healthcare remains an expensive alternative, far removed from the reach of the ordinary people in Kenya.

To cope with stress when faced with the deteriorating health of a sick or elderly family member, programs and solutions have been developed to enable the care-givers to maintain their own emotional and physical health, while at the same time providing adequate care for the sick. Studies show that while the level of deterioration of health in the ailing relative may not be directly correlated to the level of care-giver stress, outside factors such as financial burden, pressure from work or occupation, and added responsibilities for other family members greatly increases the amount of stress associated with caring for the sick or the elderly (Starrels, Ingerssol-Dayton, Dowler, & Neal, 1997).

In communities where the responsibility for family members is shared among kin, caring for the sick or the elderly may not be too daunting a task. However, movement away from the rural areas to urban areas in search of jobs and better opportunities has scattered family units, leaving fewer people to care for the old and ailing relatives in the home. The massive death toll caused by HIV/AIDS has also left a large gap in the demographics, where younger, able bodied, more productive members of the family are dying off faster than the elderly, causing a large and foreboding problem for families.

To tackle these issues, programs to provide care for the sick at a lower economic cost have been started across the country. These programs aid in the alleviation of the financial burden that is associated with the care of the sick. Educational programs established at the community and district level to inform people about the dangers of unwise sexual activities and the suffering and death caused by HIV/AIDS have had measurable success in some communities around the country (UNICEF, 2004). While these programs still need to be increased in breadth and depth and the message broadcast across the nation, the efforts to eradicate HIV/AIDS are gathering momentum.

Public health efforts to educate people about new threats to community health have been championed by the Ministry of Health and other organizations in the public health arena. Efforts to educate women, who are more often the primary care-givers have been established and are proving to be worthwhile as more and more women become knowledgeable not only in family health, but also in their reproductive health care (UNICEF, 2004).

CHILD AND FAMILY-FRIENDLY LEGISLATION

Legislation and implementation of family-friendly laws is a source of knowledge strength for families. Recent implementation of child and family-friendly legislation and policies such as free primary education in 2003, the Children's Act of 2001, and the family law of inheritance and succession of 1999 have had a positive input in strengthening families. Government legislation promotes family strengths by serving as a point of reference for family obligations to treat their members in a fair and desirable way. The Kenyan constitution recognizes the traditional culture and practices governing marriage and family life; however, the constitution states that the tradition shall be honored when it is deemed not to be repugnant in the light of the existing secular legislation. For instance, the traditional law of inheritance and succession did not consider single and married daughters as heirs of the parent's property upon the latter's death. The secular law takes cognizance of children of both sexes, whether they are married or not. This is an example of a family-friendly legislation that is used in case of disputes between sons and daughters over their deceased parents' property.

Kenya ratified the United Nations Convention on the Rights of the Child in 1990. Since then, tremendous gains have been made toward meeting the rights of children for survival and development in the provision of basic social services, such as health and free primary education, among other services. Kenya has developed a special program to target children with disabilities in order to improve interventions. District Rapid Response Units, popularly known as Crisis Desks, have been established in children's departments throughout the country to meet the needs of children at accessible locations to both children and families in distress. The government has set up a fund for the upkeep of orphans and other vulnerable children. Parents and guardians looking after orphans are given a little stipend of Kenya Shillings 500 (equivalent to USD $7.00) per month to provide for these children's basic needs (Kenya, 1999).

Women as Sources of Family Strength

Research has shown that women across the globe sustain human life beyond bearing children (Rombo-Odero, 2004). They provide nurturing socialization by meeting holistic needs of their families socially, economically, emotionally, and physically. They engage in relationships with notions more holistic than their male counterparts. This enables women to nurture individuals for survival even in very harsh living situations. It is not uncommon to find women living and fending for their children in the rural areas, while their husbands reside in town earning a salary that cannot sustain the family. The husband may visit and/or send monetary support, but the day-to-day survival of the family largely falls on the woman, who has been socialized to take the burden on the family.

Women's groups are one way of pooling women's resources together for family development. These organizations are found in every part of the country, both rural and urban areas and across social economic status. In 1994 there were 23,614 registered groups, 80% of the groups were established in the 1980s, compared to 4% in the 1960s and 1% in the 50s (Kabaji, 1997). There are numerous groups that are not registered, but still serve women and their families through direct and indirect provision of moral, social, and economic support. The women's group meetings provide for their recreational needs as they entertain and serve food. Some undertake educational or self-enhancement skill development in such groupings. The outcome can be therapeutic to the women by boosting their self-esteem which subsequently influences their parenting and interactions with family members positively.

Combating HIV/AIDS

This includes strategies established by government and local communities for HIV/AIDS prevention, management, and control. The government has recently developed a policy to promote and strengthen non-institutional care of people living with AIDS and distribution of anti-retroviral drugs at an affordable cost. In every constituency there is an HIV/AIDS support committee set up by the government to supplement resources for care giving by the extended family. There is also a policy guideline on HIV and infant feeding to prevent and reduce mother-to-child transmission through breastfeeding. At the family level, members continue to provide care for the infected and affected family members at great social-emotional and economic cost. Other strategic solutions include establishing alternative mechanisms for providing care to infected and affected populations through community-based, faith-based, and non-governmental organizations.

Poverty Eradication Programs

Of the United Nations' 8 Millennium Development Goals, the first is to eradicate extreme poverty and hunger in the world. Kenya is struggling to achieve this goal by increasing the minimum wage to the equivalent of two dollars (US) a day (Ministry of Labor, 2005) and by improving access to basic social services, particularly education and primary health care. There has been a concerted effort over the last few years to reduce government domestic borrowing. Efforts have been made to negotiate with donor communities on debt rescheduling and cancellation. For the first time in 2005, the national budget was prepared without factoring in donor support (Ministry of Finance, 2005). The economic growth rate has been estimated at 4.3% in 2005. Measures have been established to reduce the domestic interest rates, improve infrastructure, and promote increased agricultural production.

At the family level, men, women, and children living below the poverty level apply enormous strength and creativity to solve their persistent practical problems of daily living. They use their physical energy, skills, values, and culture for family survival. They work hard to earn their livelihoods and they are thrifty when it comes to spending incomes on the essentials of living. They establish their own local cooperatives and credit societies as a strategy of savings and investments. They exchange labor on rotational basis in cultivating their small-scale farms, and they use barter trade instead of their scarce money incomes. Given the necessary support, families can be the main actors of sustainable development and beneficiaries of an improved quality of life (Kenya, 200b).

Role of Religion in Family Life

The practice of religion–belief in the existence of a supreme being who directs life–provides spiritual balance and psychological wellness by providing a channel through which one can direct their beliefs in the sacred and the spiritual. There are several different religions practiced in Kenya, the largest one being Christianity, which accounts for 82% of the population, followed by Islam, 6%, Hindu, 1%, and traditional African religions, 11%. Kenyans are deeply religious people and religion is regarded as a source of family strength which cuts across kinship, ethnicity, social status, age, and sex. While affiliation with a selected religious group is a matter of one's choice, religion is a unifying factor among people of diverse backgrounds (Kenya, 2002 Vol I).

Religious rituals are intertwined with family rituals across the lifecourse from birth to death (Mugambi, 1989). For instance, the traditional naming ceremony for a newborn child is linked with the practice of infant baptism; the adolescent rite of passage into adulthood often coincides with confirmation as a full member of a church or religious association; and premarital negotiations and payment of bride wealth is linked to modern premarital counseling and marriage preparation. Even in death there are funeral rites that link the dead and the living across time with the belief in life after death. Strong religious beliefs bring stability and meaning to people's lives during times of hardship and stress. Religion is a driving force behind the will to live and overcoming challenges in life, which gives hope for a better future.

The role of the religious institutions in Kenya has been multifold: from participating in educational forums and community activities, such as building settlements, schools, and orphanages, to raising awareness about diseases like HIV/AIDS and providing health care across the country. Religious forums are not confined to the spiritual arena only, but use a holistic approach in meeting human needs.

CONCLUSION

Despite the myriad challenges facing Kenyan families, the family as an institution has passed the test and proven itself to be resilient. The Kenyan family has adapted to a diverse array of challenges, situations, and opportunities by adopting new and varied forms, new functions, and creative strategies. Strong families exist and respond positively and effectively to contemporary challenges, such as poverty and HIV/AIDS pandemic. The strategies that families employ may be summarized as communitarianism. These include promotion of family values such as familism and collectivism, use of extended kin and family social networks, communal childrearing practices, and collective care giving of vulnerable family members, such as the elderly, sick and members with disability. Women, as sources of family strengths, have continued to provide windows of hope for family survival in the face of adverse living conditions. The role of religion cannot be overemphasized in a society that is regarded as highly religious. Strong religious beliefs bring stability and meaning to individual's lives, the family institution and society as well. Religion is the driving force behind the will to live on and to search for solutions to the persistent and perennial practical challenges facing Kenyan families.

The secular arena has also played a part in providing child- and family-friendly legislation, publicly-funded poverty eradication, and HIV/AIDS prevention, management and control programs, as well as rural development efforts aimed at improving the livelihoods of Kenyan families. Kenyan families can therefore be termed as resilient: they have the capacity to face, overcome and be strengthened by the contemporary challenges of life.

REFERENCES

Barnett, T., & Whiteside, A. (2002). *AIDS in the twenty first century: Disease and globalization.* New York: Palgrave Macmillan.

Draper, P. (1989). African marriage systems: Perspectives from evolutionary ecology. *Ethnology and Sociobiology, 10*, 145-169.

Frederiksen, B. F. (2000). Popular culture, gender relations and the democratization of everyday life in Kenya. *Journal of Southern African Studies, 26*, 209-222.

Hiltz, S. (1978). Widowhood: A roleless role. *Marriage & Family Review, 1*, 1-10.

Kabaji, E. (1997). Women in development in Eldoret, Kenya. http://www.ossrea.net/eassrr/jan00/review/review.htm

Kabeberi-Macharia, J., Kameri-Mbote, P., & Mucai-Katambo, V. (1995). Law and the status of women in Kenya. In J. Kabeberi-Macharia (Ed.), *Women, law, customs and practices in East Africa: Laying the foundation.* Nairobi: Women and Law in East Africa.

Kariuki, T. (2005, April). *Personal communication on qualities of strong marriages and families in Kenya.* Juja, Kenya.

Keller, S. (1980). Does the family have a future? In A. Skolnick & J. Skolnick (Eds.), *Family in transition: Rethinking marriage, sexuality, child rearing and family organization.* Boston: Little, Brown and Company.

Kenya (1999). *AIDS in Kenya: Background, projections, impact and interventions.* Nairobi: Central Bureau of Statistics, Ministry of Planning and National Development.

Kenya (2000a). *National report for the special session of the UN General Assembly on follow up to the World Summit for Children.* Nairobi: Government Report.

Kenya (2000b). *Poverty in Kenya.* Nairobi: Central Bureau of Statistics, Ministry of Finance and Planning.

Kenya (2002a). *Republic of Kenya: 1999 population and housing census: The popular report.* Nairobi: Central Bureau of Statistics, Ministry of Planning and National Development.

Kenya (2002,Vol. I). *Republic of Kenya: 1999 population and housing census Vol. I: Population distribution by administrative areas and urban centers.* Nairobi: Central Bureau of Statistics, Ministry of Finance and Planning.

Kenya (2002, Vol. II). *Republic of Kenya: 1999 population and housing census Vol. II: Social-economic profile of the population.* Nairobi: Central Bureau of Statistics, Ministry of Finance and Planning.

Kenya (2002 Vol. III). *Republic of Kenya: 1999 population and housing census Vol. III: Analytical report on Population dynamics.* Nairobi: Central Bureau of Statistics, Ministry of Finance and Planning.

Kenya (2002,Vol. IV). *Republic of Kenya: 1999 population and housing census Vol. IV: Analytical report on fertility and nuptiality.* Nairobi: Central Bureau of Statistics, Ministry of Finance and Planning.

Kenya (2002, Vol. V). *Republic of Kenya: 1999 population and housing census Vol. V: Analytical report on mortality.* Nairobi: Central Bureau of Statistics, Ministry of Finance and Planning.

Kenya (2002,Vol. VI). *Republic of Kenya: 1999 population and housing census Vol. VI: Analytical report on migration and urbanization.* Nairobi: Central Bureau of Statistics, Ministry of Finance and Planning.

Kenya (2002,Vol. VII). *Republic of Kenya: 1999 population and housing census Vol. VII: Analytical report on population projections.* Nairobi: Central Bureau of Statistics, Ministry of Finance and Planning.

Kenya (2002, Vol. VIII). *Republic of Kenya: 1999 population and housing census Vol. VIII: Analytical report on education.* Nairobi: Central Bureau of Statistics, Ministry of Finance and Planning.

Kenya (2002, Vol. IX). *Republic of Kenya: 1999 population and housing census Vol. IX: Analytical report on labor force.* Nairobi: Central Bureau of Statistics, Ministry of Finance and Planning.

Kenya (2002, Vol. X). *Republic of Kenya: 1999 population and housing census Vol. X: Analytical report on housing conditions and household amenities.* Nairobi: Central Bureau of Statistics, Ministry of Finance and Planning.

Kenya (2002, Vol. XI). *Republic of Kenya: 1999 population and housing census Vol. XI: Analytical report on gender dimensions.* Nairobi: Central Bureau of Statistics, Ministry of Finance and Planning.

Kenya (2003). *Demographic and Health Survey Report.* Nairobi: Central Bureau of Statistics and Ministry of Health.

Kimani, F. K. (2005, April). *Personal communication on qualities of strong marriages and families in Kenya.* Thika, Kenya.

Kenyatta, J. (1953). *Facing Mount Kenya: The tribal life of the Gikuyu.* London: Secker & Warburg.

Ministry of Finance (2005, June 9). *Excerpts from the National Budget Speech read by the Minister for Finance.* Nairobi: Ministry of Finance.

Ministry of Labor (2005, May 1). *Excerpts from the Labour Day Speech read by the Minister for Labor in Nairobi.* Nairobi: Ministry of Labour.

Mugambi, J. N. K. (1989). *African heritage and contemporary Christianity.* Nairobi: Longman, Kenya.

National Aids Control Council (2000). *The Kenya national HIV/AIDS strategic plan 2000-2005.* Nairobi: National Aids Control Council Report.

Ngige, L. W., Njue, J., & Rombo, D. (2005). *Case studies of strong marriages and families in Kenya.* Unpublished manuscript. Nairobi: Kenyatta University

Ngige, L. W., Ondigi, A. N., & Wilson, S. M. (2005). Family diversity in Kenya. In C. B. Hennon (Ed.), *Handbook of families in cultural and international perspectives.* (Chapter 9). New York: The Haworth Press.

Olson, D. H., & DeFrain, J. (2006). *Marriages and families: Intimacy, diversity, and strengths* (5th Ed.). New York: McGraw-Hill Higher Education.

Oppong, C., & Bleek, W. (1982). Economic models and having children: Some evidence from Kwahu, Ghana. *Africa, 52*(4), 15-33

Rombo-Odero, D. (2004). Families of Kenya. *Family focus on international perspectives.* Issue FF24. Minneapolis, MN, USA: National Council of Family Relations. Retrieved June 20, 2006, from http://www.ncfr.org/pdf/Focus1204.pdf

Starrels, M., Ingerssol-Dayton, B., Dowler, D., & Neal, M. (1997). The Stress of caring for a parent: Effects of the elder's impairment on an employed adult child. *Journal of Marriage and the Family, 59,* 860-872.

State sets up scheme for orphans' upkeep. (2005, June 17). Retrieved June 20, 2006, from http://www.nationmedia.com/dailynation/nmgcontententry.asp?category_id=1&newsid=51235

UNICEF (2001). Paternity leave, births and evils spirits. *The state of the world's children.* New York: United Nations.

UNICEF (2004). *Report on combating childhood diseases in Kenya.* Nairobi: UNICEF.

United Nations Development Program (2003). *Human development report 2003 on millennium development goals.* New York: United Nations.

Wamugunda, C. M. (April 2005). *Personal communication on qualities of strong marriages and families in Kenya.* Nyeri, Kenya.

Wilson, S. M., & Ngige, L. W. (2005). Marriages and families in Sub-Sahara Africa. In B. Ingoldsby & S. Smith (Eds.), *Families in global and multicultural perspectives.* (pp. 247-273). Thousand Oaks, CA: Sage.

doi:10.1300/J002v41n01_04

Strengths in Somali Families

Hawa Ibrahim A. Koshen

SUMMARY. Somalis populate an area on the Horn of Africa which includes the country of Somalia and parts of Djibouti, Kenya and Ethiopia. They share the same language, religion and culture. The majority of Somalis are pastoralists, although urbanization is a growing modern phenomenon. They belong to stratified clan or tribal structures and follow time-honored traditions based on Islamic practices and customary law, called *xeer*. The civil war, which began in 1988, pitted the state against certain clans and then degenerated into inter-clan fighting, followed by intra-clan fighting. Throughout the conflict the population was subjected to atrocities: slaughter and rape was widespread, property and livestock were pillaged, infrastructure was ruined. The turmoil sent shock waves through the society, causing tremendous changes which stretched traditional coping strategies to the limit. doi:10.1300/J002v41n01_05 *[Article copies available for a fee from The Haworth Document Delivery Service: 1-800-HAWORTH. E-mail address: <docdelivery@haworthpress.com> Website: <http://www.HaworthPress.com> © 2007 by The Haworth Press, Inc. All rights reserved.]*

Hawa Ibrahim A. Koshen is Faculty Affairs Specialist, Office of the Provost, Zayed University, P.O. Box 19282, Dubai, United Arab Emirates (E-mail: hawa.koshen@zu.ac.ae).

[Haworth co-indexing entry note]: "Strengths in Somali Families." Koshen, Hawa Ibrahim A. Co-published simultaneously in *Marriage & Family Review* (The Haworth Press, Inc.) Vol. 41, No. 1/2, 2007, pp. 71-99; and: *Strong Families Around the World: Strengths-Based Research and Perspectives* (ed: John DeFrain, and Sylvia M. Asay) The Haworth Press, Inc., 2007, pp. 71-99. Single or multiple copies of this article are available for a fee from The Haworth Document Delivery Service [1-800-HAWORTH, 9:00 a.m. - 5:00 p.m. (EST). E-mail address: docdelivery@haworthpress.com].

Available online at http://mfr.haworthpress.com
© 2007 by The Haworth Press, Inc. All rights reserved.
doi:10.1300/J002v41n01_05

KEYWORDS. Family challenges, family strengths, peace, social progress, Somali families, family stability

Somali proverb: *Awr heeryadiis cunay.*
Literal Translation: The camel ate its own shelter.

INTRODUCTION

This chapter will concentrate on the common family strengths shared by Somalis in general, dealing in particular with communities that were affected by the civil war that took place in Somalia, the home of the majority of Somalis. The Introduction focuses on the geography, demography, and the events which triggered the civil war. In the pastoral environment in which the Somalis live, livestock are kept in shelters made from cut bushes and tree branches. "The camel ate its own shelter" is a Somali metaphor and, in this context, describes the destructive, self-defeating nature of the civil war.

Ethnic Somalis live in the horn of Africa occupying territories in Djibouti, eastern Ethiopia, northeastern Kenya, Somalia, and Somaliland. Recent unofficial estimates quote the size of the ethnic Somali population as approximately 10 million, whereas the 2001 United Nations Development Programme (UNDP) estimates of the population in Somalia and Somaliland as 6.38 million, the majority (59%) of whom are nomadic or semi-nomadic. Other relevant social indicators quoted by UNDP reveal that the average life expectancy as 47 years, with one of the highest infant mortality rates in the world (132 per 1,000 live births); 20% of children die before the age of five and less than one fifth of all children attend primary school; adult literacy rate is 17.1%, and access to health services and clean water is only available, respectively, to 28% and 23% of population. Nearly half of Somalia's population lives on less than $1 a day with GNP per capita quoted as $200 (UNDP Human Development Report, 2001).

The division of the Somali territories took place in the early twentieth century when the French, Italian, and British colonialists carved up the region, thus dividing a homogenous population that shares the same language, religion and culture. Recent post-colonial history began in 1960 when former British and Italian Somalilands united to form the Republic of Somalia, run by a democratically-elected government. During the 1969 electoral process, political turbulence resulted in a bloodless coup d'etat, leading to the 22 years rule of President Mohamed Siyad Barre. Barre manipulated tribal differences and allowed corruption and nepotism to be practiced with impunity by the ruling clans. The inevitable disillusionment led to civil disobedience in the northwestern region which was brutally repressed. Direct attacks by the Government on the main cities in that region to contain the insurgency caused an unprecedented exodus of the population.

The civil war then spread to other parts of Somalia, resulting in the ouster of Siyad Barre in January 1991. Somaliland (the northwestern region) seceded and declared itself a sovereign state in May 1991. In southern Somalia famine caused by drought and insecurity in 1992 led to the United Nations effort to mitigate the death and destruction. The United Nations Operation in Somali (UNOSOM) intervention failed in a debacle that killed thousands of Somalis as well as dozens of peace-keeping troops. UNOSOM troops withdrew in late 1993 and the ensuing territorial battles led by warlords continue in some parts of the country until today. The relative stability of Somaliland allowed for the voluntary repatriation of refugees organized by the United Nations High Commissioner for Refugees from camps in Ethiopia and Djibouti. So far, an estimated 800,000 people have returned.

Farther south in Somalia, lack of security is still considered a serious threat despite peace efforts. For this reason the voluntary repatriation of hundreds of thousands of refugees in camps in Kenya, Yemen, and Ethiopia cannot take place until an adequate level of peace and stability is established.

Recent events such as the civil war and the collapse of the central government have resulted in human loss and large-scale destruction of assets. Notwithstanding claims of having one of the longest coastlines in Africa (approximately 3,000 miles) and abundant marine resources, Somalia's fragile economy is based on the livestock resources with pastoralism governing the lifestyle of the majority of Somalis. Currently, despite the obvious difficulties associated with lack of formal government structures, trade and commerce are the main engines of economic activity and are flourishing through the entrepreneurship of individuals and private investors. Services such as utilities, telecommunications, transportation (roads, aviation, and maritime), health, and education are provided by the business community with a significant number of women involved in micro enterprises.

Financial services are provided by private (*hawala*) companies, which efficiently transfer funds across continents. In the absence of internationally-recognized and functional banking systems in their homeland,

Somalis working and resident abroad send funds to their families via the *hawala* companies. Such remittances are an essential part of people's livelihood system, with a significant number of urban households receiving between $50-200 monthly. The Somaliland Ministry of Planning and Coordination estimates an amount of $20 million received in remittances monthly. Apart from meeting household needs, the remittances also contribute to financing basic social welfare needs, trade, infrastructural investment, and political projects (Ahmed, 2000). High unemployment and lack of livelihood opportunities are the main hindrances to development. This is exacerbated by the exploitation of natural resources such as deforestation, due to the charcoal industry and overgrazing of pastureland.

FAMILY LIFE

In this section we will focus on the culture, religion, and traditional family life among Somalis. Family roles and coping strategies will be examined in response to evolutionary challenges, such as urbanization, modernization, environmental changes, and so forth. Intergenerational relationships will also be described.

Culture

Somalis belong to a patrilineal society, in which their clans and sub-clans, often linked to specific geographic areas, identify everyone. This clan identity and affiliation form the basis of social structures defining relationships, rights, and obligations. Hence the clan and extended family provides protection, emotional and economic support, and identity. To perpetuate this tradition, children are taught to memorize their genealogy backwards along the male line (father, grandfather, and so forth) until the founding father of the clan is reached, often up to 20 generations back. Honor and pride in the patrilineal lineage is a strong factor in the everyday lives of Somalis. The clan also demands loyalty in both allegiance and in material support. This is illustrated by the fact that rural and pastoral families seek help and sustenance from their urban brethren during periods of drought. Conflict in urban areas reverses the process, instigating families to move to rural areas for protection and assistance. While the male clan members dominate the hierarchy, women retain their legal rights with their agnatic group even after marriage. This forms the most important institution which protects their basic rights and safeguards their interests and welfare. For example, a woman in distress is given moral or material assistance by her kinsmen. If she commits any crime, only her agnatic kinsmen are liable to pay compensation. If she is wronged, the sub-clan may claim compensation on her behalf. Upon marriage, the woman's reproductive and productive roles are transferred to her husband. Cross-clan marriages were in the past widely encouraged to create links which act as diplomatic bonds between clans. The rationale was that the more marriages there are between the clans, the stronger the relationship between them. However, one of the consequences of the civil war has been the tendency for young people to prefer matrimony within the clan, tribe, and sub-tribe, hence reducing the chances of falling victim to inter-clan conflicts. It is evident, therefore, that clannism has a range of virtues: it provides its members physical security, a social welfare safety net, and a rich body of customary law designed to minimize and manage conflict. However, when manipulated for personal or political purposes, clans can also be a force of division and fragmentation.

Religion and Traditional Justice Systems

Religion transcends the clan system. Islam, practiced by 99% of Somalis, provides moral sustenance and acts as a unifying force to some degree. Islamic conservatism guided by the *Holy Quran* and the teachings of Prophet Mohammed (may peace be upon him) permeates both pastoral and urban life. The basic pillars of Islam which testify that there is only one God and Mohammed is his prophet (*shahada*), five daily prayers at prescribed times (*salat*), payment of alms (zakat), pilgrimage to Mecca (*haj*), and fast during the month of *Ramadan* (*sawm*) govern the lives of all Muslims. The five Islamic prescriptions regarding the family which are identified apply to the Somali context: marriage as a religious duty and social necessity; prohibition of sex outside marriage and the husband's obligation to provide for his wife; the wife's obligation to obey her husband; the obligation to be kind to one's relatives and have concern for their well-being (Houseknecht & Pankhurst, 2000, p. 92). In addition, nurturing Islamic values in children is of primary importance. In many cases, however, circumstances prevent the husband from meeting his obligation to provide for his wife and family, due to unemployment and lack of income. Spiritually, in Somali society, the simple belief that whatever happens is pre-ordained by the Almighty provides the resolve to persevere through adversity.

Materially, despite the fact that poverty is relatively widespread, the obligatory payment of alms (*zakat*) and other charitable acts (*sadaqa*) benefit those who are less fortunate. The influence of religious leaders guides the daily lives of most Somalis and they are often quoted to justify behavior or to advocate for social change.

According to a United Nations International Children's Emergency Fund (UNICEF) study, the nomadic population constitutes 80% of the total population of Somalia, a figure significantly higher than other estimates. The study states that nomads define themselves as "someone who owns livestock and follows the rains." Harsh environmental conditions govern the nomadic way of life for the majority. Arid land with competition for water resources and pasture by different clans often lead to conflict. In cases of conflict or social misconduct, elders of the warring clans convene a council which negotiates peace and rules on matters such as causes of the conflict, compensation, and sharing of resources. Parallel to functional government systems, customary or *xeer* law administered by clan elders is observed. This traditional form of law borrows heavily from Islamic *Shari'ah* law and is a unique blend of conventions and procedures with precedents passed down orally through generations, enshrining basic values of Somali society. It is binding to all parties who opt for that recourse and includes elements of protection as well as covering day-to-day issues such as management of communal land and pastures, conflict management and prevention, family law and justice, *diya* (blood money), and compensation for defamation.

The 2002 Socio-Economic Survey for Somalia published by UNDP and the World Bank reported that, on the question of availability and functional status of justice systems, respondents perceived their clan/community based justice systems as far exceeding those of Islamic *shari'ah* or the judiciary. Violation of this code of social conduct can evoke condemnation and antagonism between tribes until compensation is agreed upon. The practice of collective liability renders male members of the tribe (or the smallest political unit called *diya*-paying group) jointly responsible for the wrong-doing of its affiliates. Each unit has a collective obligation to honor certain debts and make claims for restitution for wrong deeds against its members. Even those living abroad are liable to pay their share of the compensation. Traditional arbitration strategies include marriage between tribes for securing peace, joint use of pasture and grazing, and sharing of communal resources. Strong agnatic ties and *diya* obligations are chiefly responsible for the cohesion and guarantee protection of life and property (UNDP &World Bank, 2002). During mediation meetings elders recite poetry and use their oratorical skills to express their concerns. Somali women are not openly involved in the decision-making process, which is the domain of men, although their opinions are sought privately by the menfolk. Their participation in such gatherings is not unusual; they encourage the dialogue by reciting poetry or *buraanbur*, and providing food.

Families

Numerically large families are favoured and women are encouraged to have many children. Six is considered average. The congratulatory message at marriage ceremonies is *"Wiil iyo cano,"* which literally means "Sons and milk," representing fertility and prosperity and reflecting the importance of males in the patrilineal society. The enactment of this tradition takes place when a newly-wedded couple steps into their conjugal home for the first time, the bride carrying a baby boy (borrowed from a relative or neighbour) in one arm and a container of milk in her hand. The bride and groom also dip their right foot in water to signify purity as they cross the threshold of their new home.

Household composition (urban and rural) includes a number of extended family members, and often exceeds ten persons. Extended family includes paternal and maternal relatives, aunts, uncles, and cousins, including those several times removed who may belong to other clans or tribes.

Division of labor in pastoral life is clearly defined. The male head of the family, with his animal-husbandry skills, is responsible for the safety and security of his herd and travels great distances scouting for water and pasture. He is responsible for watering the livestock as well as transporting water to the homestead. The women, on the other hand, are responsible for the domestic work such as cooking, searching for firewood, caring for children and elderly, loading and offloading the camels, erecting and dismantling the traditional shelter (*aqal*), keeping count of the livestock and managing the consumption and sale of its by-products, and crafting mats and utensils for the household. Children, in traditional pastoral families, are proud to be granted incremental responsibilities, divided on gender lines. The boys and young men are responsible for the camels, whereas the girls are responsible for domestic chores and the sheep and goats.

Descriptive of family relationships, the story below is recounted by a father on his daughter's failed marriage:

A young man whose family I know asked for my beautiful daughter's hand in marriage. For her bride price, he gave me ten gorgeous female camels and I gave the couple my blessing. After some years my daughter came to me crying and looking very old, claiming that her husband had been beating her and she could not take it any more. So I promised not to return her to him if she did not want to go. A week later, the husband came to me claiming that my daughter had abandoned her children and the livestock and that she should come with him at once. To which I answered, "Son, my daughter no longer wants to be married to you and I am not one of those fathers who force their daughters into unhealthy marriages." The husband then argued that if not the woman, he should have his camels back. I agreed and went into my camel stock, selected the ten oldest and weakest camels and brought them to him. When he saw this he went into a rage, arguing that he gave me ten young camels and that he should get those and their offspring which should have multiplied by now. "Son," I answered, "I gave you a young, beautiful girl for the bride price of ten she camels, I have in front of me a used, beaten and tired old woman. If you want your camels and their offspring, bring back to me my daughter's youth and her offspring. (War Torn Societies Program, p. 20)

This story demonstrates the father's concern for his daughter and how he carries out his paternal duty in protecting her from an abusive husband. However, while the perception may be that it depicts the marriage process as a transaction between two men, it should be remembered that in Islam a women may choose her husband and that she is always under the protection of her father or, if married, under the protection of her husband. Her dowry is shared with her family members and can be pledged in camels or gold jewelry. (The author herself has a marriage certificate which certifies 20 camels as the dowry.) Descriptive of the material value placed on a camel is this Somali proverb: *"Geel nin aan lahayn, geeridii war ma leh,"* which translates into "The death of a man without camels is no news," indicating the importance of camel wealth.

Thus, pastoral and traditional influences are pervasive in towns and villages also where the responsibilities are greatly reduced for men in particular. Instead of scouting for water and pasture, the men go in search of news which they get from interaction with other men at the ubiquitous coffee and tea shops and in *khad*-chewing cliques described later in the chapter. As a consequence of urbanization and the high unemployment rate, young men and boys are left to their own devices with nothing to fill the vacuum of their traditional pastoral chores. Women, however, continue to carry out their domestic roles and responsibilities with the help of young girls.

TRANSITIONS

The complexities of change can better be understood by exploring transitions between rural/urban and traditional/modern Somali society. Recent events and multiple crises, such as conflict, recurrent drought, environmental degradation, and poverty, have hastened transitions.

In the rural/urban context, significant changes in circumstances overwhelm the predominantly nomadic population, whose independence and pride in owning and nurturing their livestock have sustained their rigorous lifestyle for hundreds of years. One of the coping strategies in times of hardship is migration to urban areas in search of better opportunities. While the move to urban areas helps to relieve pressure on poor households, it also reduces the labor and expertise available for the rural community. Nomadic families are not willing to abrogate their responsibilities; however, they are sometimes forced to send their children to urban relatives for educational opportunities or because of their inability to provide appropriate care.

Another factor contributing to urbanization is the tendency for destitute returnees from refugee camps, who were previously pastoralists, to settle in towns and villages. Lack of access to basic services, harsh environment, diminished livelihoods, and appropriation of communal land has caused rural communities to become largely marginalized, hastening the trend towards urbanization. This marginalization is substantiated by a UNDP and World Bank study (2002) which revealed that the poverty rate for nomads is more than double that for the urban population (53.4% compared to 23.5%). Other statistical indicators (except household income and unnatural causes of death, such as war and accidents) support the dichotomy of disadvantaged rural and privileged urban lifestyles. The primary differences are educational opportunities; the distance, affordability, and availability of health facilities; the distance to water sources; the distance to markets; and access to durable and nondurable possessions.

Similarly, the dichotomy of tradition versus modern is mainly due to increasing exposure to different cultural environments as a result of migration. The perception that the benefits of modern life far outweigh those of traditional life has been fueled by the availability of consumer goods as well as the advantages of technology. While some traditional practices could be considered detrimental to society–particularly those that relate to gender such as female genital mutilation (FGM)–there are modern influences which are also harmful.

Khat. One example is the habit, indulged in by most men, of chewing the narcotic leaf *khat*, which has reached endemic proportions. The *khat* plant contains cathinone, an active brain stimulant that acts much like an amphetamine. *Khat* ingestion results in decreased appetite, euphoria, and hyper-alertness. Chronic use of *khat* often produces sleeplessness, nervousness, impotence, constipation, and nightmares. It is chewed during lengthy sessions which take place in *mefrishes* or rooms where men lounge on cushions and drink black tea and soft drinks. Most habitual chewers claim that it is a way of socializing and exchanging news and gossip. However, it can be considered almost as serious as alcohol and drug abuse in the West–both which Islam prohibits–with similar triggers such as frustration, unemployment, helplessness, loss of authority, stress and distress, nostalgia for the simple and secure past life, trauma, and loss of family members. Other social effects include antisocial behavior, neglect of families, and use of much needed-household income to sustain their habit. The effect on the economy includes low productivity and scarce capital used to import the plant from the neighboring countries of Kenya and Ethiopia.

Employed wives. Another feature which has far-reaching consequences is the fundamental change in family dynamics, which occurred as women were pushed to the forefront in the role as income-earners due to the absence of male family members during and after the civil war. While men widely recognize and appreciate this positive development, some perceive it as erosion of their authority and a precursor to a breakdown in family structures. This trend is further described in the next section.

Generation gap. The previously unknown *generation gap* is another phenomenon, which has crept into relationships as a result of displacement from the extended family, causing misunderstanding and alienation. Previously, intergenerational interaction was a natural part of the extended family environment. Children and youth felt a close affinity to other members of the family regardless of age. Urbanization and modernization has removed the previous communal spirit of openness and sharing, with the younger generation more possessive of their privacy and less willing to share. Despite this trend, Somalis still value their traditions and it is not uncommon for youth who have grown up in Western countries and who have become too *foreign* to be sent home for reorientation. All in all, family values and priorities, while appearing to adapt to modern influences maintain a symbiotic and mutually supportive relationship with the traditional way of life.

A quote from a traditional leader during a workshop aptly portrays how people perceive the socio-environmental changes that are taking place:

> A bird is wondering, a horse is wondering and an old man is wondering: The bird thought it was the only one that could fly, but a plane flew over it. The horse thought it was the fastest, but a car passed it along the road. The old man used to solve the problems brought to him because he had seen every problem in the world. Nowadays he is being told, "But you are not a politician." They are all wondering." (Danish Refugee Council, 2004)

This depicts the general opinion among elders that their social and public roles have been compromised, leaving them with little authority or influence.

ADVERSITY

In this section the focus will be on the impact of the civil war on families. It describes the trauma precipitated by violence and displacement, and the changes in family roles and relationships in the struggle to survive.

Even the harsh nomadic way of life, which evolved over centuries, did not prepare Somalis for the trauma of protracted civil war. Hundreds of thousands of people were killed and maimed (the UNDP Human Development Report (UNDP-HPR) in 2001 estimates the number of deaths due to killing and starvation at 370,000 between 1988 and 1992); 1.5 million fled the country, and as many as 2 million were internally displaced. Death, starvation, destruction of social and economic infrastructure, asset stripping, and forced displacement are but a few of the consequences of civil war. The UNDP-HDR (2001) also states that in 1988 when the war erupted in the northwest (now known as Somaliland), over 600,000 people fled to Ethiopia, one of the fastest and largest forced population movements ever recorded in Africa. Since then, the Rwanda conflict has the dubious distinction of the fastest mass exodus. Subsequent to that, over 1 million people fled from southern Somalia in 1991. UNDP-HDR (2001) also reports that over one million landmines were laid by government forces as weapons of terror against civilians on agricultural land, roads, around water resources, and in people's homes. To this day, in spite of having cleared thousands of mines, there are reports of civilian casualties, not to mention the loss of livestock assets of pastoralists.

Situations preceding the conflicts were as stressful for families as the on-going conflict. Depending on their perceived loyalties, families were targeted if menfolk were involved in the conflict: they were held hostage, detained, kidnapped, raped, or harassed. The mere presence of adult males gave rise to suspicions that they were party to the insurgency either by force or voluntarily.

Evacuations themselves were chaotic. Resources were squandered in the search for security; families separated; the physical constitution of the elderly and the young irreparably damaged; accumulated family savings were quickly exhausted; movable property was often sold (or destroyed); there was a lack of food, clean water and proper sanitation; and an increase in mortality rates, to name but a few.

Life in the refugee camps presents its own challenges, such as inadequate basic services and food, as well as the high incidence of communicable diseases. Families suffered economic distress due to loss of income, and women resorted to selling their gold jewelry to buy necessities. Despite having crossed borders in search of safety, the refugees' security was not guaranteed. They were still vulnerable, and even the simple search for firewood beyond the safety of their camps exposed women to sexual violence. Families were separated because males who could not submit to the humiliation of camp life preferred to seek their fortunes elsewhere.

The International Committee of the Red Cross (2001) reports that armed conflicts uproot families, and that women and children form the majority of the world's refugees and displaced persons. In cities, large numbers of female-headed households are being created where men have been conscripted, detained, displaced, have disappeared, or have died. Furthermore, OXFAM reports that, in extending their roles to cover that of absent males, women may discover new capabilities which neither they nor their menfolk thought they had. This gives them the confidence to challenge and in some cases redefine the cultural and social perception of themselves and their former boundaries in society (O'Connell, 1993).

Such was and is the case in Somalia. Circumstances have completely changed women's roles in the family, the community, and the public domain. The breakdown or disintegration of the family and community networks has forced them to assume new roles, to bear greater responsibility for their children and their elderly relatives, as well as for the extended family. They have had to find ways and means of feeding and sustaining their wards, while maintaining a modicum of stability for their families in an environment where their safety and security is at risk. UNICEF (2002), in its report on women and children in Somalia, notes that women often develop a sense of assertiveness over time as a pre-condition for survival since becoming refugees. The report states that in developing characteristics to cope with the increased demands of camp life, some of the women have been forced to assume these more assertive patterns of behavior that can often have dramatic implications for the marital relationship. This occurred to the extent that the traditional role of men as providers became severely altered. Thus, as refugees, cultural constraints broke down in the face of critical changes in life circumstances and some women have assumed both a greater role for themselves within the family and have exercised more power within the marriage. This may be a positive change, but if viewed through the lens of loss, poverty, and deprivation endemic to war, the cost is enormous. The changing and redefining of family roles and responsibilities may be a temporary coping strategy or it may be a fundamental change with far-reaching consequences.

In an effort to explain the predicament of men, an elderly man stated during a workshop, "Fathers have faced unprecedented crises where they have been victimized, tortured, robbed, and killed. We cannot expect them to heal and recover so soon and at the same time to provide for their families. In order for the father to fulfill his family obligations he has to be provided with income-generating opportunities." Yet another complained, "We have been supporting the family for years before the war, and if today women somehow become the breadwinners, they shouldn't disgrace us, but they should become considerate and sensitive to our feelings" (Academy for Peace and Development, 2002). Such sentiments indicate the helplessness men feel in being unable to carry out their obligations.

Disruption and chaos caused by the civil war placed extraordinary stress on families, straining the social fabric and sewing seeds of mistrust in communities. Traditional conventions which granted immunity to the elderly, the sick, women, and children were violated. In contravention of all norms of society, gender-based violence and rape became a common weapon. The collective responsibility of clans for wrongdoing of individuals was overtaken by events where the scale of killing and maiming spiraled out of control. Rules governing retribution and compensation were not respected. Neither the tribal elders nor the government were able to exert their authority and influence to check the violence. As a result of the mayhem, poverty is widespread. Mutual support systems and coping mechanisms have been undermined by economic hardships, such as high unemployment and scarcity of resources. Absence of male family members due to war has weakened traditional structures and increased the number of female-headed households. For those who have sought asylum, exposure to foreign influence and lifestyles are additional issues which lead to frustration and tension within families.

RECOVERY

This section deals with the reconciliation process and rebuilding of lives: healing and reintegration for those who are repatriated; in the case of émigrés, adapting to new environments; and for those in refugee camps, their hopes for returning home. Also discussed are families' strategies for adapting to new environments, and the importance of maintaining their links with home.

According to the United Nations High Commissioner for Refugees (2005), in the last decade an estimated 700,000 refugees have returned to "Somaliland" alone, while an estimated 150,000 or more went home to the northeastern part of Somalia, also known as Puntland. This leaves some 350,000 Somali refugees still in exile worldwide.

Despite the overwhelming costs of civil war, peace brings its own challenges: healing and reconciliation, restructuring of relationships and communities; rebuilding of livelihoods and reconstruction of homes; restitution of land and property. In mobilizing for peace, women alongside men have been at the forefront of activities ranging from spontaneous demonstrations to *Allah bari* prayer meetings so as to help in the process of reconciliation and mobilizing the community. At such meetings women use their oral skills by reciting poetry *burambur*, urging peace and reconciliation which include rhetorical questions such as:

Why is this section of the town not speaking to that section?

Why is my right arm not talking to my left?

Why is my brother fighting my son?

Why is my son fighting my brother?

Why is my husband fighting my brother?

The Diaspora. This refers to the Somali population living outside the country (mostly in Europe and North America) who have emigrated in search of asylum.

Nomadic tendencies coupled with a spirit of adventure have made Somalis intrepid travelers. Even before the civil war, sizable communities were to be found in the north and east of Africa, in the Middle East, the United Kingdom, Italy, and the United States, where several generations have assimilated. In the years preceding the civil war, harassment and persecution drove thousands of Somalis to the Gulf where they found employment and sent remittances to their families. The civil war brought violence, insecurity, and displacement, and with it an exodus of civilian populations even further afield: Australia, Canada, Scandinavia and other European countries.

Resettlement in Europe and North America is a very much sought after option. Apart from security and stability, it offers opportunities such as social welfare, education, health services, employment, and a higher standard of living. In desperation, people risk their lives to relocate abroad, not only to secure the future for themselves and their children but, just as importantly, to find the means to financially support their family back home. More often than not, those same family members contributed to financing their travel abroad, an investment which usually brings financial rewards. Those who have achieved legal status and have settled in the Diaspora embrace their new life abroad and at the same time maintain strong links with the homeland. They try, in their new surroundings, to foster ways of sustaining bonds with values, customs, kin, and the community left behind. A direct result of emigration is the life-line of financial remittances that sustain families and the economy of Somaliland.

Families in the Diaspora have their own set of challenges associated with new environments. Faced with cultures that have different family structures and where permissiveness is widespread, integration becomes extremely difficult. The fear is that fraternization and peer pressure will lead children to abandon their religious roots and cultural values. Hence, the main drawbacks reported by émigrés are the absence of religious guidance and family networks. Added to these troubles, most families are headed by the mother who is often frustrated by not being familiar with the language of the adopted country, and therefore is unable to communicate her concerns. A common refrain relating to role-reversal is, "Our inadequacy is such that our children have to accompany us everywhere and translate for us, how can we command respect when we are so dependent on them?" It must be mentioned here that single parenthood is usually a result of abandonment, divorce, or widowhood, and cases of children born out-of-wedlock are uncommon. In another interview, a woman expressed her concern about crime in the West where many children are victims, compared to Somalia where children can walk around freely and safely on their own. She also quoted negative social influences to which children are exposed, e.g., substance abuse, and the absence of the safety net provided by the extended family. Children and youth also find the transition stressful in trying to adapt to their new homes and in meeting the conflicting expectations of their Western peers and their families.

In a study of Somali children in Nordic countries, a social worker in Denmark observed that, "Somalis in Africa know the suffering of war and destitution in refugee camps, but not the suffering of isolation and loneliness," which other Somalis experience abroad. Parents undergo great sacrifices to facilitate the migration of their children to Western countries, instilling in them the mission of making a success of their lives in order to support the family back home. The social worker sympathizes with the predicament of Somali émigré children by stating, "Parents don't understand the loneliness of the West . . . they can't imagine what it's like to go a whole day without seeing someone you know." The researcher notes that families in Somalia are concerned that their children in Christian countries are being exposed to lax influences, feeling that it is important that they should, "pray, receive Quranic instruction and maintain Somali customs," while living abroad (Ayotte, 2002).

Similarly, in the event of divorce, women can resort to the welfare safety net, therefore the stigma for divorced women and single parenthood is diminishing. This empowerment has created the perception in men that they are dispensable, or that a woman is "too big for her boots." Despite all these challenges, older generation males prefer to return to their homeland, assured that the family's material needs will be met by welfare benefits, but effectively depriving their families of the paternal presence and role model. In the few households where the father is present, he also acts as a community elder, performing *xeer* duties within the framework of local law. In the absence of gainful employment, this role is often enthusiastically embraced to offset his diminished status in the family. Here again, men spend time in other pursuits, such as frequenting coffee shops or in *mefrishes* chewing *khat*, and discussing social issues and politics or just plain camaraderie. Recent global events related to 9/11 have further marginalized Somali communities, leaving young men in particular feeling vulnerable and insecure because of their religion and immigrant status, and causing them to yearn for the *safety* of their war-torn country. Thus, women have to struggle to raise their children in an alien environment with little moral support. To offset these challenges, many families prefer to live in clusters where there are other Somalis settled so as to benefit from the communal social safety net. In such communities there are also facilities offering religious lessons for children and interested adults in local mosques or in private homes.

There are still hundreds of thousands of people living in refugee camps in the neighboring countries of Kenya, Ethiopia, Djibouti, and Yemen. They have lived in miserable conditions for over ten years and they face a grim future of uncertainty due to the continuing insecurity in Somalia. On a positive note, the camps offer safety, access to basic necessities, and an environment which is not altogether alien since they are in close proximity to their kith and kin. The very conditions that are considered life-saving are also paradoxically considered detrimental to social norms. As quoted by a seminar participant in the study on the impact of war on the Somali family, "The first bombshell of the war initially dispersed the family into different directions in search of safety; but the most serious dispersion of all took place in the refugee camps where food rations were distributed on an individual basis, thereby granting unprecedented independence to each member of the family. Upon return from the camps, family unity was never restored and individualistic patterns have ultimately prevailed" (Academy for Peace and Development, 2002, p. 13). In the Kenyan Dadaab refugee camp, residents expressed different opinions on the prospect of return. Men were concerned about their role as providers and lack of income-earning opportunities. Women expressed reservations about the availability of basic services such as food, shelter, education, and health facilities. Youth were despondent about their future. A young man lamented to the author,

> The youth are the most disaffected group; some of us have completed our schooling and have no other opportunities. The daily grind of life in a camp is depressing—nothing to do and nowhere to go. Some of my friends could not bear it and went back to Somalia in desperation, and now they are members of militia, manning roadblocks, since this is the only source of revenue. (Interview in Dadaab Refugee Camp, Kenya, March 2005)

Coping Strategies

How do families remain cohesive units in the face of change? The International Family Strengths Model (DeFrain, 2000; DeFrain et al.,

2006) posits six general qualities that describe strong families world-wide. These will be discussed in the Somali context of extended families, clans and communities.

Having described the conditions facing contemporary Somali families, we can summarize that the political, civil, and social upheaval have placed unprecedented pressures on Somali families. Death, destruction, and displacement have been the fate of millions. Internal tensions within the family are also emerging as a consequence of the drastic alternation of the traditional role of men as providers. Given the patriarchal nature of the society, this change in the delicate balance of gender roles, has nullified the image of men as breadwinners and absolved them from providing material support for their families. In defiance of their cultural and religious obligations, many men opt to abandon their families rather than be an additional burden. Even though they recognize that families rely on the income earned by women and that this has allowed them to become major decision makers at home, fathers and husbands nevertheless believe that their authority is being eroded. Thus, this is considered one of the main causes of breakdown in family structure both at home and abroad. In a study to examine the impact of the war, an elderly man is quoted as saying, "We have lost our cultural and religious identity because of the working mother who is trying to make a living in the market place. The family will not be the same as before–unless we reinforce our cultural and religious values and return mothers to their homes." Women, on the other hand, challenge men to be diligent and regain their authority and respect by providing for the family and surrendering their *khat* habits. A common refrain was articulated by a middle-aged woman interviewee when she said, "A father controls his family by maintaining their daily life. He would not be able to do so if he is not providing for them." This contentious issue will only be settled when fathers and husbands can meet the needs of their families, thereby allowing women to adjust their roles. Related to this, is the rising incidence of polygamy which, although permitted in Islam, could be recognized as a coping strategy for men in an attempt to regain respect and authority. While it may satisfy their egos, it further alienates the father and husband from his other wife and children (Academy for Peace and Development, 2002).

Despite the calamities and their consequences, the extended family institution remains strong. Extensive research carried out by John DeFrain, Nick Stinnett, and many colleagues around the world, identifies six major qualities shared by strong families across many cultures: enjoyable time together, appreciation and affection, positive communication, commitment, spiritual wellbeing, and the ability to manage stress and crisis effectively (DeFrain, 2000; DeFrain et al., 2006). We now consider these *strengths* in the Somali context. To add a cultural dimension, Somali proverbs germane to each quality are quoted. This will allow readers to appreciate both the context in which the discussion takes place and the richness of Somali language and tradition. The writer regrets that sometimes the meaning is lost in the translation, due to the cryptic nature of the proverbs.

Enjoyable time together

Somali proverb: *Laba kala bariday, kala war la.*
Translation: Spend a night apart and neither knows
how the other is faring.

Contrary to the commonly espoused Western ideas of *quality time* and making time to enjoy together, Somalis adopt what is more like an easy rhythm in a family-oriented setting that implies you are "welcome to join whatever is going on." The social structure is such that nuclear families very rarely enjoy time together as a separate unit. In extended families the norm is for peer groups divided along gender and age lines to spend time together, thus forming close and ever-lasting relationships. The adults are normally satisfied with this arrangement, assured that trusted members of the family who share common values are at hand to fulfill each other's emotional and material needs. Similarly, eating arrangements are communal and divided on the same lines, with separate groups of males, and females with children. Standard etiquette is followed with several people in a circle, and eating from the same large platters of food (everyone using their right hand for eating after thoroughly washing). Prime time for enjoying family interaction is in the late afternoons and early evenings in both urban and rural settings. While satellite TV has usurped this slot in towns and villages, rural families still enjoy time together. They gather, young and old, male and female, under the stars and around the camp fire to engage in conversation. Other occasions for doing things together include going to the mosque for prayers at prescribed times or, where there are no mosques, group prayers indoors or outdoors led by the eldest person–men and women separately. The *khat*-chewing habit reduces the amount of time families spend together, since male members prefer to spend leisure time with their peers chewing *khat* and discussing issues of common interest. In this respect, women form their own group networks which serve as safety and support systems. Poverty and lack of leisure facilities prevent family outings. Paradoxically, in refugee camps, time is a commodity which is always available–apart from queuing for relief supplies, there is not much else to do. Deprived of material comforts, time spent together in confined quarters and in a cheerless atmosphere does act as a bond.

Appreciation and affection for each other

Somali proverb: *Gacmo is dhaafa gacalo ka timaadda.*
Translation: To love is to give.

In a society where love and affection are valued, physical demonstration of such feelings are not encouraged across gender lines. Their importance is, however, evident in poetry, folklore and popular contemporary love songs. In spousal relationships, intimate moments are confined to the bedroom because outward gestures of affection between couples are considered awkward and embarrassing in public. Lack of privacy in the home further limits the degree of affection married couples can display. However, care for each other manifests itself in a number of ways such as being attentive to each other, care for personal appearance, courteous relationships with in-laws and extended family members, and other subtle acts. Kissing and hugging are acceptable only between the same gender or across gender lines between adults and young children. Non-physical ways of appreciation and affection can be shown by acts of kindness, praise and indulgence of children, or in the manner of addressing one another. Using humor and teasing in a non-offensive way are very common. Occasions which are observed in many countries to express sentiments of love and affection between individuals, such as birthdays, Valentine's Day, and so forth, are not observed by Somalis. Religious holidays, however, are marked by buying new clothes and celebrated by events such as feasts where sheep are sacrificed. The family head usually presents gifts or money to the whole household rather than intimate exchanges between individuals. In refugee camps this is practiced on a very modest scale, conditions being such that poverty and deprivation do not allow generosity. Such residents are keenly aware of their predicament–helpless and without any means. Moral support becomes the currency of love and affection, a reflex strengthening of bonds within and beyond family structures. The few people who are more privileged are very discreet and sensitive about flaunting their good fortune. Intergenerational relationships are sustained by the confidence and regard shown to each other and the desire to live up to expectations. This tenderness and indulgence toward elders and to younger members of the family, in particular, signifies their special status. Love and affection are therefore symbolized by generosity, by kind acts and by mutual support.

Positive communication with each other

Somali proverb: *Hubsiimo hal baa la siistaa.*
Translation: To know something for sure,
one would part with a she camel.
Somali proverb: *Af jooga looma adeego.*
Translation: Do not speak for someone who is present.

Somalis belong to an oral society with a language that is rich and expressive. Although Somali language is not in itself a polite means of communication, its harshness is attributable to the tough way of life where there is no ambiguity. For example, the word *please* does not exist in the vocabulary. To offset the absence of courteousness, the manner of speaking and the body language are important: deference to elders and respected people is shown by modifying behavior and by being attentive. Communication within the family very much depends on the age and standing of the communicants. A child would be spoken to in a more patronizing manner, while communication with older children serves to reinforce pride, responsibility, and confidence. Within families, the manner of communication with the head of the family (usually the patriarch), is usually formal and respectful. It is not unusual for another family member to approach the patriarch as an advocate or mediator when the situation so warrants. Quick wit and repartee is admired within and beyond family circles, united in enjoying light humorous moments. The penchant for story telling and exchanging life stories is one of the favorite pastimes. Everyone can relate to adversity and hard times, while at the same time harboring hopes for good fortune. This coping strategy facilitates the integration of varied experiences into the fabric of their lives.

Poetry is a much-admired oral tradition which is often repeated and quoted. Most poems expound wisdom and bravery and generate lively discussion by the listeners, young and old. Important conversations take place in a formal manner and other family members are invited to attend so that they can contribute opinions. The quoting of verses from the *Quran* normally precedes discussion. Poetry and other relevant stories also serve to put the topic of discussion into perspective and gain attention. Information flows freely within the inevitably large households where lack of privacy and space make any attempt at secrecy futile. In the event of misunderstandings and disputes, there is no shortage of family members who go to great lengths to intervene and mediate. For Somalis in the Diaspora, secluded lifestyles force them to seek out other Somalis who become surrogate extended families. Tensions are apparent in such families where the younger generation do not share the same perspectives and often have difficulty understanding the *open house* attitude, leading to the perception that the Western environment is not conducive to this way of life.

Valuing each other and demonstrating commitment

Somali proverb: *Iskaashato ma kufto.*
Translation: Mutual support never fails.
Somali proverb: *Meel "hoo" u baahan, hadal wax kama taro.*
Translation: Where material help is needed, words do not suffice
Somali proverb: *Ilko wadajir bay wax ka gooyaan.*
Translation: Teeth can only bite when they work together.

Commitment and responsibility is inculcated in children from a young age. Strength of character is emphasized by training children to fend for themselves and become productive members of the group. Children are nurtured with the knowledge that they will one day assume the duty of caring for their parents as well as elder and needy family members. They understand what is expected of them in the traditional setting where responsibilities are clearly delineated, foremost of which is to maintain the family and clan's reputation. Indicative of this sense of belonging is the typical call for help: "*Tolay, tolay*," which literally means, "Oh my kin, oh my kin." The obligation to respond to this call is incumbent upon all capable family members.

As far as conjugal commitment is concerned, fidelity is usually broken when a husband decides to get another wife, as casual liaisons are not common within the community. Despite the fact that it is permissible in Islam, polygamy is often a source of disagreement and disharmony, with the different wives competing for the attention and resources of the husband.

The extended family structure also places importance on grandparents, aunts, uncles, cousins, and so forth, both maternal and paternal. The role of grandparents is particularly important. They are respected and cared for in old age, they provide guidance and wisdom, they teach the younger children traditional values, and often act as confidantes as well as arbitrators in family matters.

Demonstrating commitment is the core value of the extended family network and this is one of the main strengths which have helped in overcoming multiple challenges presented by social and civil strife. Typical occasions to show solidarity and support within the extended family include happy occasions such as weddings and births, as well as for misfortunes such as sickness and death. On such occasions and wherever they may be–towns, villages, rural areas, refugee camps–the family rallies and extends their assistance. In so doing, the interests of those in need are put above their own, sacrificing time, effort, and material items including money. Patterns of flight in times of war or drought illustrate very clearly the significance of familial ties, since people always choose to move to safe areas where they are assured of receiving protection and assistance from their kin. Commitment can also be measured by financial support for relatives, and none is as demonstrative as that of remittances sent by those who are living abroad to their families back home. The United Nations reports that such remittances are a crucial part of the Somali economy, quoting an estimated annual value of $800 million where, in some cities, it can represent 40% of the income of urban households. The UN further reports that while remittances are fairly regular; they increase in times of economic stress, such as drought or times of inter-clan warfare. It can also be noted here that remittances increase during the *Eid* festival periods. Most Somalis in the Diaspora make it a point to send the obligatory alms or *Zakat* payment to their homeland for distribution to the poor. In the absence of the extended family network, Somalis living abroad seek and develop alternative support systems, usually other Somalis who are not necessary related. These relationships substitute for the extended family and provide the mutual commitment and support otherwise not available. Residents of refugee camps resort to the extended family and create bonds with others in the same position, such as neighbors and the community.

Spiritual well-being

Somali proverb: *Allow, nimaan wax ogayn ha cadaabin.*
Translation: O Lord, do not punish one who acts through ignorance.
Somali proverb: *Salaad walba waqtigeedaa la tukadaa.*
Translation: Every prayer should be offered at its prescribed time.

(Note: By referring to the five daily prayers at prescribed times, this proverb can also mean that things should be done at the appropriate time.)

Somali proverb: *Roonaa Rabbaa og.*
Translation: Only God knows what is best.

Spiritual sustenance is one of the few *strengths* that have not fallen victim to the social changes in the Somali context. Islam is the guiding force for all families and acts as the primary social safety net, particularly in times of stress and strife, encompassing all aspects of their lives. The belief that everything is preordained and that humans should persevere in the face of adversity is strongly upheld. Hence, Somalis draw upon their inner resources to endure all hardships with a stoicism and dignity widely recognized (Drysdale, 2000). The power of God and the strength of faith are manifested by constantly evoking His name–*Bismillah* (in the name of Allah), *Alhamdulilah* (thanks to Allah), *InshaAllah* (if Allah wills)–are but a few phrases which are always on their lips. The name of Allah is invoked to seek help and to offer thanks both for their successes and failures. The obligation to offer prayers five times daily is foremost in most peoples minds and they interrupt whatever they are doing to do so at the prescribed times. Going to the mosque (mostly men and a few women) at prescribed times, praying collectively shoulder to shoulder, meeting regulars and welcoming newcomers, these very acts make people feel good. Teachings of the Prophet Mohammed (peace be upon Him) are often quoted when dealing with family matters and followers are urged to emulate his exemplary behavior. Prayer and meditation groups spring up wherever there is a sizable community, providing solidarity and comfort. Even in camps, refugees garner their resources and build a makeshift structure which serve as a local mosque, appointing the most learned among them as the *sheikh*. Other elders support him in counseling and mediating in disputes, with the community contributing to the *sheikh's* salary in cash or kind. As corroborated by an elder from the Dadaab refugee camp in Kenya, families or individuals in distress approach the local mosque for assistance. Undoubtedly, Somalis everywhere turn to spiritualism as a source of faith and hope. This belief system has been a powerful influence in overcoming the multiple crises experienced by Somali families.

Managing stress and crisis effectively

Somali proverb: *Eebbe ma naxee, waa naxariistaa.*
Translation: God allows us to experience adversity, but he is merciful.

Somali proverb: *Belaayo kaa sii jeedda layskuma soo jeediyo.*
Translation: If misfortune shows its back,
do not force it to show its face.

   Famine, drought, civil war, and displacement are external factors which
have combined to make Somalis resilient people, hence the remarkably
common ability to handle stress and crisis effectively. Stressors as a
consequence of civil war include the high number of injured and traumatized men, women, and youth. Without any medical facilities, the
victims are cared for by the extended family that provide for them,
watch over them, and when necessary, physically restrain the increasing
number of mentally disturbed people. Tacit understanding and support
from the community contribute to providing assurance and solidarity.
Similarly, in other crises such as death, communal rituals assist surviving
family members in coming to terms with their loss and grief. Mourning
presents an opportunity for relatives and friends to provide moral and
material help to the family of the deceased. This takes the form of arranging for the burial, hosting all the mourners for a period of three
days, providing and cooking food for the poor and giving alms, reading
of the *Quran* and praying for the deceased. As a spiritual strength, Islam
assists in overcoming stress in ways described above and by fostering
strong values, faith, and compassion which help families rise above the
barriers of poverty, loss, and despair. Other unconventional coping
strategies include resorting to clairvoyants who are also sometimes religious mystics, in the hope of getting advice, relief, and cures from illnesses and other misfortunes. Socio-environmental changes are causing
confusion of roles and expectations throughout the family structure,
with gender roles being the main cause of tensions. Where men are the
traditional decision-makers and providers, rampant unemployment
coupled with urbanization deprives them of the role, making them feel
marginalized and ineffective. Pragmatically, women are filling the role
as breadwinners in the hope that the status quo will change and that men
will regain their status.
   The aspiration of most refugees is to seek asylum abroad as a *solution*.
They are inspired by stories of Somali individuals and families who successfully established themselves professionally, financially, or socially
in their new environment. To achieve that goal and thereby escape from
the despair and uncertainty, potential émigrés take great risks. A case in
point is the jeopardy in which the Somali *boat people* place themselves
with their ultimate destination being to reach a Western country. They
often clandestinely traverse perilous seas in rickety boats and trek across

borders in search of safety, freedom, and a promising future. Once they reach safety abroad, they sometimes face culture shock, loneliness, and disillusionment. They consequently turn to other Somalis for mutual support in the absence of family or clan. These clusters of support systems, sharing the same culture, religion, and language, are almost as effective as having tribal backup. They pull together in times of need, they intervene and mediate when called upon to do so, and they watch over each other. Stress in camp life is somewhat different from what it is outside the camp. Since residents are provided with basic necessities such as food, shelter, health care, and education to a certain level, their physiological needs are met. However, conflict and tension are common in family relationships, caused by perceived expectations and guilt in not being able to meet those expectations. In Dadaab Camp in Kenya, a young man expressed his inadequacy, saying that he had completed his schooling up to the level available, and without any other opportunities, spent all day wandering around the camp with his friends. He described the anxiety and helplessness he felt when he had to look into his mother's hopeful eyes in the evenings, with nothing positive to offer her. Beyond the borders of Somalia, the author was impressed to observe the readiness of people to offer assistance and perform services such as translation and mediation. Lacking foreign language skills, other Somalis who are familiar with the bureaucracy consider it their civic duty to assist and advise their compatriots. Hardship and struggle seem to be the realm in which most Somalis exist. Their remarkable ability to handle stress and crises effectively has served them well in multiple crises.

CONCLUDING REFLECTIONS

The civil war has been a catalyst which has severely altered the lives of most Somalis. It is evident from the foregoing that families negotiate change and stressful life events by clinging to tradition and religion. Extended family and clan members depend on each other for moral and material assistance. This is an arrangement which assures a system of cooperation and mutual support built on religious and cultural values.

Everyone has their own story about what is literally referred to as the *qab* or catastrophe, which has wrought untold hardship directly or indirectly. Despite this, with minimal resources and sheer determination, families in the three different categories–returnees, émigrés, and camp residents– have gone about re-defining priorities and readjusting. For the returnees, priorities are reconciliation, reintegration, and self-reliance under the ever-present threat of renewed violence. For those who have resettled abroad, the struggle is to adjust without surrendering religion, tradition, and culture. For those incarcerated in refugee camps, religion, tradition, and culture are survival strategies to overcome anxiety, uncertainty, and despair. These challenges and the inevitable evolutionary socio-economic changes have had a profound effect on Somali society as a whole. Somali families have been tested to the extreme by the multiple stresses which present themselves. With tools for coping severely limited, the innate qualities described in this chapter have proven to be their salvation.

This exploratory study validates the hypothesis of researchers, Stinnett and DeFrain, that strong families often share six major qualities: enjoyable time together, appreciation and affection, positive communication, commitment, spiritual wellbeing, and the ability to manage stress and crisis effectively. Two qualities in particular emerge as the bedrocks of the Somali family: spiritual well-being and commitment. However, the author also notices inter-linkages: core values of spirituality and commitment lead naturally to appreciation, communications, and enjoyable time together which all promise successful management of stress.

Parallel to the characteristics mentioned above, interviewees and informants identified the following critical strengths they consider unique to Somalis:

• Strong religious faith
• Close attachment to culture, rituals, and traditions
• Strong kinship bonds including filial responsibilities
• Readiness to meet obligations and provide help to extended family
• Belief in helping people less fortunate
• Unity during adversity and pulling together in difficult times
• Aspirations to success and wealth
• Commitment to invest in their homeland

International law recognizes that the family is a fundamental unit of society requiring special protection such as Article 16(3) of the Universal Declaration of Human Rights which declares that the family is the "natural and fundamental group unit of society and is entitled to protection by society and the state." In the Somali context, on the one hand the state, in the midst of trying to emerge as a credible entity, cannot provide *protection* or security nor can it provide institutional social services, such as disaster mitigation, health care, education, and so forth. On the other hand society, itself in crisis as an aftermath of the civil war, is witnessing new family dynamics. The main manifestation of this, as perceived by the author, is the empowerment of women: as breadwinners in Somalia, as recipients of welfare benefits in countries of asylum, and as recipients of aid in refugee camps. Such fundamental changes in social structures and roles is evidently causing internal tension within the family over and above the struggle to cope with external challenges. Strong family relationships can only be nurtured in an environment where no one feels threatened or marginalized, where individuals feel that they are worthy members of society. Therefore it is critical that steps be taken to overcome ideological biases by educating people on the potential of women, alongside their men, as a resource in the development of the nation.

In closing, the author cannot but note the paucity of information on such an important topic. Having survived 15 years of turmoil, reeling from crisis to crisis, Somali families need some respite to come to terms with the changes. At this critical juncture where the focus is on national recovery and rehabilitation, reliable data and in-depth examinations of family strengths are needed to guide and enhance development policies and strategies.

REFERENCES

Academy for Peace and Development. (2002). *The impact of the war on the family*. Hargeisa, Somaliland: APD.

Ahmed, I. (2000). *Disasters: Remittances and their economic impact in post-war Somaliland*. Oxford, UK: Blackwell.

Ayotte, W. (2002). Separated children: Exile and home links: The example of Somali children in Nordic countries. Copenhagen, Denmark: Save the Children.

Danish Refugee Council. (2004, August). Human rights and peace advocacy impact on Somali customary law: The Togdheer experience. Copenhagen, Denmark: DRC.

DeGenova, M. K. (Ed.). (1997). *Families in cultural contexts: Strengths and challenges in diversity*. Mountain View, CA: Mayfield.

DeFrain, J. (2000). What is a strong family, anyway? University of Nebraska-Lincoln for Families website: http://unlforfamilies.unl.edu.

DeFrain, J., et al. (2006). *Family treasures: Creating strong families*. Lincoln, NE: University of Nebraska Extension.

Drysdale, J. A. (2000). *Stoics without pillows*. London: Haan Associates.

Drysdale, J. A. (2004). Study of the Somali Hybrid Insurance System and the consequences of its rejection by Southern Somalia's political leadership. Unpublished report.

Gardner, J., & El Bushra, J. (2004). *Somalia, the untold story: War through the eyes of Somali women*. London, UK: Pluto Press.

Hassan, D. F., Amina, H. A., & Amina, M. W. (1995). *Somali poetry as resistance against colonialism and patriarchy*. London, UK: Zed Books.

Houseknecht, S., & Pankhurst, J. (Eds.). (2000). *Family, religion and social change in diverse societies*. New York: Oxford University Press.

International Committee of the Red Cross (2001). ICRC study on the impact of armed conflict on women: Executive summary. Geneva, Switzerland: ICRC.

Kapchits, G. L. (2001). Somali proverbs: A study in popularity. Unpublished report.

LeSage, A. (2005, July). Stateless justice in Somalia: Formal and informal rule of law initiatives. Geneva, Switzerland: Centre for Humanitarian Dialogue.

Lewis, I. M. (1999). *A pastoral democracy: A study of pastoralism and politics among the Northern Somali of the Horn of Africa.* Hamburg, Germany, and Oxford, UK: Verlag, and James Currey Publishers.

Ministry of Planning and Coordination. (2004). *Somaliland strategy for economic recovery and poverty reduction plan 2004-2006.* Hargeisa, Somaliland.

Mocellin, J. S. P. (1993). *Psychosocial Consequences of the Somalia Emergency on Women and Children.* Somalia: UNICEF and WHO.

O'Connell, H. (Ed.). (1993). *Women and conflict.* Oxford, UK: Oxfam.

United Nations Development Programme. (2001). *Human development report, Somalia.* Nairobi, Kenya: UNDP.

United Nations High Commissioner for Refugees. (2005, January). Introduction to the comprehensive plan of action. Unpublished preliminary document. Nairobi, Kenya: UNHCR.

United National International Children's Emergency Fund. (1991). *An analysis of the situation of children and women in Somalia.* Nairobi, Kenya: UNICEF.

United National International Children's Emergency Fund (2002). *Assessing the current status of the nomadic population in Somalia.* Nairobi, Kenya: UNICEF.

United Nations Development Fund for Women. (UNIFEM). (1998). *Somalia between peace and war: Somali women on the eve of the 21st Century.* Nairobi, Kenya: UNIFEM.

United Nations Press Release. (2005, March). 25 million civilians displaced by war are unprotected. Geneva, Switzerland: UN.

Universal Declaration of Human Rights. (1948, December). Article 16(3). United Nations, New York website: http://www.un.org/Overview/rights.html

War Torn Societies Programme. (2000). The role of Somali women in post-conflict reconstruction. Nairobi, Kenya: WSP Somali Programme.

World Bank/United Nations Development Program. (2004, January). *Socio-economic survey, Somalia.* Nairobi, Kenya: World Bank/UNDP.

doi:10.1300/J002v41n01_05

THE MIDDLE EAST

The Resilience of Families in Israel: Understanding Their Struggles and Appreciating Their Strengths

Maha N. Younes

SUMMARY. This article reveals the mystifying reality, enduring struggles and uncertain future facing families in Israel. The compelling literature shortage of inclusive and fair scholarly representation of the various ethnic groups in Israel inspired the focus of this work on the commonalities, including the shared sense of suffering as well as manner in which life is celebrated. Of significance are the factors that generate divergence among the various ethnic groups while supporting their family strengths.

Maha N. Younes is Professor of Social Work, 2014 Founders Hall, Department of Criminal Justice and Social Work, University of Nebraska-Kearney, Kearney, NE 68849 (E-mail: younesm@unk.edu).

The author wishes to acknowledge the valuable contribution of Yoav Lavee, Professor of Social Work in the School of Social Work, University of Haifa, Israel, to this paper.

[Haworth co-indexing entry note]: "The Resilience of Families in Israel: Understanding Their Struggles and Appreciating Their Strengths." Younes, Maha N. Co-published simultaneously in *Marriage & Family Review* (The Haworth Press, Inc.) Vol. 41, No. 1/2, 2007, pp. 101-117; and: *Strong Families Around the World: Strengths-Based Research and Perspectives* (ed: John DeFrain, and Sylvia M. Asay) The Haworth Press, Inc., 2007, pp. 101-117. Single or multiple copies of this article are available for a fee from The Haworth Document Delivery Service [1-800-HAWORTH, 9:00 a.m. - 5:00 p.m. (EST). E-mail address: docdelivery@ haworthpress.com].

Available online at http://mfr.haworthpress.com
© 2007 by The Haworth Press, Inc. All rights reserved.
doi:10.1300/J002v41n01_06

Family and cultural resilience is a mere derivative of the commitment to family and traditions, faith, communication styles, and a strong recuperative energy that unite all groups. doi:10.1300/J002v41n01_06 *[Article copies available for a fee from The Haworth Document Delivery Service: 1-800-HAWORTH. E-mail address: <docdelivery@haworthpress.com> Website: <http://www.HaworthPress.com> © 2007 by The Haworth Press, Inc. All rights reserved.]*

KEYWORDS. Families in Israel, family strengths, Israel, Palestinian, Arab-Jewish

INTRODUCTION

Israel is the "Land of Milk and Honey," the "Holy Land," and honored as the cradle of Judaism and Christianity. Israel refers to a land that is most noted in religious scriptures, and whose soil is so precious religiously and historically that it conjures up images of spirituality, ancient traditions, and peace. Yet, peace is most elusive to this land that has witnessed endless controversy and bloodshed for hundreds of years and countless generations. Understanding the underlying sociopolitical dynamics of this country is crucial for appreciating its rich diversity and the resilience of its families. It is simply impossible to separate the history of the land from the story of its people and the strong traditions that underlie family life and functions.

The Land

Israel is located in the Middle East with the Mediterranean Sea to the west. Neighboring Arabic countries include Lebanon to the north, Syria to the northeast, Jordan to the east, and Egypt to the southwest. Despite the country's small size, the scenery varies with the Negev desert in the south, a beautiful coastline, and a central mountainous region. In fact, in approximately ninety minutes one can drive across the country from west to east, and a six-hour drive is enough to cross the country from north to south. The Dead Sea represents the lowest point on the earth's surface and is located between Israel and Jordan (Hirsh, 1998). The geographic beauty of the country along with its historic and religious significance makes it an ideal tourist destination.

Israel's climate varies but has two prevailing seasons: a rainy winter extending from November to May and a dry season extending the following six months. However, regional conditions differ. The coastline enjoys humid summers and mild winters. The mountain region enjoys hot summers but moderately-cold temperatures in winters. Hot summers and pleasant winters are the rule in the valleys and desert conditions predominate in the Negev (Hirsh, 1998).

The People

Arabs and Jews inhabited the land before the establishment of Israel under previous occupations. The land, which was known as Palestine was part of the Ottoman Empire from 1840-1918 and granted as an administrative mandate to Great Britain in 1920. At the time, the majority of the population was Palestinian with a growing Jewish minority group. Following World War I, the British assured the Palestinians a homeland while making a similar pledge to the Jews (Stephan et al., 2004). In 1947, the British Commission with approval of the United Nations divided the Palestinian region into an Arab and a Jewish state.

The Jewish population accepted the division; however, the Palestinians rejected it leading to subsequent wars and ongoing tensions (CIA, 2005). Israel was then established as a nation in 1948 following the withdrawal of the British from Palestine. As a result, seven Arab countries attacked Israel but were defeated by Jews who gained additional land but lost old Jerusalem. The West Bank and Gaza regions were placed under Egyptian control. This bitter war of 1948 is etched into Palestinian consciousness as it led many Arabs to flee their homes and land to become refugees in Gaza, the West Bank, and Jordan. Through this fight for land a demographic shift occurred almost overnight. Saouli (2001) reports that more than 700,000 Palestinians fled their homeland and became refugees in surrounding Arab countries. The 160,000 remaining Palestinians very quickly became a minority with the Jewish minority becoming the new majority. The new minority, which was mostly composed of the poor and peasants since the elite had fled, was left without leadership and placed under Israeli military rule for control purposes from 1948-1966 (Saouli, 2001). While military rule ended as soon as Israel was fully merged, control over the Arab minority continued. Thus the term *Israeli Arab* differentiates the Arabs who remained in Israel from other Palestinians (Stephan et al., 2004). This brief but important summary describes the birth of a young nation and the beginning of what is known as the Palestinian-Israeli or Arab-Jewish conflict.

Arabs and Jews continue to coexist in Israel and the size of the population has grown from the 873,000 at the nation's inception to the current 6,276,883. The Jewish percentage is 80.1 with the following breakdown: Europe/America-born 32.1%, Israel-born 20.8%, Africa-born 14.6%, and Asia-born 12.6%. The non-Jewish percentage made up mostly of Arabs is 19.9% (1996 estimate) (CIA, 2005).

It is important to note inter-group diversity, as not all Jewish or Arab people share the same backgrounds. Since the 1948 declaration of Israel's independence, large waves of Jews immigrated from Europe, North America, and Islamic countries such as Iraq, Syria, Yemen, and North Africa. Beginning with 1970, large numbers of Jews migrated from Russia and Ethiopia. As noted in Katz and Lavee (2003), the Jewish population is generally divided into two categories. The Sephardim (Spanish) migrated from the Near East, North Africa, Yemen, Ethiopia, and other Islamic countries and the Ashkenazim migrated from America and Europe.

A breakdown of the Jewish population reveals the percentage of children who were either born or are children of the following groups: 33.5% of Asian-African origin, 40% of European-American origin, and 26.5% of Israeli origin (Central Bureau of Statistics, 2002) The median age among Jews is 30.3 with 996 men per 1,000 women (Bureau of Statistics, 2003). Jewish families average 3.5 members per family, with 10% of all Jewish families having more than five members.

The Israeli Central Bureau of Statistics (2003) indicates that Arabs in Israel comprise 1.302 million, or as noted previously 19% of the population. Muslims represent the majority of Israel's Arabs at 82% or 1.073 million, Christians account for 9% or 116,000, and the Druze 9% or 111,000. While information about the Christian and Muslim religion is widespread, the Druze religion remains unknown to outsiders. What is known is that they maintain the philosophy of *taqiyya*, which stresses loyalty to the government and country of residence.

The high fertility rate among Arabs results in a generally younger population with a median age of 19.7, and 1,035 men per 1,000 women. On average, Arab families are comprised of 4.9 persons and an overall average of three children. Thirty-six percent of Arab families have more than five people and at least 76% have at least one child. While the overall Arab population is projected to grow to 2.32 million by 2025, that increase is occurring among Muslims. The number of Druze is showing a slight decline with a noticeably continuing decline among Christian Arabs.

Other groups exist within the Arab minority, such as the Bedouins who comprise 10% of the Muslim population and reside within 30 tribes that live in northern Israel. Traditionally, the Bedouins maintained a nomadic life style but are currently transitioning into a permanent housing style and slowly joining the labor force. The Circassians, who are Sunni Muslims, number 3,000. They maintain a separate ethnic identity from the Arabs, Muslims, and Jews but participate in Israel's labor force.

While the above statistics accurately represent different groups in the population, it is important to examine the social and economic reality of Israeli families and its impact on their quality of life. The Israeli Central Bureau of Statistics (2001) reports that participation in the labor force between Arab and Jewish men is "almost identical" at 60%. The lower participation rate of Arab women in the labor market, at 17% compared to Jewish women at 55%, results in an overall lower participation rate among Arabs at 39%. Of Arabs with academic degrees, 84% of Arab men and 62% of Arab women have jobs, as compared to 76% of Jewish men and 79% of Jewish women. On average, the income of Arab workers is 69% of the amount earned by Jewish workers, with females earning slightly higher incomes due to education. This discrepancy reflects the multidimensional social, economic, and political reality confronting minorities and their continuing efforts to achieve economic security and political equality.

CHALLENGES FACING ISRAELI FAMILIES

Violence, Terrorism, and War

Although the impact of wars, political and economic instability, and ever-changing demographics penetrates and transcends all family dynamics and societal structures, common challenges confront Israel and its overall population. First and foremost, violence resulting from terrorism, war, or the threat of war is a part of daily life in Israel. The devastating impact of this kind of violence is ubiquitous, powerful, and inescapable. It infiltrates all societal structures and population groups while simultaneously tearing and binding them in this fragile yet enduring country. The social, economic, and political dynamics generated by terrorism and war influence family functioning, childrearing practices, and overall familial well-being. The common threat of violence due to war and terrorism "doesn't distinguish between Jewish and Arab children" and should be acknowledged as "collective distress" (Efrat et al.,

1998, p. 59). This fact seems lost on the international media. Depending on the media's country of reference, each group tends to be presented either as a victim or villain and martyr or terrorist without regard for the excessive price paid by both sides.

All eligible Jewish and Druze women are drafted into compulsory armed services at the age of 17; however, service is voluntary for Christians, Muslims, and Circassians. Men serve for a period of three years, while women serve for 21 months. Upon completion, men serve their army duty for 39 days a year up to age 51 (CIA, 2005). This policy makes war a family concern and with the small size of the country, war or terrorist acts have immediate consequences on Israeli families who are vulnerable to loss of a family member. Wysman and others (1993) indicate that combat stress reaction (CSR) and post-traumatic-stress disorder (PTSD) impact family and marital well-being. Their findings indicate, "Wives of traumatized veterans have to contend far more often than other wives with conflict and rigidity in family functioning" (p. 104). Regardless of combat experience, the threat of violence is ever-present and the subsequent anxiety is experienced by all population groups.

The Palestinian Intifada or resistance, which began in 1987 and re-emerged in 2000, continues today as a constant source of stress that is impossible to ignore. In addition to fostering personal and national insecurity, it intensifies the already present sense of resentment between Arabs and Jews. The Intifada involves Palestinians of the West Bank and Gaza who are offspring of the refugees that fled the land upon the establishment of Israel. They perceive themselves as refugees in their own land and have increased greatly in number since 1948.

Stephan and others (2004) note that as of 2000, most of the approximately four million Palestinians residing in Gaza and the West Bank continue to live in refugee camps. Their high fertility rate is viewed as a threat to Israel's viability, as some fear that their population rate could exceed that of the Jews in Israel (Kahn, 2000). The likelihood and timeline of this happening is debated. Soffer of Haifa University believes it could happen by 2020 but others such as Zimmerman, Seid, and Wise (2006) of the Begin-Sadat Center for Strategic Studies in Israel stress the exaggeration of such figures and note that demographic concerns of Israel are comparable to those of 1967. Moreover, their continued struggle for a homeland and resistance against Israeli forces complicate the coexistence of Israeli Arabs. They are caught between their ancestral heritage and current reality as a minority group in a Jewish nation. They sympathize with the Palestinian struggle but dislike the toll it creates on their general well-being and the intensification of Jewish mistrust and discrimination against them.

Diversity and Ethnic Tension

The continuous tension between and among the different groups is another major challenge that Israeli families have to contend with. Examples are the Arabs versus Jews, secular versus devout Jews, Ashkenazi versus Sephardim Jews, and political left versus political right (Efrat et al., 1998). The outcome is "significant segregation, racism, negative stereotypes, suspicion, animosity, rejection, feelings of alienation, anger, and marginalization of some groups" (Efrat et al., 1998, 59). The struggles and tensions noted among the various groups ravage families socially psychologically, and economically.

The two major minority groups in Israel are the Arabs and Orthodox Jews. As a group Arabs face discrimination at multiple levels, such as employment, education, reduced government assistance, and in terms of substandard services. They also maintain a more traditional and conservative ideology than the Jewish population (Haj-Yahia, 1995). Arabs in Israel experience inter-group conflict in addition to conflict with the majority Jewish population. Little if any attention has been given in the literature to the conflict between Muslims and Christians. Additionally, when questioned by outside forces about the ongoing tensions between the two groups, most Arabs would either deny or minimize its existence. Some Arabs even assert that such conflict is mere propaganda promoted by a majority Jewish government that aims to divide and conquer. However, such claims fade when each Arab segment debates the issue within the safety of their own group. This reality contributes to the declining number of Christians who immigrate to Europe and America in search of religious freedom, as well as more equitable educational, economic, and political opportunities. The wide-ranging discomfort of Christian Arabs and their subsequent abandonment of the Holy Land is regrettable not only to them but to Christians throughout the world.

Nethe (2002) notes, "Muslims represent the largest and fastest-growing religious group" and adds that "with 1.2 billion practitioners, Islam represents roughly one-fifth of the world's population" (p. 1). The growth of Islamic fundamentalism that began in the Middle East and is experienced in many regions of the world has also influenced Arab Muslims in Israel. Peled (2001) explains that, "A wave of Islamism swept the Middle East following the Iranian revolution of 1979, inspired by its anti-Western platform. Muslims in Israel joined the bandwagon by lashing out against the rapid Westernization and modernization that characterized Israeli society" (p. 380). The fundamentalist Islamic trend promotes a form of conservatism and tradition that rejects modern forces and enforces a strict code of conduct on the part of individuals, families, and communities. It represents a significant force, which advanced the tensions among Arab Christians and Muslims, and is not lost on a Jewish nation that understands the threat of a growing Arab Muslims minority.

Despite the extensive prejudice and discrimination experienced by Arab Christians within Israeli society, assertions exist that they still receive a more favorable treatment than their Muslim counterparts for the appeasement of Christians in the West. Arab Muslim associations are monitored by the Israeli government carefully due to fears of "the linking of Israeli Muslim concerns with strands of Arab nationalism in the broader Arab world" (Smith, 2003, p. 201). Smith notes that while Israeli Muslims are granted religious and cultural independence, they are denied the prospect of national Muslim leadership or the establishment of an Islamic education system.

The ultra-Orthodox Jews share the same dynamics as Arabs, but are more conservative than both Arabs and Jews and tend to separate themselves from the "formal state of Israel" (Ben-Arieh et al., 2004, p. 775). While facing challenges of their own, this group defies national expectations of Jews to participate in building and defending their own country. This discourse is linked to the refusal of ultra-Orthodox people to follow modern trends and go along with Western lifestyles (Stadler, 2002). They maintain their own communities, stress traditionalism and religion, and lead their lives in accordance with the strictest interpretation of sacred texts. Since work is "interpreted as a potential threat to human salvation, individual ties and group solidarity," most males withdraw totally from the work force until the age of 40 on average (Stadler, 2002, p. 455). This rationalization, which effectively exempts them from the work force and military service, is highly controversial for most secular Jews. Furthermore, it has immense implications on these families where norms, roles, and overall functioning take the backseat to staunch religious ideology and practices. These families counter expectations of husbands being economically prepared to support a family as precedence for marriage (Shai, 2002). Early marriages, highly fertility, and strong extended family networks characterize these families. In addition females are the economic supporter of the family until the male spouse is prepared to work. Shai (2002) states that, "The woman's primary role is that of a wife and mother as she is 'working only to support the family and to enable the husband to learn'" (p. 113).

Poverty

Poverty rates in Israel are reported to be higher among Arabs, Jewish ultra-Orthodox, and immigrants with large numbers of children, one working spouse, and single-family households (Gal, 1997). A 2001 estimate, reports that 18% of the Israeli population is below the poverty line (CIA, 2005). A 1999 report indicated, "One in every four Israeli children is living below the poverty line, a fourfold increase within 20 years" (Xinhua News Agency, 1999). The consequences of poverty are especially noticeable in children as their development, educational achievement, and health status are affected (Gal, 1997). The "worsening economic situation, characterized by growing unemployment, relatively high inflation levels and a lack of growth" is not likely to change especially since demographic trends are unlikely to change (Gal, 1997, p. 66).

Immigration exacerbates the issue of poverty further, as new immigrants confront numerous adjustment issues and the threat of unemployment. The 700,000 of immigrants from the former Soviet Union and the 56,000 from Ethiopia face numerous challenges as they adjust to the Israeli way of life (Katz & Lavee, 2004). Children in these families make up 12% of all children in the country. Families of Ethiopian origin tend to have a large number of children, whereas families from North America tend to have a higher rate of single parents (Ben-Arieh et al., 2003). Needless to say, this changes the general cultural and social landscape of families in Israel.

Family Instability

Israeli families can be described as somewhat large due to the birth rate among Arabs and ultra-Orthodox Jews. Marriage is an expectation in Middle Eastern societies and Israel is no different. Families tend to be traditional with a rate of 8.6% being single parents (Ben-Arieh et al., 2004). Regardless of background, issues of marriage and divorce are left in the hands of religious organizations. These highly conventional societies value family systems as reflected in the fact that only 5% of Arab families and 6% of Jewish families are single parents with at least one child between the ages of 0-17. Furthermore, childless Arab couples comprise 4% of the general population and childless Jewish couples 7% (Central Bureau of Statistics, 2003).

Despite this focus on families, the divorce rate is gradually increasing, but remains significantly lower than that of most Western nations. This is a concern as it signifies a rise in family instability. Israel is unique in that matters of marriage and divorce are assigned to the religious courts for each population group. Jews are accountable to rabbinical courts, Shari'a courts for Muslims, churches for Christians, and so forth (Lavee & Katz, 2003). The involvement of religious institutions maintains traditionalism and makes marital dissolution more challenging. Courts also intercede in matters of child custody and property.

FAMILY STRENGTHS IN ISRAEL

The Family Strengths Model as created by Stinnett and DeFrain highlights six qualities of strong families. These are: commitment, appreciation and affection, positive communication, enjoyable time together, spiritual well-being, and the ability to manage stress and crisis effectively (DeFrain, 1999). The fact that the family strengths perspective recognizes challenges confronting families while emphasizing the elements that promote their endurance is critical.

Due to the social and political nature of the region, Israeli families, regardless of affiliation, are continually challenged to overcome adversity of all sorts. Yet, the aforementioned elements of the Family Strengths Model seem naturally interwoven into the cultural and social fabric of families. It seems paradoxical that the same elements that create cultural division and promote social, economic, and political instability also unite families and illuminate their resiliency. They share many attributes including loyalty and commitment to family and traditions; unfaltering religious convictions; passionate communication styles; and an endless recuperative energy to cope with a seemingly never-ending stream of social, political, and economic turmoil. Each sector of the population is passionately engaged in familial, communal, and national affairs; indifference and apathy is not an option in Israeli society where there seems to be too much at stake.

Diversity of Strengths

It is important to discuss some of the differentiating factors between Arab and Jews as they contribute to family strengths and resilience factors. Arabs maintain a more collective orientation and Jews a more individualistic one (Hofstede, 1991). Arabs maintain group affiliation, commonality, collaboration, trust, and a strong sense of belonging that is noted in nuclear and extended family and community (Haj-Yahia, 1997). Familial support is important as "the traditional Arab society is seen as defending the individual and providing for the individual's needs by utilizing a wide social network of family members" (Pines & Zaidman, 2003, p. 467). The prevalent belief that destiny is predetermined and their reliance on the will of God promotes their fortitude. Arab families maintain hierarchal family structures with roles and functions delineated accordingly.

Jewish families maintain more democratic family structures resembling Western societies. Democratic values within the family and a socialist belief system promote egalitarianism and little regard for authority and status (Griffel et al., 1997). In their review of existing literature, Pines and Zaidman (2003) found that Arabs underutilize formal services due to lack of trust in governmental agencies, desire to keep family affairs private, and the fact that extensive informal supportive services exist within the family to address personal issues.

Commitment

Commitment to family is an unquestionable expectation of all population groups in Israel and is central to their resiliency. As noted in Lavee and Katz (2004), marriage is highly valued as less than 3% of all Israeli population are unmarried by age fifty. They confirm the aforementioned information in this chapter about the divorce rate being much lower than that of Western nations but on the rise from the 13% rate found in the 1990s. Marriage brings children that are cherished by society and raised with the expectation that they will marry and form their own families. While it is typical for children in most Western societies to leave their parents as they enter adulthood, this is the opposite case scenario for Israeli families, where in most cases children reside in their parent's home until marriage.

Parents and extended family play a pivotal role in supporting children through compulsory military service for Jews, preparing adult children for marriage, getting them married, encouraging procreation, caring for offspring, and providing wanted or unwanted parenting advice. The circle of social responsibility continues as adult children maintain close contact with their family, reinforce family loyalty, and care for aging parents and relatives.

Israeli society can be described as *child oriented* (Lavee & Katz, 2003). Moreover, "Political and civil institutions influence fertility through redistribution of resources that subsidize procreation" (Fargues, 2000, p. 441). Fertility is considered a right, especially in light of concerns that the Arab population in Israel will outgrow that of the Jews. Toren maintains, "In this respect, the goal of bearing and rearing of many children is to maintain the 'demographic equilibrium' and the 'Jewish character' of the nation state" (2003, p. 65). Thus, infertile couples have the right to receive government-supported medical treatment that would enable them to have children. Beyond politics, parents, extended family, and the wider community value children who are raised to be independent at a young age. It is a common practice for young children at seven or eight to take public transportation on their way to school or to run errands for their family. Lavee & Katz (2003) note, "The welfare of children is considered a collective responsibility" (p. 6).

Growing old in Israeli society brings about a sense of distinction and respect for the elderly as they become a source of experience and wisdom for the younger generation who are obligated to care for them. The majority of elderly resides close to their children, have daily contact, and are actively involved in their lives (Lavee & Katz, 2003). This enables them to maintain their own residence as evident by statistics that show 95% of healthy elderly and 76% of those with disabilities being able to do so (Brodsky, 1998).

For Arab families, the strong sense of tradition and social obligation compels adult children to have their elderly parents reside with them as necessary. Multigenerational living arrangements are also common among Jewish immigrants from the former Soviet Union where economic reasons necessitate two-thirds of the elderly to reside with their family (Strosberg & Naon, 1997).

Spiritual Well-Being and Practice

A second critical element that promotes the strength of Israeli families is religion and the related spiritual practices that allow families to express their faith. Religious organizations regulate issues of marriage and divorce, reinforce traditional values and social norms, and address the spiritual needs of all families. However, religion also presents a complicated bittersweet reality that divides Arabs Muslims, Arab Christians, and Jews, while promoting inter-group unity and solidarity. In examining the historical sociopolitical conflicts, religious scriptures are used to justify the sense of entitlement that Arabs and Jews have to the Holy Land and the endless sacrifices for its sake. Whereas the Western world seems obsessed with race and skin color, religion dominates life in the Middle East, and especially in the Holy Land. It is a divisive factor in the Arabic community where Muslims outnumber the Christians, whose percentage in the population continues to decline due to a decreasing birth rate and immigration to western countries where they can enjoy more freedom and equality.

Christians tend to reside in urban areas and belong to various denominations such as Greek Catholic (42%), Greek Orthodox (32%), and Roman Catholic (16%) (Hirsch, 1998). Muslims are mostly Sunni, reside in small towns and villages, and maintain a conservative ideology that stresses traditional and Muslim beliefs. Religious practices also distinguish among observant and non-observant Jews. The ultra-Orthodox Jews tend to maintain a closed community separate from secular Jews, and rely on extended family networks and the community for support and belonging. With prohibition on dating and emphasis on bride purity, marriage tends to be arranged and occurs at a young age for both genders as it is the only outlet for sexual activity. For them, religion plays a central role in life, family, and career planning. The withdrawal of males form the workforce until later in life also compels the government to provide economic subsidies as needed.

Religion provides each group with highly-spiritual customs that are celebrated elaborately and extensively during holiday events. For Christians and Jews, the joy of celebrating the holidays in the one of the holiest lands on the face of the earth, in the bosom of history, is unsurpassed spiritually. It is like being transformed hundreds of years back in time to the historical birthplace of religion. The word of God as each group knows it is predetermined and unquestionable, and every related religious expression is laden with meaning.

Open Communication

Israelis, like other Middle Easterners are passionate people who come across to outsiders as overly expressive, assertive, and emotional. Since each Israeli group continues to fight for its own right to exist and be recognized, apathy is a luxury that no one can afford. This contributes to the strength of these families that tend to maintain a unique communication style, which for the most part is open, straightforward, and somewhat dramatic. Even the friendliest conversation can seem emotionally charged to an observer who is unfamiliar with Middle Eastern customs. Israelis tend to be assertive or having a lot to say about most things, affectionate and are unafraid to show it, and maintain a minimal social space compared to Western cultures. Occasions such as weddings and funerals are intense and prolonged, typically extending over a several days and involving extended family and community. For example, funerals, which usually extend over a few days may involve open wailing and extended mourning periods. Israelis are generous with emotions and material possessions and can rarely be accused of being emotionally restrained or stingy. They love life and celebrate it to its fullest through food, music, dance, and a wide array of traditions that will sustain them for generations to come.

Coping Skills and Support

The strength of Israeli families is also manifested in the way they cope with the stream of violent attacks within the country's borders. In the midst of intense conflict lies the desire for peace, stability, and acceptance. The Israeli-Palestinian conflict continues to erupt like an angry volcano that spews destruction, hatred, and senseless killings and sacrifices on both sides.

Security issues are a main concern for all Israeli families–Arabs and Jews–since both are impacted by the aftermath of violent attacks. One of the most hideous effects of violence is the divisiveness it engenders among Arabs and Jews who have to coexist within Israel. Stephan and others (2004) define coexistence as, "the word used in Israel to signify the peaceful existence of two peoples–Jewish and Arab–living side-by-side within Israel" (p. 237). They further explain that, the "Jews perceive the actions they take against the Palestinians and other Arabs as self-defense against an enemy that seeks their extermination," while "the Palestinians feel they have been dispossessed of their rightful homeland by war, annexation, and Jewish colonization," thus justifying their political behavior (p. 237).

Since this ongoing conflict sabotages the well-being of both sides, national efforts have been extended to improve the nature of their coexistence. Education has been an arena where progress has been made as Hebrew is taught in Arabic schools and spoken by all citizens regardless of ethnicity, and Arabic is spoken by 40% of the Jews (Stephan et al., 2004). Coexistence education programs have also been created in some areas to encourage intergroup cooperation and acceptance between groups.

Recognizing the vulnerability of Jewish families, the Israeli government has also supported a wide range of community-based interventions that support Jewish families following violent attacks. The number of families affected by violence, directly and indirectly, represents a sizeable proportion of the population. Services supporting families and promoting their resilience are common for Jews and are found in various settings such as education, social services, and hospitals. Katz and Lavee (2004) report that following attacks, response centers equipped with trained personnel are set up to provide information and referrals. Intense professional services are also made available to families that are impacted directly by the loss and injury of members. Short and long-term services are supplied by the National Insurance Institute, and include a wide array of services such as medical, therapeutic, rehabilitative, financial, and more (Katz & Lavee, 2004). These services play a pivotal role in stabilizing families and supporting their strengths. While the government focuses on the needs of Jewish families in the aftermath of violence, it continues to neglect the direct and indirect implications of such violence on Arab families. This compels Arabs to rely on informal family networks and local community resources for support and acceptance.

CONCLUSION

There is a saying among Arabs of the Middle East: "I am against my brother, my brother and I are against my cousin, and my cousin and I are against the stranger." Despite the diversity of Israeli families, they share the same bittersweet reality and a hopeful but uncertain future. They are brothers in many ways, and definitely cousins in that they share ancestors; thus what may be needed is the recognition of common and unfulfilled needs that undermine their collective well-being as people sharing one society. These families are united in their strengths, their devotion to the long forgotten traditions they firmly uphold, and their willingness to endlessly honor commitments to their heritage, families, and children. They appreciate the frailty of life and vigorously celebrate its gifts within their families and communities. They are passionate communicators who are actively engaged in private family matters and public national affairs. Their spirituality is linked to ancient religious practices that continue to dominate their personal ideology and lifestyle, as well the social and political landscape of the country today.

Most inspiring though, is the manner in which these families cope with crisis by utilizing spiritual guidance, family support, and community collaboration. Israelis recognize the supremacy of the family unit above all other social institutions, and understand the critical role it plays in socializing and maintaining cultural heritage. Despite the confounding elements that may blemish their portrayal, their beauty shines through as they truly exemplify the worthwhile elements of the Family Strengths Perspective.

REFERENCES

Ben-Arieh, A., Boyer, Y., & Gajst, I (2004). Children's welfare in Israel: Growing up in a multi-cultural society. In A. Jensen, A. Ben-Arieh, C. Conti, D. Cotsar, M. Ghiolla Phadraig, & H. Warming Nielsen (Eds.), *Children's welfare in ageing Europe: Vol. 2.* pp. 771-811. Trondheim, Norway: Norwegian Center for Child Research, University of Science and Technology.

Ben-Arieh, A., Zionit, Y., & Krizak, G. (2003). The state of the child in Israel: A statistical abstract. Jerusalem: National Council for the Child.

Brodsky, J. (1998). The elderly in Israel. In G. Fridman & J. Brodsky (Eds.), *Aging in the Mediterranean and the Middle East* (pp. 67-80). Jerusalem: JDC-Brookdale Institute of Gerontology and Human Development. (Hebrew).

Central Bureau of Statistics (2003). *The Arab population in Israel* (statistic-lite). Retrieved on June 20, 2005 from: http://www.cbs.gov.il/statistical/arab_pop03e.pdf.

Central Intelligence Agency (CIA) (2005). *World Fact Book: Israel.* Retrieved on June 21, 2005 from http://www.cia.gov/cia/publications/factbook/geos/is.html#People.

DeFrain, J. (1999). Strong families around the world. *Family Matters, 53,* 6-13. Retrieved on December 20, 2005 from http://www.aifs.gov.au/institute/pubs/fm/fm53 jdf.pdf.

Efrat, G., Ben-Arieh, A., Gal, J., & Haj-Yahia, M. (1998). Young children in Israel: A country study prepared for the Bernard Van Leer Foundation. Jerusalem, Israel: National Council for the Child.

Fargues, P. (2000). Protracted national conflict and fertility change: Palestinians and the twentieth century. *Population and Development Review, 26,* 441-482.

Gal, J. (1997). Issues in poverty among children in Israel. In J. Gal (Ed.), *Poor children in Israel: Multi-disciplinary review* (pp. 1-17). Jerusalem: National Council for the Child, Center for Research and Public Education, and The Movement for War on Poverty. (Hebrew).

Griffel, A., Eisikovits, A., Fishman, G., & Grinstein-Weiss, M. (1997). Israeli youth survey 1997: Patterns of help seeking in times of distress (Report Number 4). Haifa: University of Haifa, Minerva Center for Youth.

Haj-Yahia, M. M. (1995). Toward culturally sensitive intervention with Arab families in Israel. *Contemporary Family Therapy, 17,* 429-447.

Hirsch, E. (Ed.). (1998). *Facts about Israel.* Jerusalem: Hamakor Press.

Hofstede, G. (1991). *Culture and organizations: Software of the mind.* London: McGraw Hill.

Kahn, S. M. (2000). *Reproducing Jews: A cultural account of assisted conception in Israel.* Durham, NC: Duke University Press.

Katz, R., & Lavee, Y. (2004). Families in Israel. In B. Adams, & J. Trost (Eds.), *Handbook of World*. Sage Publications, Inc., Thousand Oaks.

Lavee, Y. & Katz, R. (2003). The family in Israel: Between tradition and modernity. *Marriage & Family Review, 35*, 193-217.

Nethe, R. H. (2002). The demystification of Islam. *The Humanist, 62*, 28-30.

Peled, A. R. (2001). Towards Autonomy? The Islamist movement's quest for control of Islamic institutions in Israel. *The Middle East Journal, 55*, 378-402.

Pines, A. M., & Zaidman, N. (2003). Israeli Jews and Arabs: Similarities and differences in the utilization of social supports. *Journal of Cross-Cultural Psychology, 34*, 465-480.

Saouli, A. (2001). Arab political organizations within the Israeli state. *The Journal of Social, Political and Economic Studies, 26*, 443-460.

Shai, D. (2002). Working women/cloistered men: A family development approach to marriage arrangements among Ultra-Orthodox Jews. *Journal of Comparative Family Studies, 33*(i1), 97-116.

Smith, C. D. (2003). Debating Islam in the Jewish state: The development of policy toward Islamic institutions in Israel. [Book Review]. *Shofar, 21*, 201-203.

Stadler, N. (2002). Is profane work an obstacle to salvation? The case of Ultra-Orthodox (Haredi) Jews in contemporary Israel. *Sociology of Religion, 63*, 455-475.

Stephan, C.W., Hertz-Lazarowitz, R., Zelniker, T., & Stephan, W. G. (2004). Introduction to improving Arab-Jewish relations in Israel: Theory and practice in coexistence educational programs. *Journal of Social Issues, 60*, 237-253.

Strosberg, N., & Naon, D. (1997). The absorption of elderly immigrants from the former Soviet Union: Selected findings regarding housing, social integration, and health. *Gerontology, 79*, 5-15 (Hebrew).

Toren, N. (2003). Tradition and transition: Family change in Israel. *Gender Issues*, 60-76.

Waysman, M., Mikulincer, M. Solomon, Z, & Weisenberg, M. (1993). Secondary traumatization among wives of posttraumatic combat veterans: A family typology. *Journal of Family Psychology, 7*, 104-118.

Xinhua News Agency, Nov 18, 1999. Israel drafts plan to fight child poverty. News Provided by COMTEX (http://www.comtexnews.com).

Zimmerman, B., Seid, R., & Wise, L. M. (2006). The million person gap: A critical look at Palestinian demography. The Begin-Sadat Center for Strategic Studies, Bar-Ilan University, Israel. http://www.biu.ac.il/SOC/besa/perspectives15.html

doi:10.1300/J002v41n01_06

The Omani Family:
Strengths and Challenges

Thuwayba A. Al-Barwani
Tayfour S. Albeely

SUMMARY. To gain a better understanding of the Omani family, the paper first presents an overview of significant attributes that characterize Omani society and its people which include: the foundation of the Omani state, the strong influence of Arabic and Islamic heritage, the influences of tribalism, the emergence of modern Oman, and the challenges that confront the Omani family today. Through analysis of field research and relevant literature on measures of cohesiveness, the authors establish that the Omani family can be considered to be highly cohesive. As well, they assert their confidence that the power of the Islamic and Arabic traditions and heritage will continue to support and sustain the Omani family, thus enabling it to confront both current and future challenges. doi:10.1300/J002v41n01_07 *[Article copies available for a fee from The Haworth Document Delivery Service: 1-800-HAWORTH. E-mail address:*

Thuwayba A. Al-Barwani is Associate Professor, Sultan Qaboos University, Department of Curriculum & Instruction, College of Education, P.O. Box 32, PC 123, Alkhod, Muscat, Sultanate of Oman (E-mail: Thuwayba@squ.edu.om). She is also a member of the State Council (Oman's Upper Chamber). Tayfour S. Albeely is Associate Professor of Psychology, and The Minister's Advisor for Family Affairs, Ministry of Social Development, P.O. Box 560, Muscat, PC 113, Sultanate of Oman (E-mail: talbeely@omantel.net.om).

Address correspondence to: Thuwayba A. Al-Barwani.

[Haworth co-indexing entry note]: "The Omani Family: Strengths and Challenges." Al-Barwani, Thuwayba A., and Tayfour S. Albeely. Co-published simultaneously in *Marriage & Family Review* (The Haworth Press, Inc.) Vol. 41, No. 1/2, 2007, pp. 119-142; and: *Strong Families Around the World: Strengths-Based Research and Perspectives* (ed: John DeFrain, and Sylvia M. Asay) The Haworth Press, Inc., 2007, pp. 119-142. Single or multiple copies of this article are available for a fee from The Haworth Document Delivery Service [1-800-HAWORTH, 9:00 a.m. - 5:00 p.m. (EST). E-mail address: docdelivery@haworthpress.com].

Available online at http://mfr.haworthpress.com
© 2007 by The Haworth Press, Inc. All rights reserved.
doi:10.1300/J002v41n01_07

<docdelivery@haworthpress.com> Website: <http://www.HaworthPress. com> © 2007 by The Haworth Press, Inc. All rights reserved.]

KEYWORDS. Family change, family challenges, Islamic heritage, modern Oman, Omani history, Omani family, Omani family cohesion, Omani family strengths

INTRODUCTION

The Sultanate of Oman claims a land area of 212,460 sq. km (roughly the size of Kansas) and shares land borders with the Republic of Yemen, the Kingdom of Saudi Arabia and the United Arab Emirates (UAE). It is the third largest country in the Arabian Peninsula and lies at the crossroads of three continents and four seas. Oman is a member of the Gulf Cooperation Council States (GCC) and it shares a number of common features like language, religion, and culture with these countries. However, when one talks about the Arab Gulf Countries, whether at present or in history, one finds that there is need for qualification as far as Oman is concerned. Unlike other countries of the gulf, Oman's coastline of 1,700 km is situated entirely on the Gulf of Oman and the Indian Ocean, while only 50 km of its coast on the Musandam Peninsula is washed by the Arab Gulf. Yet Oman's minute, detached enclave at the tip of Musandam puts the strategic Strait of Hormuz within its territorial sea. This combination of being geographically outside the Gulf and being strategically essential to it gives Oman a unique place in the regional setting of the Gulf Cooperation Council and the industrial countries of the west as well. It is through the Strait of Hormuz waterway that oil tankers can access the other gulf countries (Pridham, 1987).

Oman is different in a number of other respects; among them is its topography. It is the only country in the gulf that receives monsoon rainfalls (mainly in the southern part of the country) and has mountain ranges rising over 3,000 meters. Its cultural and traditional composition is also unique because it enjoys a multiculturalism that has come about as a result of its dominions in some parts of East Africa, now part of the United Republic of Tanzania and Gwadur, which is now part of the Islamic Republic of Pakistan. Ibadhism, a moderate sect of Islam that is practiced mainly in Oman, is another source of distinction between Oman and the other Gulf countries. Oman also differs politically because it is the only Gulf country that has remained fully independent and

under the same ruling family for the last 250 years (except for comparatively brief periods of occupation by the Persians and Portuguese around
the 16th century). All the above factors serve to give Oman distinctive
features and characteristics that have shaped the life of its people over
the years (Pridham, 1987).

Wrapping itself around the southeastern corner of Arabia, Oman's
inland consists of successive zones of coastal plain, mountains and interior plateau, and desert. The geography of Oman has historically exercised a strong influence on the development and lifestyle of its people.
In a broad sense, Oman falls into two very distinct divisions: the coast
and the interior. The coast, relatively cosmopolitan and vulnerable, was
always open to invasion and to a myriad of foreign influences. The interior, traditionally the Arab and Ibadhi stronghold, clung to its traditions
and the society remained inaccessible to the outside.

The foundations of the Omani State date back to the eastward migration of various Arabian tribal groups into the area several millennia ago.
These people reached the southeastern region in about the second century AD and then moved north to challenge the Persian supremacy. The
subsequent displacement of Persians came as a result of the conversion
of the Arab tribes to the new religion of Islam in the seventh century,
and was followed by the introduction of Ibadhism to the country and the
development of the spirit of the Omani community. Ibadhism was introduced to Oman by returning Omani Ibadhi residents in Basra who were
escaping persecution. The Ibadhi state was established in the mid eighth
century by Al Julanda bin Masoud who was elected as its first *Imam*
(leader) (Peterson, 1978).

Religion and Politics

Ibadhi is a sect of Islam that has fewer adherents than Sunni or Shi'i
Islam, but it is generally considered to be the third Islamic tradition.
Ibadhiya takes its name from the seventh century Abd Allah ibn Ibadh
who was one of its founders, and it was later organized by Jaber bin
Zaid, a native of Oman.

The Ibadhiya sect was founded as a breakaway sect from the Khariji
movement in the seventh century. Ibadh and his followers differed from
the more radical Khariji groups over the question of the relationship
with non Khariji (Khariji followers claim that all non-members of the
sect were infidels who merited death). Thus, the new sect was characterized as being moderate and less demanding of its followers and
was able to live in relative peace until the seventh century when they

were harassed and sent to exile in Oman. The Imamate (Ibadhi leadership) is based on the theory established at the death of the Prophet Muhammad that the Muslim community selects the man that the members of the community consider best able to serve as a leader.

An Imam combines political and religious functions. He is responsible for supervision of tax collection and the distribution of state revenues. He appoints governors and judges, enforces the law and provides for social welfare for his people. Ibadhi Islam has also been characterized to be a sect of *refuge*, adhering to republican, democratic, puritan, and fundamentalist religious and political beliefs (Eickelman, 1987). The largest Ibadhi community today is in Oman where its population is estimated to constitute 55-60% of the total Omani population. Other sects found in Oman are Sunni and Shi'i. Smaller Ibadhi communities can also be found in the North African Arab countries of Algeria and Libya, and in East Africa.

Followers of the Ibadhi sect often refer to themselves as "the people of consultation," because the principal tenet that distinguishes them from both Sunnis and Shi'is is their belief that the spiritual and temporal leader (Imam) of the Muslim community is selected by religious scholars and tribal notables and then elected by the people in the community. The selection is based on the individual's mastery of religious knowledge, his moral qualities, and his capacity for governing exclusively according to Islamic principles. If the leader is perceived as diverging from these principles, then the community removes him from office and another is elected to replace him.

The rise of the Al Busaid dynasty was unique in Oman's history. It started with the election of Ahmed bin Said Al Busaid to the office of Imam. As a result of his charisma, courage and strong leadership in leading his army to resist the Persian siege and later, in the expulsion of the Persian invaders from Muscat in 1744, Ahmad remained Imam until his death in 1783. To show respect for Ahmad, his son Said was elected Imam to replace him and he then subsequently abdicated the responsibility to his son Hamad, due to incompetence. Thus, the seed of succession was planted and the establishment of the Al Busaid dynasty that remains in power in Oman up to the present time was established.

Oman is an Arab country in which traditional Arab tribal organization serves as the basis of society. Oman's Arab population is divided into hundreds of tribes of varying size and cohesiveness which regulate social, territorial, economic and political relationships. Conceptually, a tribe is defined to be a clan or a group of clans that are organized around a common ancestor. In practice, however, all members simply agree that they are a tribe and have obligations to one another. The tribe is a pragmatic institution that can be fragmented when there is loss of consensus about an ancestor or joined together to form a single larger tribe.

Omani tribes have historically had a great deal of local autonomy. They have a formal structure led by a *Sheikh,* whose chief duties are to mediate disputes within the group and to lead when conflict arises with outsiders. The office is not necessarily hereditary, but Sheikhs are normally selected from an elite family within the tribe. Thereafter, the family's choice is presented to other members of the tribe for acceptance. Consensus rather than election is the rule, and legitimacy to continue is conferred upon continued tribal satisfaction with duties performed (Allen, 1987). It is important to note here that patrilineal descent ascribes membership to one or another of the many tribes in Oman.

The fundamental distinction of the Omani life patterns has always been the dichotomy between urban and Bedu or rather, between the sedentary population of the towns and the nomads of the desert. It was as nomads that the first Arab tribes entered Oman; only later did they adopt the sedentary lifestyle of the Persian inhabitants (Peterson, 1978). This interplay between subsistence farming and nomadic lifestyle continues to be an important feature of the Omani population.

Oman's rough terrain and hot dry climate is not well suited for a settled population but for thousands of years the majority of the people have tapped the meager water resources and practiced agriculture while others turned to the sea to earn a living either as fishermen or as merchants. Thus, they established a rich seafaring tradition that has given Omanis remarkable ingenuity, entrepreneurial flair, and spirit of adventure as they spread their wings to explore far off lands to market and barter their wares. Such is the heritage and tradition that Oman's forefathers have handed on to successive generations (McBrierty & Al Zubair, 2004).

MODERN OMAN

Oman's modern history can be said to have started in 1970 with the accession of His Majesty Sultan Qaboos bin Said to the throne. He is the 14th Sultan in the Al Busaid dynasty that has ruled Oman since 1744. With his rule came the great renaissance that transformed Oman and its people.

Oman is a nation in transition. Just 35 years ago, it was an isolated country unknown to the world. A number of scholars had rightly described

Oman as "the Tibet of the Arab World." However, the last 35 years have witnessed the unprecedented transformation of the country from isolation, illiteracy, disease and economic stagnation to a thriving modern nation that is internationally recognized for its progress in the eradication of illiteracy, primary health care provision, eradication of childhood diseases, reduction of infant mortality rates, reduction of gender gap in education and training, to mention only a few. Since 1970 Oman used its natural resources of oil and gas to steer the country on a fast track of rebirth and recovery but ever mindful of its culture, heritage, traditions and beliefs (McBrierty & Al Zubair, 2004).

Like its Gulf neighbors, Oman has been transformed by oil wealth during the last three decades. Oman currently produces 750,000 barrels a day and its oil income accounts for 40% of its GDP (McBrierty & Al Zubair, 2004). For a long period oil wealth was considered to be sufficient to sustain a decent standard of living for the citizens. In fact, oil wealth was used to provide basic infrastructure like roads, electricity and water and to provide essential services like free school education and primary health care for the people. However, Omani oil reserves are expected to last no more than 20 years and with the realization that oil is a depleting resource that will not be able to sustain the increasing demands of a growing population. Thus, government began to seriously consider the diversification of its economy in order to reduce its dependency on oil. Oman's abundant natural resources, coupled with its beautiful mountains and valleys together with its long coastline, provide viable alternatives to oil dependence. Thus, natural gas, mining and tourism are poised to be the next highest contributors to Oman's economy, followed by manufacturing, small industry, agriculture and fisheries.

Oman's population census of 2003 estimates its population to be slightly over 2.3 million people of whom 75% are nationals and 25% are expatriates who have come to Oman for employment purposes. The Omani population is among the fastest growing in the world and is characterized as being youthful. Its distribution shows an estimated 40.6% being less than 15 years of age, 52.2% under the age of 18, and 56% under the age of 25. The gender distribution of the total Omani population is 50.5% males and 49.5% females (Ministry of National Economy, 2003).

Education

The provision of free education has greatly contributed to the improvement in the general welfare and standard of living of the Omani people. Having just three schools enrolling 900 boys in 1970, Oman now boasts almost universal school education with student numbers reaching over 576,000 and almost half of them are girls. The provision of gender equality in education dates back to the early 1970s and as a result of the sustained national commitment to girls' education, the ratio of female students in general education increased from 12.7% in 1971-1972 to 33% in 1980-1981 to 48.6 % in 2001-2002. Current statistics show females representing 48.4% of the total school population. Table 1 below shows net enrollment of Omani students according to gender and level of education.

Efforts to eradicate adult illiteracy were initiated in 1973-1974 with the help of the United Nations Educational, Scientific, and Cultural Organization (UNESCO) and the World Bank. Ministry of Education Statistics show that there are 117 centers operating in different regions of the Sultanate with a total enrollment of 6,622 learners of whom 94.2% are females. A comparison of census data between 1993 and 2003 reveals that there was a significant drop in illiteracy among the Omani population of 15 years and older. Table 2 shows a drop in the illiteracy

TABLE 1. Gross enrollment by gender and education level, 1994-1995 to 2003-2004.

Level	1994-1995			2003-2004		
	Female	Male	Total	Female	Male	Total
Basic education	–	–	–	67,863	71,219	139,082
Cycle 1	141,669	151,973	293,642	78,036	81,931	159,967
Cycle 2	53,393	63,100	116,493	69,675	79,362	149,037
G11+G12	31,201	28,513	59,714	63,606	64,780	128,386
Total	226,263	243,286	469,849	279,180	297,292	576,472

Cycle 1 = Grades 1-4, Cycle 2 = Grades 5-10, G11 + G12 = Grades 11 & 12.

TABLE 2. Illiteracy rates by age group 1993-2003.

Age group	1993			2003		
	Female	Male	Total	Female	Male	Total
15-19	8.4	2.1	5.2	2.5	1.2	1.8
20-29	32.5	6.6	19.2	5.6	2.0	3.8
30-39	75.1	26.6	51.9	32.7	6.2	19.4
Total population	53.9	28.9	41.2	29.4	14.6	22.0

rate from 41.2% to 22% within a period of ten years. It is important to note that illiteracy among females is notably higher than for men and that for the 15-to-19 age group illiteracy is significantly lower than other age groups for both sexes.

Widening access to higher education is considered to be an important foundation of sustainable development and economic stability. Based on Oman's Vision 2020 (Ministry of Development, 1995), the government started to implement an economic strategy which has human resource development as its focus. Budgets were mobilized to provide access to free higher education to every Omani who qualifies, irrespective of gender. As a result, both public and private higher education institutions dramatically increased as escalating demand for higher education put an ever-increasing strain on public funds.

A look at recent higher education statistics shows a total of 55,413 students engaged in some form of higher education or training. Of these, 55% are females. Table 3 shows enrollments in higher education according to type of institution and gender. It is important to note here that females not only outnumber male students in most specializations, but they also outperform them in most instances. Needless to say, this phenomenon has both social and economic implications.

The progress made in education has had a significant impact on the socio-demographic situation in Oman. Results of the Family Health Survey conducted in 1995 revealed the following:

- A substantial trend toward later marriage among Omani women, with the educated urban females showing the strongest tendency.
- Women of lower educational status were found to be more likely to be married in polygamous unions when compared to those of higher educational levels (13% among illiterate women compared to 6.4% among women with secondary education or higher).
- Women with low educational status were more likely to be divorced and also more likely to remarry compared to their literate counterparts.
- Better educated women tend to favor smaller families and do not normally continue child bearing beyond the age of 35 years.
- Fertility rate was seen to decline from 7.8 in 1987 to 4.7 in 2000 to 3.12 in 2004 with younger women showing significantly lower rates compared to the older generations.
- Use of contraceptives was found to be higher among the educated and older women (Ministry of Health, 1995).

TABLE 3. Enrollments in higher education according to gender and type of institution.

Institutions	Girls	Boys	Total	Girls as % of the total
Sultan Qaboos University	6,208	6,229	12,437	50
Colleges of education	4,565	3,304	7,869	58
College of *Sharia* and Law	166	494	660	25
Technical colleges	3,520	4,796	8,316	42
Other government colleges	2,192	690	2,882	76
Private colleges	5,201	4,838	10,039	52
Universities and colleges abroad	8,647	4,563	13,210	65.5
Total	30,499	24,914	55,413	55.0

The past three decades saw significant progress in health-care services, both in terms of quantity and quality. Women received a fair share of these services resulting in positive outcomes with regard to life expectancy at birth and in maternal and childhood mortality rates. According to the Reproductive Health Survey conducted by the Ministry of Health in 2000, 97% of women in the age range of 15 to 49 years received pre-natal medical care mainly by trained health workers and 99.3 % of these had this service delivered by a government health facility. Further analysis of health data shows a steady reduction in the maternal mortality rates between 1990, 1995 and 2000 (27, 22 and 16.1 respectively). Similarly, life expectancy rates for females rose from 48.5 years in 1970, to 61.2 years in 1980, to 71 years in 1990 and reaching 74.3 years in 2000 (Al-Barwani, 2005).

Fertility rate has often been used as a good proxy indicator to measure the empowerment and advancement of women. Surveys conducted by the Ministry of Health in 1995 and 2000 have shown that the mean number of births dropped significantly for younger women and those who have had some kind of an education. This seems to suggest that the observed drop in total fertility rate is a result of the delay in marriage for a large percentage of girls who pursue their education at the secondary school level and beyond. Table 4 shows the fertility rate of Omani women in 1995 and 2000 according to age and level of education.

Women in the Workforce

Economic participation rates of females have steadily increased as more and more women gain access to education and training. Labor

TABLE 4. Fertility rates according to age and level of education.

Age	Oman family health survey, 1995	National health survey, 2000
15-19	0.98	0.60
20-24	2.20	1.68
25-29	4.23	3.46
30-34	6.53	5.54
35-39	7.95	7.49
40-44	8.69	8.76
45-49	8.56	8.60
Education		
Illiterate	7.36	7.70
Some Primary	5.88	5.47
Primary	4.34	4.10
Preparatory +	4.76	4.56
Total	5.53	5.00

statistics show the participation rate of females of age 15+ to be 6.7% in 1993, 10.1% in 1996, to 10.8% in 2000 and reaching 34.4 in 2003 (Ministry of National Economy, 2003). This increase has been largely attributed to increasing participation rates of females in education. Preliminary results of the labor force survey of 1996 (Ministry of National Economy, 1996) found that the economic activity of females was positively correlated to educational status. Similarly, results showed that the educational level of the female Omani workforce was higher than that of males. In 1996, almost three quarters (71.2%) of economically-active Omani females had a secondary school certificate or higher. Out of these, two thirds (63.6%) were employed either as professionals (40.2%) or as clerks (23.4%).

The 2003 census (Ministry of National Economy, 2003) results showed further evidence of the relationship between the educational status of women and their labor market participation rates. The highest rates of economic activity among Omani women were found among those with Ph.D.s (95%), with bachelor's degrees (93.6%), post secondary and master's degrees (89%), followed by secondary school certificates (36%) and dropping to 7.3% for preparatory school certificate holders and 3.5% for illiterates.

Chatty (2002) reports in her study of working women in Oman, that there is a significant trend of illiterate women seeking employment in simple unskilled occupations. She points out that women classified as working within elementary occupations are older: 30% in their 30s, 36% in their 40s and 19% in their 50s. This seems to indicate among other things that even illiterate and rural Omani women are beginning to seek employment away from their homes.

The bulk of the Omani female civil servants are clustered in health and education professions, as these are traditionally considered to be jobs appropriate for females. However, this is changing gradually as more and more women are forcefully entering professions such as engineering, marketing, banking, legal, academic and other such professions which were once considered to be exclusively for males. It is also not uncommon to see Omani women engaged in the armed forces, police force, radio and television, which were once seen to be unsuitable jobs for females (Chatty, 2000). It is important to note here that public sector employment is still favored by both genders because of job security, lucrative salaries, long vacations and availability of jobs near home (see Table 5).

For the reasons mentioned above, the private sector seems to show a slower growth with regard to female employment. In 2003, females represented 17.6% of the total workforce in the private sector, with two thirds of them being in the range of 20-29 years of age. (Ministry of National Economy, 2004).

The availability of services and increased employment opportunities have brought material gains that would have been unimaginable two generations ago. Despite the oil wealth and modernization that is taking place in the country, Oman continues to be described as a country that retains many of the features of its traditional organization in which the family is the central and pivotal institution. However, like the rest of the world, Oman has not been immune to some of the challenges associated with rapid economic development and globalization. Naturally, the issues

TABLE 5. Public sector employment according to gender.

| | Employment in the Government sector | | | |
	1985	1990	2001	2003
Number of Employees				
Male	30,941	47,293	46,381	51,886
Female	2,831	20,946	10,678	27,213
Total	33,772	68,496	57,059	79,099
Percentage				
Male	91.6	69.4	81.3	65.6
Female	8.4	30.6	18.7	34.4

of concern are the threats that seem to confront the Omani family as it struggles to balance between its proud heritage and its need to survive and prosper in a rapidly globalizing world.

THE OMANI FAMILY:
INFLUENCES OF THE HERITAGE

Oman has often been described as a nation that is proud of its Arab Islamic heritage. The government of the Sultanate of Oman has painstakingly and consistently taken measures to ensure that Omani people retain their identity of which they are very proud. Balancing modernity and tradition has always been a goal that Oman sought to achieve. Therefore, an appreciation of the Omani social structure in general, and the Omani family in particular, could not be achieved without looking first at its most influential Islamic/Arab heritage.

Traditionally a family has been defined to be a social institution whose major function is to reproduce and ensure the survival and the general well-being of its members. Operationally defined, a family is people living together who are connected by blood and sentiment. They have defined roles and normally share the same goals, as well as mutual expectations of each other (Olson & DeFrain, 2006; Peterson, 2000). However, the definition of the family in Islam seems to have unique characteristics that may perhaps distinguish an Islamic family from others. 'Abd al 'Ati (1997) offers an operational definition of a family in Islam to designate "a special kind of structure whose principal members are related to one another through blood ties and/or marital relationships, and whose relatedness is of such a nature as to entail mutual expectations that are prescribed by religion, reinforced by law and internalized by the individual" (p. 1). 'Abd al 'Ati's definition is based on the mutual expectations that follow from membership in such a structure. The membership may be realized through natural blood ties, or acquired through marriage, or be both ascribed and acquired if the membership unit includes, as it may, more than a married pair. It is to be noted here that this definition of family makes no reference to the residential factor because the family members may or may not occupy the same residential place. With reference to the mutual expectations of the family members, it makes no difference how or where they reside. The family members may share the same residential confines, or they may be living separately and independently. This indicates therefore that according to the universal definition, the nuclear families in Islamic societies cannot be considered to be truly nuclear.

According to Lemu and Heeren (1978), the Muslim family's main characteristics are those by which it provides a secure and healthy environment for its members, guards against passions of whims and desires, and channels them to wholesome and meaningful pursuit. The Muslim family, they assert, embraces and proliferates human virtues such as love, compassion, sacrifice, justice, etc., so as to provide a refuge against life's difficulties and hardships. Lemu and Heeren further assert that the Islamic family system brings the rights of the husband, wife, children and relatives into a fine equilibrium. It nourishes unselfish behavior, generosity, respect and love within the framework of a well-organized family system. Hence, the peace and security offered by a stable family unit is highly valued by Islam and the Muslims and is seen as essential for the spiritual growth of its members and the cornerstone for establishing a harmonious social order. The rights and obligations that are shared by the family members pertain to lineal identity and maintenance; succession and affection; socialization of the young and security and respect for the aged; and maximization of efforts to ensure the family continuity and welfare. Further, the mutual expectations of the family members are not established only by familial relationship, but also by the membership in a larger social system which derives from a common religious brotherhood. This brotherhood has its own implications. It is so conceived as to reinforce family ties, complement them and prevent their abuse.

Abbas (2001) argues that the Islamic family is better designed to stand up to contemporary and Western pressures and influences. It is based on a detailed and rigid set of rules about interpersonal relationships; therefore, the Islamic family is a well-ordained institution. The creation of man and woman and the marriage relationship permeated with tranquility, love and mercy have been described as "signs of God" and the institution of marriage and the family have been commended as the *Sunnah* or way of the Prophet Mohamed. However, and in another line of thought, Abu-Sulayman and A Abdul (1993) point out that most Muslim scholarship on family and gender relationships is restricted by and confined to the formative years of Islamic law, "approximately the first four centuries of Islamic history from around the 7th to the 11th centuries," a period during which Islamic Law (or *Sharia*) developed, and when Muslim society reached the zenith of its political, social, legal and economic maturity. The end of this period marked the culmination of a religious-legal process to which nothing of significance has since been added. Abu-Sulayman claims that this is also the period that culminated in stifling any further development of intellectual, social, philosophical and legal thought by Muslim minds in light of the faith's revealed text, the *Holy Quran*.

In support of Abu-Sulayman's position, Valiante (2003) claims that most of the classical and contemporary Muslim scholars have studied families only from a religious point of view. Accordingly, the family is viewed exclusively from a religious perspective that is held as both normative and idealized. Valiante argues that such a normative view of the family presents a version of sociological and ideological reality that contradicts the actual state of the family in most of Muslim society. Further, Valiante argues that the classical body of Muslim knowledge restricts the world view of the *Quran* itself to certain socio-cultural, behavioral, and historical time-space factors. Consequently, it limits family study to idealized versions instead of existing reality and avoids seeking solutions to correct the existing situation.

While the researchers cited above, among many others, present views and perspectives that might be considered by many as disputable, one can still confidently state that the basic Islamic principles governing the establishment of family by marriage and the principles defining the roles and the methods by which to maintain the family are of universal conviction among Muslims. This is true wherever they are (particularly in the Arab World) since they are dictated by the *Holy Quran* and the teachings of the prophet Mohamed. Nevertheless, it is imperative to clearly state here that like in other parts of the world; the family in the Muslim world is similarly undergoing dramatic changes.

Changing Non-Islamic Attitudes and Behaviors

In considering the challenges faced by the Arab/Muslim family, Badran (2003) analyzed the changes which the Arab family experienced in the last 50 years focusing on Egypt, Jordan, Iraq, Lebanon, Palestine and Syria. She notes that globalization has its effect on the life and work of people, and on their families and their societies. It affects employment, working conditions, income and social protection, culture and identity, inclusion and exclusion, and the cohesiveness of families and societies. It is believed that globalization has opened doors for millions of women to enter the labor force, which in turn undermined and revolutionized the traditional understanding of family roles. Some observers believe that the patriarchal family, which is the cornerstone of the Arab-Islamic society, is undergoing a crisis brought about by globalization.

Besides women's employment, other factors are seen to have contributed to the crisis. Increased economic power of women undermines the legitimacy of men's domination as providers for the family. The second factor is contraception, which has given women growing control over the timing and frequency of childbearing. The third factor is mass education, which has given equal opportunity to women for education and training. While these trends are more pronounced in industrialized countries, it is believed that much of the world, including the Arab world, is moving in the same direction.

Clearly, the image and characteristics of the traditional family prevalent in the Arab world is changing. The father as the provider and the mother as the housekeeper, and an average family size of seven or eight children is no longer the only model existing in Arab society. Several indicators reflect the changes that have occurred to the traditional model of the Arab family. These include delayed marriage, single-parent households, a smaller number of children, and increased urbanization and material consciousness (Nosseir, 2003).

The current profile of the Arab region is one of diversity and demographic change in terms of the structure and composition of the Arab family as a social unit. One can argue that globally and within the Arab world, the family is undergoing change in which the traditional model of two parents and a large number of children tied together in a patriarchal form is being challenged. It is clear that the challenge has been brought about by the increasing number of women joining the labor force, by the advancement in pharmaceutical technology facilitating the control of reproductive behavior, and by the facility to link and communicate electronically between women within a given country and across the world. This has resulted in observable changes that have been reflected in statistics on fertility, marriage, divorce, migration, and new types of disease (The Organization of the Arab Family, 2004).

Variety in conjugal arrangement. Other non-traditional or rather non-Islamic attitudes and behaviors have also been reported. Unheard of just a few years ago, Muslim scholars are now debating the legality of a variety of conjugal arrangements that are beginning to reappear on the Arab Islamic front. It is the opinion of some prominent Islamic scholars that *Sharia* (Islamic Law) permits other types of marriage contracts like *Almita'a* and *Almisiar* as alternatives to the single partner, long term commitment marriage contract that has been elevated and made sacred in Islam. These alternative arrangements are governed by specific rules and conditions which make marriage a temporary commitment for both parties with limited risks or sacrifices (Al-Huseini. 2002). While these alternative arrangements were being practiced in the early years of Islam, they virtually disappeared over the years. However, their recent popularity has opened heated debates about their legitimacy.

Divorce. Divorce is another issue that is undergoing change. A divorce arrangement called *Khalaa*, which enables the wife to divorce her husband, is also gaining popularity in some Arab countries. Similarly, it is no longer uncommon to find young adults defying their parents and asking the court to certify their marriage in the event of the disapproval of their parents, or for a woman to ask the court to divorce her from her husband. What all this seems to indicate is an increased intolerance of norms and traditions, nonadherence to religious rules and codes of conduct, pragmatism, and adoption of a global culture that is transmitted through the mass media.

Characteristics of the Traditional Omani Family

Omani society is basically traditional and it retains most of the characteristics that constitute an Islamic society: tribal identity and loyalty, male dominance, a strict code of conduct and social support. In keeping with these social characteristics, the Omani family is also said to be traditionally tracing its characteristics to the Islamic/Arab definition of a family.

An anthropological study conducted by Barth (1983) of the culture and society in an Omani town gives insight about life in *Sohar* that can be considered to be representative of a typical Omani town. Barth describes the Omani household as constituting the following categories: incomplete households (single parent as a result of death or divorce), solitary couple, elementary family plus dependents, polygynous household, patrilateral joint households and matrilateral joint households with members of the household ranging between 6 and 15. In all these households, the husband, father, or older son is invested with ultimate authority in all normative and moral matters. Barth explains that men have ". . . the final power of decision in all questions concerning wife and children, as well as the responsibility for their behavior and training" (p. 117). However, women see themselves as autonomous and morally responsible individuals involved as equals with their husbands in a relationship that both sides shape. Barth goes further to explain that gender roles are complementary and not based on the division of labor. Women normally do all housework and men are responsible for all work that is related to the outside, but most tasks can be done by either sex. For example, cooking is women's work only as it relates to domestic use but when it comes to larger feasts and collective occasions, men are the cooks.

With regard to family relations, Barth says that in most everyday matters "husband and wife tend to meet roughly as equals and many couples seemed to exercise a fairly balanced control over each other in matters of mutual concern" (p. 121) . It is clear from this description that the Omani family is generally an extended family that is characterized by a large number of children. It is normal to have between three or four generations living under one roof and that the father is the main provider and is therefore the most powerful figure in the family. The mother is the homemaker and wields a lot power over her children making her the main agent of socialization. However, it is to be noted that other members of the extended family have an equally important role in the socialization of the children. Family problems and crises are normally managed and resolved within the family. Women and girls have limited freedom of movement and their interactions are often limited to their own gender. Marriages are therefore mostly arranged by the parents and often with a cousin, a distant relative, or a non-relative who is known to the family including neighbors. Al-Harthi (2003) conducted a sociological field study about family and marriage in the Sultanate of Oman. One of his findings indicated that 59.1% of the male participants did know their wives before marriage, since they are mostly close or distant relatives. At the same time, most of the other 40.8% indicated that although they did not know their wives before marriage, their wives were known and/or recommended by family members. Barth's study indicated, however, that a larger percentage of the unions in *Sohar* were between strangers (86%) compared to those with first or second cousins (14%). It is important to note here that *strangers* are considered to be anybody other than a first or second cousin.

THE CHANGING ROLES OF THE OMANI FAMILY

The last decade has transported Oman from a traditional and conservative society to a modern society that is beginning to experience the winds of change and some of the negative effects of globalization. While these changes are relatively modest compared to other countries, they are nevertheless notable.

The availability of education for all, an improved standard of living, females' access to the job market, access to the mass media, information technology and communication, among other things, have reshaped the construct of the Omani family. With education, the Omani woman is becoming more confident and independent in her opinion about things that affect her life. Accessibility to the job market has given her economic independence that is changing her position from a dependent consumer to an independent co-provider. Education has given the Omani woman spending power and therefore exposure to the material world. Driving licenses, mobile telephones, shopping malls and wider mobility have all contributed to breaking the walls of tradition and exposing the woman to the external arena that was traditionally men's domain.

With the woman's movement to the outside came the weakening of her role as the agent of socialization. One could venture to say that the emancipation of the Omani woman, while positive in itself, has had a domino effect on the family. This worry is confirmed when one analyzes the results of the national census conducted in 2003 (Ministry of National Economy, 2003). Available data reveal some new trends that were not apparent in the 1993 census. Among these are changes in the fertility rate (from 6.87 in 1993 to 3.64 in 2002), an increase in the number of nuclear family structures and higher divorce rates (3,291 reported cases in 1993 and 3,830 cases in 2003). Similar changes can be seen in the rapid increase in women's participation in the labor market and an increase in the mean age of marriage for both males and females (Ministry of Development, 1993; Ministry of National Economy, 2004).

Other notable changes can be observed in the overall increase in cases of juvenile delinquency, substance abuse and sexually-transmitted diseases (Ministry of Health, 2002). Radio and television talk shows and newspaper articles have expressed concern regarding what they describe as the weakening of family ties, reduced authority over the welfare of individual members of the family, a loss of effective communication between family members and a decrease in the norms and values that bind members of the family together. It is important, however, to reiterate that these changes are minor and do not as yet constitute a major threat to the closely-knit fabric of the Omani society.

COHESION AND STRENGTH OF THE OMANI FAMILY

As the world moves further into the new millennium, social scientists question the family's ability to cope with multiple stressors and demands that are placed upon it. Based on his review of the literature on family cohesion and the interviews he conducted with members of 20 Omani families (males and females), Albeely (2003) identified two types of threats to family cohesion. The first is internal and the second is external. According to Albeely's findings, internal threats to family cohesion are manifested in the following: lack of adjustment between parents, lack of proper economic management, lack of positive communication between members, absence of free expression and exchange of sentiments between family members, lack of democratic ideals and practices, lack of commitment to family roles, lack of cooperation and support between members, inflexibility of decisions and self-centeredness of the members. The external threats, on the other hand include: economic conditions, societal influences, peer pressure, influence of external media and influences of the global popular culture of consumerism and materialism. It is to be highlighted here that all of Albeely's interviewees have indicated that when their problems get out of hand between the wife and the husband and the threat of disintegration increases, they usually revert to the elders in their extended families for solutions and support. In fact, the majority of the marital problems that married couples cannot handle are resolved with help from members of the extended family. It is to be highlighted also that the Islamic way of settling family disputes as stated by *Allah* (God) in the *Holy Quran* dictates the intervening of arbiters from both the husband's and the wife's families: "If ye fear a breach between them twain, appoint arbiters, one from his family, and one from hers; If they seek to set things aright, *Allah* will cause their reconciliation: for *Allah* hath full knowledge and is acquainted with all things" (*The Holy Quran, Surra 4*, Verse 35).

Al-Barwani (2005) conducted extensive interviews with 15 young women from three main regions in the Sultanate representing different educational and socio-economic levels. All the interviewees were married with children and enjoying a stable family life. The purpose of the interviews was to probe the strengths and challenges confronting today's families, giving special attention to the changing family roles, changing relationships, and changing behaviors, practices, and traditions in family life.

Changing Family Roles

Interviewees indicated that they had the major responsibility for the children: their care, education and general well-being. Discipline, however, was generally the responsibility of the father. While the father continues to be mostly responsible for external matters and the mother mainly internal, it is clear that there is an encroachment into each other's territory. It appears that many roles are beginning to get diffused as women take up the role of partner, contributing equally to the family budget and getting involved in decisions that affect the family. While discussion and dialogue seem to be the approach used to deal with issues, solve problems and make important decisions, it appears that the father is the one who makes the final decision and bears the responsibility for its outcomes.

Changing Relationships

Interviewees felt that compared to their parents they were closer to their husbands and their children. It appears that there is more openness than was ever possible before. One interviewee said, "Our children can talk to us freely and sometimes question our decisions and give us their opinion about things. They respect us but they are not afraid of us. When I was growing up, I couldn't talk to my father, he was not approachable. I could talk to my mother but I couldn't possibly question her."

Families of spouses seem to continue to have an important role, especially in issues related to the welfare of the children. It appears that grandparents and other close relatives are often consulted and their opinions are valued. Moreover, the grandparents seem to retain respect, status and power over their children. Two of the interviewees, however, felt that living in close proximity to the in-laws invited interference, especially with regard to raising the children. Even though the younger generation seems to generally prefer to live independently after marriage, they normally do not opt to live far from their parents. In situations where husbands work in the city or in neighboring countries, the preference is to leave the wife and children in the village to be cared for by the extended family. Those who lived in extended family arrangements felt that it was very useful because there was a lot of help and support, especially when the family faces difficulties. It is important to point out here that both the interviews and personal observations have confirmed that the extended family is still very strong in Oman and the support of the members of the extended family in ensuring their wellbeing is the prime duty and responsibility of all members.

Changing Behaviors, Practices and Traditions

Interviewees unanimously agreed that today's children are self-centered, materialistic and easily influenced by the media and peers. On the other hand, they are smart, expressive and tend to be free in their speech and behavior. Nevertheless, they felt that they still have full control over their children's lives and that in most cases children obeyed and respected their parents' wishes.

All interviewees indicated that they try to balance between inculcating Islamic principles and Omani traditions with the need to survive in the modern world. They all confessed that the biggest challenge was to bring up the children with proper Islamic values and traditions while they are constantly being defied by the popular culture.

Ten of the fifteen interviewees indicated that their marriages were arranged and their spouses were either cousins or members of their respective tribes. Others indicated marrying a neighbor, a friend or relative of a close member of the family. In most cases, the bride would know the groom and would be approved by the family. One of the interviewees said about arranged marriages, ". . . they are more stable because they have strong support of the two families. Also, the bride and groom go into the marriage without prior expectations and they get to establish a bond between them as they share and experience life together."

Considering that the Omani family is essentially built on Islamic principles, Al-Barwani and Albeely (2004) conducted a study aimed at investigating the cohesion and strength of the Omani family across known broad areas of strength that strong families tend to share (DeFrain, 1999; DeFrain, Cook, & Gonzalez-Kruger, 2005). Specifically, the study explored the differences between sub-samples in their expression of cohesiveness relevant to such variables as gender, marital status, position in the family, family size, educational level, type of work, income and region. The research also explored whether the study sample exhibited aspects of family disintegration and the extent to which these families comply with the general definition of a Muslim family. The findings confirmed that the Omani family is generally highly cohesive and can be said to be in compliance with the general definition of an Islamic/Arab family. No significant differences were noted between men and women with regard to their global perception of their family's cohesion. However, males whether married, divorced or single perceived their families to be more cohesive than their female counterparts. Results also showed that parents tended to perceive their families to be more cohesive than their children did and that those having between one and nine children perceived their families to be more cohesive than those with ten or more children. While some differences were found within the level of education and type of work variables, no significant differences were observed with regard to region and income level.

CONCLUSION

Through the analysis of literature on families in Oman, census statistics, interviews and personal observations, the authors made an effort to present insight into the Omani family. In order to have a better understanding of the Omani family, it was deemed necessary to first present significant elements that characterize the Omani society and its people.

Oman's rich history, its Arab/Islamic heritage and the Islamic way of life and code of conduct were presented as a way of establishing the extent to which these elements have contributed to the formation of the character of the Omani person and the Omani family. It was also shown how Oman's tribal system, its monarchical system, and its overseas dominions have added to the distinct characteristics of the Omani person.

It is clear that there is notable effort, both at the governmental and individual levels, to balance between tradition and modernity. Census data and the results of some surveys conducted have indicated some changes with regard to some social indicators, especially those related to women and youth. Over the last 35 years, Oman succeeded in closing the gender gap in education, thus empowering the Omani woman to make important decisions that affect her life. Education and good health services have given the Omani woman the option to delay marriage and childbearing, thus reducing both the fertility rate and family size. It also gave her the option of employment, thus giving her economic power that she had never experienced before. With employment and economic power came her mobility and purchasing power which gave her the option to buy services that reduced her role as a homemaker. Rising divorce rates, increasing youth restlessness and distance from religion and traditions are some of the negative indicators that may reflect on the absence of tolerance, communication, support and clear role definitions.

One cannot dismiss the fact that globalization and the information technology and communication revolution will continue to present themselves as potential challenges to the Omani family in the coming years. However, we are confident that the power of Islam and the Omani Arab traditions and heritage will continue to have the capability to sustain the family and give it the strength it requires to survive future challenges.

REFERENCES

'Abd al 'Ati, Hammudah (1997). Foundations and boundaries of the family in Islam. In *Family Structure in Islam*, Chap. 2, pp. 19-49. Indianapolis, IN, USA: American Trust Publications.

Abbas, N. (2001). *The Muslim family's role in building a righteous society.* Manila, The Philippines: The Wisdom Enrichment Foundation, The Ideal Muslims. Retrieved November 9, 2005, from http://www.wefound.org/texts/Ideal_Muslims_files/Family.htm

Abu, S., & A. Abdul, H. (1993). *Crisis in the Muslim mind.* Translated by Y. T. DeLorenzo. Herndon, Virginia, USA: International Institute of Islamic Thought.

Al-Barwani, T. (2005, Sept). Distinct features of social development in the Sultanate of Oman. Paper presented at the Center for Contemporary Arab Studies, Georgetown University, Washington DC.

Al-Barwani, T., & Albeely, T. (2004, Aug). Cohesion of the Omani family: A solution to the threats of globalization. Paper presented at the 31st International Conference on Social Welfare, Kuala Lumpur, Malaysia.

Albeely, T. (2003, Nov). Family Cohesion. Paper presented at the Ministry of Social Development Seminar on "The effects of globalization on the family's social and psychological cohesion," Muscat, Oman.

Al-Harthi, S. (2003). *Family and marriage in the Sultanate of Oman.* Unpublished master's thesis., Rabat, Morocco: Mohamed Alkhamis University.

Al-Huseini, M. (2002). *The truth about Almisiar marriage, and the legality of Almita'a.* Retrieved November 12, 2005, from http://www.hashem.150m.com/zaw.htm

Allen, Jr., C. (1987). *Oman: The modernization of the Sultanate.* Boulder, Colorado, USA:Westview Press.

Badran, H. (2003). Major trends affecting families in El Mashrek El Araby. In *Major trends Affecting families: A background document,* Report for United Nations. New York, USA: United Nations Department of Economic and Social Affairs, Division for Social Policy and Development, Program on the Family.

Barth, F. (1983). *Sohar: Culture and society in an Omani Town.* Baltimore, USA and London: Johns Hopkins University Press.

Chatty, D. (2000). Women working in Oman: Individual choice and cultural constraints. *International Journal of Middle East Studies, 32,* 241-254.

DeFrain, J. (1999). Strong families around the world. *Family Matters: Journal of the Australian Institute of Family Studies, 53*(Winter), 6-13.

DeFrain, J., Cook, R., & Gonzalez-Kruger, G. (2005). Family health and dysfunction. In R. J. Coombs (Ed.), *Family Therapy Review.* Mahwah, NJ: Lawrence Erlbaum Associates, 3-20.

Eickelman, D. (1987). Ibadhism and the sectarian perspective. In B. R. Pridham (Ed.), *Oman: Economic, social and strategic developments.* London: University of Exeter Center for Arab Gulf Studies.

The Holy Quran. (1984). English translation of the meanings and commentary. Almadina, Saudi Arabia: King Fahd Holy Quran Printing Complex.

Lemu, B., & Heeren, F. (1978). *Women in Islam.* Cambridge, UK: Islamic Council of Europe.

McBrierty, V., & Al Zubair, M. (2004). *Oman, ancient civilization: Modern nation, Towards a knowledge and service economy.* Dublin, Ireland: Trinity College Dublin Press.

Ministry of Education/UNICEF. (2000). *EFA assessment report 2000.* Muscat, Oman.

Ministry of Development. (1993). *General census of population housing and establishments.* Muscat, Oman.

Ministry of Health. (2002). *Towards a better understanding of youth: KAP survey of secondary school students.* Muscat, Oman.

Ministry of Health. (1995). *Family health survey.* Muscat, Oman.

Ministry of National Economy. (1996). *Results of 1996 labor force survey*, Muscat, Oman.

Ministry of National Economy. (2003). *National census statistics.* Muscat, Oman.

Ministry of National Economy. (2004) *Oman human development report.* Muscat, Oman.

Nosseir, N. (2003). *Family in the new millennium: Major trends affecting families in North Africa.* In *Major trends affecting families: A background document,* Report for United Nations. New York, USA: United Nations Department of Economic and Social Affairs, Division for Social Policy and Development, Program on the Family.

Olson, D. H., & DeFrain, J. (2006). *Marriages and families: Intimacy, diversity, and strengths* (6th Ed.). New York: McGraw-Hill Higher Education.

Peterson, G. (2000). Characteristics of healthy family systems. Dr. Gayle Peterson: Making Healthy Families. Retrieved November 11, 2005 from: http://www.askdrgayle.com/chfs.html

Peterson, J. E. (1978). *Oman in the twentieth century.* London: Croom-Helm.

Pridham, B. R (1987). *Oman: Economic, social and strategic developments.* London: Center for Arab Gulf Studies, University of Exeter.

The Organization of the Arab Family (2004). *A strategy for the Arab family.* Sharjah, United Arab Emirates.

Valiante, W. (2003). *Family therapy and Muslim families: A solution focused Approach.* Retrieved October 28, 2005 from http://www.arabpsynet.com/Archives/OP/OP/

doi:10.1300/J002v41n01_07

Chinese Family Strengths and Resiliency

Anqi Xu
Xiaolin Xie
Wenli Liu
Yan Xia
Dalin Liu

SUMMARY. Chinese family and marriage strengths and challenges are delineated in this article, including equity in marriage, affection, the ability to adapt to changes, mutual trust, compatibility, harmony, and family support. Despite the fact that Chinese households are getting smaller as a result of governmental policy and the broadening of housing markets, families remain crucial support networks, especially in the areas of socialization and intergenerational relationships. Current research on Chinese

Anqi Xu is Professor, Shanghai Academy of Social Sciences, People's Republic of China (E-mail: xaq@sass.org.cn). Xiaolin Xie is Associate Professor, School of Family, Consumer and Nutritional Sciences, Northern Illinois University, DeKalb, IL 60115 (E-mail: xiaolinx@niu.edu). Wenli Liu is Senior Researcher, Beijing Normal University, Beijing, People's Republic of China (E-mail: liuwenli200555@yahoo.com.cn). Yan Xia is Assistant Professor, Department of Education and Family Studies, University of Nebraska-Lincoln, Lincoln, NE 68588 (E-mail: yxia@mail.unomaha.edu). Dalin Liu is Founder, Chinese Ancient Sex Culture Museum, Tongli and Shanghai, People's Republic of China.

Address correspondence to: Anqi Xu.

[Haworth co-indexing entry note]: "Chinese Family Strengths and Resiliency." Xu, Anqi et al. Co-published simultaneously in *Marriage & Family Review* (The Haworth Press, Inc.) Vol. 41, No. 1/2, 2007, pp. 143-164; and: *Strong Families Around the World: Strengths-Based Research and Perspectives* (ed: John DeFrain, and Sylvia M. Asay) The Haworth Press, Inc., 2007, pp. 143-164. Single or multiple copies of this article are available for a fee from The Haworth Document Delivery Service [1-800-HAWORTH, 9:00 a.m. - 5:00 p.m. (EST). E-mail address: docdelivery@haworthpress.com].

Available online at http://mfr.haworthpress.com
© 2007 by The Haworth Press, Inc. All rights reserved.
doi:10.1300/J002v41n01_08

marriages and families is cited, outlining attitudinal changes regarding mate selection, divorce, and childbirth between genders, between older and younger generations, and between urban and rural residents. doi:10.1300/ J002v41n01_08 *[Article copies available for a fee from The Haworth Document Delivery Service: 1-800-HAWORTH. E-mail address: <docdelivery@ haworthpress.com> Website: <http://www.HaworthPress.com> © 2007 by The Haworth Press, Inc. All rights reserved.]*

KEYWORDS. Chinese families and marriages, family strengths, family resiliencies

INTRODUCTION TO CHINESE MARRIAGES AND FAMILIES

Chinese families have undergone tremendous changes in the past several decades as a result of socioeconomic developments, among them, the governmental one-child-per-family policy that has impacted family structure and family dynamics. The economic growth in major cities has prompted development of the housing market that gives young married couples the opportunity to purchase their own housing. Thus, the nuclear family has become the normative family structure. This chapter is an effort to delineate family strengths typical of contemporary Chinese families, and to provide current research on Chinese marriages and families that chronicle attitudinal changes on mate selection, divorce, and childbirth between genders, between older and younger generations, and between urban and rural residents.

Chinese Family Strengths

Chinese culture, being collective in nature, is well-known for its emphasis on family relationships and support. Families are described as close-knit units, manifested in three-generational households. However, the current norm of family structure today in China is no longer a three-generational household; rather, it is the nuclear family. Research shows that despite the changes, family remains the main pillar of the social support network. Families are still greatly valued by the young and the old. Intergenerational relationships are not to be undervalued or underestimated. Child care and elder care remain families' responsibilities both in urban and rural China.

The studies of family strengths among Chinese families are scant. In the West, Stinnett and DeFrain (1985) identified major six strengths among American families: affection and appreciation, commitment, positive communication, the ability to manage stress and crisis effectively, enjoyable time together, and a sense of spiritual well-being. Xie, DeFrain, Meredith, and Combs (1996) conducted the first study of family strengths in China. They found that besides loyalty, family support, enjoying time together, families in China perceived a sense of harmony being an important aspect of family strengths. Again, this may be related to the collectivist culture that emphasizes unity and togetherness in the family. One example to illustrate this is that Chinese culture, like most other Asian cultures, tends to put the family name before first name, implying that families' needs take precedence over individuals' needs.

Xie, Xia, and Zhou (2004) conducted an in-depth interview study with 40 Chinese immigrants in the US to delineate major family strengths and challenges. The following family strengths were identified: family support; social support from friends and community; communication among family members; balancing host and heritage cultures, and spiritual well-being. These two studies seem to identify the recurring theme–family support to facilitate family functioning in China.

Current Status of Chinese Marriages and Families

Mate selection. This has been a significant research topic in the study of Chinese marriages and families for the following reasons: (1) mate selection is prelude to marriage and is the foundation of future family life; (2) though mate selection is a personal issue, and hinges on one's choices and interests, in reality, it is influenced by the families of origin, society, and culture.

Research indicates the following trends in mate selection among Chinese youths today: (1) youths consider personality more important than one's family background; (2) though men still emphasize chastity more than women, on the whole, the concept of chastity is downplayed by both genders; (3) education is valued in mate selection, especially among the educated group; (4) romance and affection are highly emphasized among the young, the educated, and professional groups (Li, 1989; Liu, 1996; Fei & Xie, 1995).

In her study of 3,000 married men and women in Shanghai and Harbin, China, Xu (2000) found that the main criteria in mate selection were health (60.9%), honesty (53.4%), personality compatibility (47%), and affection (36.9%). Those with education held higher expectations for their future mates and were more careful in their selection process. Not only did they take into consideration their mate's financial status, but compatibility and affection. However, factors that influenced mate selection were multifaceted, such as gender, geographic regions, the family's financial situation, and housing conditions.

Studies in the past showed that arranged marriages were a common practice in China, with approximately two-thirds of marriages arranged in urban areas and even higher percentages in rural areas, especially those that were economically disadvantaged (Pan, 1987; Shen & Yang, 1995; Xu, 1997). However, recent trends showed that arranged marriages were decreasing in rural areas, and even more rapidly in urban areas. Friends and colleagues took over the matchmaker roles that parents, relatives and neighbors used to play (see Table 1).

As friends and colleagues were more likely to introduce a perspective mate than relatives, youths were granted more freedom to choose their own mates. Today, in rural China, arranged marriages where both couples did not know each other before marriage and were not happy with the choices represents only 4.7%, compared to 29% in 1966. Self-selection of a mate represents 56.7%, compared to 32.8% in 1966 (Xu, 1997). Table 2 shows that a majority of the couples are happy about their own mate selection.

After 1949, dating was discouraged and frowned upon for several decades. Many couples went underground when dating. Because of the lack of entertainment centers and financial resources at the times, dating

TABLE 1. How couples met (in percent).

	Cities		Rural Areas	
	Beijing and four other cities	Beijing and six other cities	Gansu	Guangdong
	1982	1992	1996	
Through Parents	17.6	4.3	60.8	2.1
Through Relatives	22.6	21.4	16.6	20.5
Through Match-Makers		7.7	0.8	25.2
Through Friends	36.0	33.4	8.4	21.4
Own Self	23.0	32.0	12.9	30.3
Through Work	0.8	1.2	0.0	0.1
Through Agencies		0.1	0.0	0.0
Others			0.5	0.4
Total	100.0	100.0	100.0	100.0
N	4878	5476	1330	1537

Sources: Adapted from Pan (1987); Shen & Yang (1995); Xu (1997).

TABLE 2. Marriage decision making among rural couples at different periods (%).

| Marriage decision making | Different Periods | | | | |
	1946-1966	1967-1976	1977-1986	1987-1996	Row average
Arranged by Elders, Not Knowing Each Other Before Marriage	25.2	13.9	8.2	3.8	12.8
Arranged by Elders, Not Happy with the Choice	3.8	1.5	1.4	0.9	1.9
Arranged by Elders, Happy with the Choice	38.2	46.7	42.4	38.5	41.4
Own Choice, Parents Happy	24.1	32.6	43.1	50.2	37.5
Own Choice, Parents Not Happy	0.8	1.0	1.4	1.8	1.3
Own Choice, Parents Deceased, or Did Not Care	7.9	4.4	3.5	4.7	5.1
Total	100	100	100	100	100
N	477	613	1013	763	2866

Source: Adapted from Xu (1997).

behavior was restricted to chatting at one's own home or strolling on the street (Xu, 1997). Su and Hu (2000) found that letter writing was the main communication instrument between couples. In their study of 20- to 30-year-old youths in China, Li and Xu (2004) revealed that 47% of the couples wrote letters to express their affection for each other. This behavior was more popular among the educated group.

As to the number of dates couples had before marriage, in a study that involved 1,600 married couples, Xu (1997) found that the average number of different partners that they dated before marriage was 1.5 for each participant. Two thirds married the first and only person they dated. Only 10.8% had dated two or more people. Li and Xu (2004) found that among youths, the average number of dates was 3.3. Sixty-eight percent had one to three people with 11% having dated six or more people. Because of the limited selection pool among the middle aged and older groups, many of them dated fewer people.

Pan and Jen (2000) conducted a random study of dating behavior among college students on 150 campuses in 1997. Results showed that 41.4% of students had kissed, 26.7% had sexual touches, and 10.1% had sexual intercourse. Another study involved 5,070 university students on 26 campuses in 14 provinces revealed similar results: 11.3% had sexual intercourse. Among those students who had engaged in sexual intercourse, gender differences were also revealed: 52.2% of male participants had one sexual partner versus 67.9% of the females; 22% of males had six or more sexual partners versus 18.3% of the females (Research on Sex Education among College Students, 2001).

Marriage. Marriage is a salient life event. Marriage attitudes are reflections of family, social and cultural values. They influence marriage behaviors and family life. It is still against the law in China to cohabit. The majority of Chinese are against this behavior, but it is becoming more accepted among the younger generation. Lu (1997) found some age differences in their consensus with the statement "No cohabitation unless married": 65% of those 36 years and younger, versus 68% of those 35 to 55 years old, and 75% of those 55 and older agreed with that statement. In another study on a similar topic, Li and Xu (2004) found that half of their 683 participants approved of cohabitation conditionally. To the statement, "It was all right to cohabit if the couple planned to get married," 51% agreed, and 25% disagreed. There was also a gender difference in response to that statement. 17% of male participants disagreed versus 33% of the females. In the same study, 49% reported kissing on a date, 35% had sexual intercourse, 11% cohabitated, and 11% got pregnant. It also was reported that the main constraints for sexual involvement were lack of passion (37.4%), fear of the consequences (20.3%), and that this behavior was immoral (4.7%) (Pan, 1995).

Chastity is considered an important value in traditional Chinese culture. Premarital sexual involvement is scorned and regarded as a social vice. However, among the youths today, it has become more acceptable. One study on sexual attitudes that involved 541 university students revealed that 48% of the students considered that "chastity was important," 33% believed that "the concept was too traditional, and should be abolished," 19% did not have an opinion one way or the other. Gender differences were found in this study with 55% of females versus 38% of males considering chastity important; 36% of males and 31% of females considered this concept too old-fashioned; 26% of males and 13% of females did not have an opinion one way or another (Zhen et al., 2000). In another study, among those 20 to 30 years of age, 34% considered chastity outdated; 64% of males and 84% of females thought the concept unfair for women (Li & Xu, 2004).

Husband-wife relationships and their role identities. Chinese culture emphasizes social stability and family harmony. Family and social needs takes precedence over individual needs. This leads some studies to posit that Chinese marriages are of high stability, but low quality (Fu, 1988;

Chui, 1994). However, studies show that the majority of married couples report high satisfaction in their relationships. In his study involving 5,000 couples in seven cities in China, 36.1% of wives versus 37.6% of husbands reported that their marriage was highly satisfying, 38.1% of wives versus 40.9% of husbands reported that they were satisfied, 24.9% of wives versus 21.3% of husbands reported an average level of satisfaction, and only .9% of wives and .2% of husbands report they were highly unsatisfied (Shen & Yang, 1995).

Another study of a similar nature revealed consistent results: 42.2% of the participants in Beijing were highly satisfied about their marriage. 49.4% reported they loved their spouse deeply, and 49.5% reported that their spouse loved them deeply (Li, 1996). Xu (1997) conducted a study on marital quality in Shanghai and its four surrounding regions. In the study, the majority of the respondents reported they were satisfied or highly satisfied with their marriage. Only a quarter of the respondents reported an average level of satisfaction. Those who described having equity in their marriage, mutual trust, and compatibility reported higher satisfaction scores. Therefore, it can be concluded that these are major characteristics in happy marriages. In the same study, 89% of the couples had not considered separation or divorce in the past year, only 0.7% thought about divorce often, 72.8% of the couples did not believe that their spouse would leave them, and only 0.7% believed that they would divorce their spouse. This shows that most Chinese marriages enjoy stability as well as satisfaction. Factors that lead to marital satisfaction include affection for each other, knowing each other well before marriage, the ability to adapt to changes, and compatibility (Xu & Ye, 2002).

Over the past several decades, women's roles have changed dramatically. Since the 1950s, the Chinese government has adopted policies that allow and encourage women to work outside the home. Today, the majority of women have jobs outside the home. These policies also help reduce the gender gap in education levels, career choices, income, and old age support. In a 2000 study of women's social status, involving 19,449 participants age 18 to 64 in 30 provinces, the majority of respondents disagreed that "women should avoid becoming superior to their husband in social status." Only 18.5% agreed with that statement. This is 3% lower compared to a similar study done in 1990 (The Second Investigation on Chinese Women's Social Status, 2001). A more recent study echoed similar results. The majority of the respondents believed that the husband and wife should share responsibilities in household chores and children's socialization and education. As to the statement, "The husband's role was to make money, whereas the wife's role was to take care of the family," only 2.8% of those 20 to 30 years old agreed, and 14.7% somewhat agreed; 2.8% agreed that the woman's careers should not supersede men's careers, and 10.1% somewhat agreed. 8.6% of the respondents agreed that "men should not do housework" (Li & Xu, 2004).

As a result of their work-force participation, women's decision-making power at home has increased. This was supported by the Second Investigation on Chinese Women's Social Status (2001): 67.4% of the participants reported joint decision making or the wife's sole decision making in career choices. This was an increase of 17.3% compared to 1990. Also, 60.7% of the wives were involved in decision making in family financial investment, and 70.7% participated in decision making about housing purchases. This was an increase of 10.2 and 15.1%, respectively. In the same study, 88.7% of women versus 90.9% of men solely decided what personal items they purchase, and 91.3% of women versus 94% of men solely decided how much support they provided their parents (The Second Investigation on Chinese Women's Social Status, 2001). Though the hours spent on daily housework were reduced for both genders, the fact that women still shouldered the majority of the housework did not change. They spent an average of 4.01 hours a day on the household, 2.7 hours more than their male counterparts. Urban women spent an average of 2.9 hours a day, 1.6 hours more than urban men (The Second Investigation on Chinese Women's Social Status, 2001).

There are concerns that globalization and market competition jeopardize women's labor-force participation and their income. In recent years, women's employment rate has been declining. At the end of 2000, 87% of urban women aged 18 to 64 years old were employed. This is 6.6% lower compared to men's employment rate. Both rates dropped compared to those in 1990, but the decrease is more visible for women than for men. Despite the fact that women's income increased in the past ten years, the gap between men's income and women's income widened. Women made 70.1% of what men made in townships, 7.4% less than what men made in 1990 (The Second Investigation on Chinese Women's Social Status, 2001).

Marital conflicts. Xu and Ye (1999) concluded that household chores, disagreement on children's education, and finances, but not extramarital affairs or family violence as depicted in the media, were the major causes for marital conflicts. Household chores accounted for 51.7% of the marital disputes, disagreements on children's education was 38.1%, financial issues, 23.7%, in-laws issues, 14%, the unhealthy habits of one spouse, 13.3%, and sexual disharmony, extramarital affairs, or giving birth to a girl together totaled only 2%. Geographic locations account for differences in marital conflicts. In a rural area in Gansu, China, an economically-depressed province, major conflicts centered on finances and division of household chores. In Shanghai, a metropolitan city, living standards were relatively higher than other parts of the country, and parents held high academic expectations for their onlies, therefore, it was not surprising to see that the main source of marital discord was disagreement on children's education. This was consistent with Sa's (1995) study that urban couples argued about children's education more than rural couples, whereas rural couples fought about finance more than their urban counterparts.

In their study about the frequency of arguments among marital couples, when asked how often they argued in the past year, 2.4% reported "often," 13.2% reported "sometimes," 36% stated "seldom," and 48% reported "never." Most of arguments and fights occurred within 3 to 7 years of the marriage, with the least occurring after 30 years of marriage. After their arguments and fights, only 2% of the couples said they made no compromises; 46.7% of urban husbands versus 30.2% of their rural counterparts made initial repair attempts. This was in comparison of 12.7% of urban wives versus 27% of rural wives. Fighting behaviors were different for husband than wives. During fights, husbands tended to do the following: yell and scream (51.2%), silent treatment (46.9%), physical violence (19.9%); while wives tended to do the following: silent treatment (77.6%), crying (70.1%), and screaming and yelling (41.1%) (Xu & Ye, 1999). Because of a lack of availability of marriage and family counseling programs, extended families or networked families tended to play a role in couple-conflict resolution: 29.5% of wives talked to their family of origin about the fight, 12.4% of wives went to stay at their own parents' place, 29.4% of parents and relatives offered help to the fighting couples at one point, 1.8% of the parents and relatives voiced disapproval of their idea of divorce, and only .4% supported it. However, in some extreme situations when families of origin were overinvolved, couples' relationships deteriorated faster than anticipated.

Marital dissolution. When marriages become unsalvageable, marital break-ups are likely to occur. Marital dissolution is influenced by different factors, such as geographic locations, social and cultural issues, family structure, and family networks. Divorce is still considered a social stigma that has a negative impact on one's reputation and on social stability.

As more people crave better marital relationships, and as the social and psychological costs related to divorces lessen, people, especially today's urban youths, adopt a more tolerant attitude toward divorce. In his study of 541 university students, Zhen et al. (2000) revealed that 44.4% of students believed that "the increasing divorce rate was a byproduct of social growth"; 68.6% believed that divorce was a private matter; 87.3% believed that divorce was a better option than a conflictual marriage. This was consistent with Li and Xu's (2004) study that reported only one third of their respondents believed that divorce had a negative impact on one's reputation and was detrimental to a child's emotional and physical health. Though single youths were less likely than married couples to acknowledge any negative impacts of divorce, when asked to respond to the statement, "Love was the foundation of marriage, and if love died, marriage should end," only 36.6% of the former group agreed.

However, married couples are more discreet about divorce than youths for fear that it will be detrimental to their children and to themselves. In a study conducted by the Shanghai Academy of Social Sciences in 2002, 53.8% agreed that for the sake of children, a couple should maintain their marriages despite the fact that they were not happy together. 70.6% agreed that divorce affected one's reputation to some degree.

The last half of the twentieth century witnessed the ebb and flow of divorce rates in China in light of political, social, and economic changes. At the beginning of 1950s after the war ended and a new political party came into power, many arranged marriages or marriages involving violence and abuse crumbled under the new Marriage Law. The divorce rate went up dramatically during that period, and decreased around the mid-1950s. The economic growth after natural disaster in the late 1950s triggered another hike in the divorce rate, but quickly cooled down. The late 1970s saw another increase in the divorce rate, but of relatively smaller magnitude compared to the previous two periods of increased divorce rates. It has maintained the same momentum till now (see Figure 1). This recent increase in divorce rate reflected people's changing attitudes toward divorce, and their higher expectations for marriage against the backdrop of an improved living environment and economic growth (Xu, 1995; Zhang, 1994). In 1980, the crude divorce rate was 0.35%, and in 2004 it was 1.28%. Geographic regions made a difference in divorce rates. In 1980, the highest crude divorce rate was 3.98% in Sinjan, the lowest was 0.16% in Shanxi; whereas in 2004, the highest was 3.51% in Shanxi, the lowest was 0.46% in Tibet.

Some studies suggest that differences in people's belief systems were likely to loosen social coherence and lead to a further increase in the divorce rate (Glenn & Supancic, 1984; Glenn & Shelton, 1985; Breault & Kposowa, 1987). In China, family structure, social coherence, ethnic

FIGURE 1. Divorce trend in China from 1980-2004.

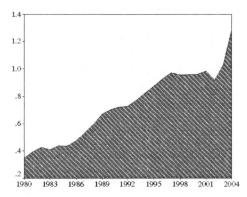

Source: Adapted from Chinese Statistics Bureau (1990, 2005).

culture, and implementation of marital law all influenced divorce rates in various locales in China. Low childbirth rates, small family structures, educational levels, job mobility, improved living standards, and membership in an ethnic minority all were associated with a higher divorce rate (Xu, 1997).

Socioeconomic growth in China has impacted people's views on marriages and families. It is anticipated that divorced families, single-parent families, singlehood, and childless marriages are likely to become more accepted and acknowledged. However, because of differences in value systems between urban and rural areas, between the coastal areas and inlands, and because of the lack of a government-sponsored social security system in rural China, many couples have only their families to rely on during crisis or transition stages.

Family structure. Traditional Chinese families are child-centered rather than couple-centered. Intimacy between couples is thought to have a negative impact on their commitment and responsibility to their extended family. The idea of the three- or four-generation family household remains a stereotype. Even in rural China, nuclear families are the main family structures with a household size of 3 to 6 persons. Married siblings no longer share a large household. The current small-scale economic model, different from the extended family structure, and conflictful in-law relationships help diminish the family size (Fei, 1983; Du, 1992). Table 3

TABLE 3. Family structures in urban and rural China.

Family structure	Urban (%)	Rural (%)	Family size (person)	Urban (%)	Rural (%)
Single	3.38	2.44	1	3.63	2.59
Single-Parents	1.13	0.99	2	10.29	6.76
Husband-Wife	8.36	5.11	3	37.48	20.27
Nuclear Family	61.17	65.58	4	22.61	31.69
Stem Family	19.51	22.79	5	14.87	20.62
Extended	2.32	0.79	6	6.26	10.28
Skipped Generation	1.23	0.49	7	2.68	4.55
Others	2.71	1.18	7 or more	2.18	3.23
Total	100.00	100.00	Total	100.00	100.00
N	3,577	9,334	N	3,578	9,335
			Mean Person	3.90	4.29
			SD Person	1.53	1.55

Source: Adapted from Shen, Chen, & Gao (2000).

lists the results of a study that involved 12,913 families in eight cities and townships, and 18 rural areas.

In light of the above discussion, the following can be concluded about the current Chinese families and marriages:

1. Despite the fact that Chinese family size is getting smaller, and extended families are not the norm, families remain a crucial part of the Chinese support network. They still play a critical role socially, economically, and emotionally. They provide mutual support in times of family crisis or during difficult family situations (Pan, 1987). Research shows that besides limited protection from government-sponsored social security and pensions from employers, many senior citizens rely on the support of their adult children and families. In rural China, because of lack of social security, family support is even more prominent and critical. Family remains the major elder-care institution. The main elder-care providers in rural areas tend to be daughters-in-law (Zhang, 2001).

2. The tight housing market has an impact on family structure, especially in the city (Fei, 1982; Pan et al., 1997). Many young-married couples move in with their parents as a result of the lack of housing for themselves. They also rely on their parents for childcare. However, as the country's economic growth continues, and the housing market broadens, the job opportunities many youths enjoy

today allow them to purchase their own housing and diminish their dependence on their parents. This is also true in rural area where the economic growth allows young families to build their separate houses and as such, many nuclear families are formed (Fei, 1983; Lei, 1994).

3. The recorded household size in each city may not be accurate because of job mobility. The purpose of recording household size in the past was to control population growth and to decide on the amount of housing each family unit was entitled to (Ding, 1992; Xu, 1995). With the economic growth and commercialization of housing market, the recorded size per household may not reflect the actual number. Therefore, it necessitates cautious interpretation when data are being used.

Childbirth. The late 1970s witnessed the influential one-child-per-family childbirth control policy with the exception that some rural families were allowed to have a second child after a four-year gap. Ethnic minority families and families in sparsely-populated areas were also allowed to have two children. The number of children per woman aged 15 to 49 was 1.51 in 1995, and it decreased to 1.17 in 2003. In 2004, 69.3% of families had one child, 27.3% of families had two children, and 3.4% of families had three children (State Statistics Bureau, 1996, 2005). The lifetime childbirth rate for fertile women was 1.81: 1.22 in urban areas, and 1.98 in rural areas; 83% of married women used contraceptives; 81% of families believed that birth control is still the woman's responsibility (see Figure 2).

Traditional Chinese culture holds that having a child protects one's old age, and the more children one has, the more blessings. However, with more women being educated and the implementation of family policy, some youths in metropolitan cities today opt for the DINC (Double Income No Children) lifestyle. Dong (2001) found that 14.1% of youths

FIGURE 2. Who is responsible for birth control.

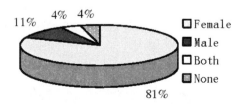

Source: Adapted from the Second Investigation of Chinese Women's Social Status (2000).

in five metropolitan cities consider a childfree marriage ideal. Lo and Fen (2001) found similar results in a survey of 681 university students: 15.9% of students said that they would not have any children after marriage. As to the response to the statement, "Childless marriages were incomplete marriages," only 11.5% agreed, 33.6% somewhat agreed, 22.8% somewhat disagreed, and 7.5% disagreed; 24.6% were undecided (Li & Xu, 2004). These studies suggested that having children was no longer considered the continuity of ones hopes and dreams. Youths' views on childbirth were becoming multidimensional.

Socialization of only children. The Chinese government implemented the one-child-per-family policy in 1979 to curtail population growth, which was predicted to reach 2.1 billion in 2080 if left uncontrolled (Tseng et al., 1988; Wang et al., 2000). Since its implementation, this policy has raised concerns about its impact on only children. Wang et al. (2000) found that attitudes toward only children remained the same over the years. Only children were reported to be overprotected by their parents and grandparents, and therefore, would experience disadvantages in their physical, social, emotional, and psychological development. Many Chinese speculated that only children, or "little emperors," would grow up to be spoiled, self-centered, non-cooperative, maladjusted, and lacking in the virtues that Chinese emphasize (Falbo et al., 1989).

Research on only children have focused on personality traits, behavior characteristics, and academic performance, and have reached mixed results. Liu et al. (2003) found in their study of psychosocial attributes that only children reported a higher level of anxiety and depression than those with siblings. This study was in sharp contrast to Yang et al. (1995) who previously found that only children reported a lower level of anxiety and depression, regardless of age, than sibling children. Tseng et al. (1988) found gender differences when they compared behavior problems between only children and sibling children. Boys who were only children did not differ from those with siblings. However, girls who were only children reported a higher level of depression. This result was compounded by the number of children preferred by parents and the dwelling-place of the families. Specifically, this effect was more pronounced in rural China. Jiao et al. (1986) compared only children and sibling children and found that the former had undesirable personality characteristics. In their study, sibling children scored higher than only children in independent thinking, persistence, cooperation with peers and behavior control, whereas only children scored higher in frustration tendencies and egocentrism than sibling children. Poston and Falbo (1990) reported similar results in their large-scale study of Chinese children in first and fifth grades from rural and urban China. The only difference between these groups was found in academic achievement, where only children enjoyed more advantages than sibling children. This result was confirmed in their subsequent study that involved 4,000 children from the third and sixth grades in four provinces in China. Only children reported a higher level of academic performance than sibling children and no significant difference was found in personality attributes or character development (Falbo & Poston, 1993).

Several factors influenced the results of the studies. These factors included methods of data collection, age of only children when data were collected, geographic locations of only children, and the use of appropriate instruments. First and foremost, methods of data collection varied from teachers' or parents' perceptions of only children to self perceptions. Second, the age of only children when data were collected varied from kindergarten to college age, with most studies focusing on elementary school students. Zhang et al. (2001) stated that a negative description of only children as "little emperors," "stubborn," "easily loses his/her temper," etc., predominated in the younger age group (3-5 years old). Once the child was getting older, those negative descriptions dropped, and positive description rose. Falbo (1982) suggested that by the time these only children became young adults, many differences reported in the research studies between only children and sibling children may have been eradicated or reduced. Third, Poston and Falbo (1990) reported that the majority (90%) of only children lived in the urban areas of China. Fourth, the use of culturally-appropriate and sensitive instruments was critical. Many studies that measured personality characteristics used instruments developed in the West, leading to issues related to validity and cultural sensitivity (Polit & Falbo, 1987; Wan et al., 1994).

The studies of only children have received much attention in the past several decades. Recent studies seemed to point to more positive results (Wan et al., 1994; Wang et al., 2000). Wang et al. (2000) posited that one must incorporate an understanding of Chinese culture when studying only children in China. Chinese families tend to live in close proximity, thus, creating opportunities for children to interact with each other. They may be only children in each individual family, but they do not lack playmates.

In sum, research studies on only children in China had inconsistent results, with some painting a negative and deficit picture of only children, and others painting a neutral or positive one. However, recent studies lean toward the latter trend. A more thorough analysis of only children has concluded that only children and sibling children were not different from each other significantly in personality, behaviors, and character development. However, one difference seems to be consistent over time, the difference in academic achievement, with only children being in the more advantageous position than sibling children. This was consistent with Fong (2005) who found that children with few siblings or no siblings receive more parental investment. There is no exception for daughters, who are also encouraged to pursue higher education and competitive careers.

Intergenerational relationships. Confucianism, a traditional philosophy still impacting Chinese families, emphasizes family hierarchy and social and family harmony (Ho, 1981; Hsu, 1985). Inherent in Confucianism is the value of filial piety, which demands respect and obligation to aging parents, honoring the family name, and emphasis on group harmony rather than individual gratification or identity (Wong, 1998). Filial piety encompasses authority, power hierarchy, and family lineage. As such, Chinese families are often described as highly cohesive, partially due to the cultural emphasis on harmony and mutual obligations, and the low tolerance for overt family conflicts (Chow, 1999).

Traditionally, the Chinese family was a very strong institution. Because of economic and social reforms, Chinese families have gone through numerous changes in the past several decades. These changes include the widening housing market, increasing divorce rates, smaller family size, and greater mobility among youths. Pei and Pillai (1999) found that 90% of rural elderly had adult children living in the same village, whereas only 44% of their urban counterparts had adult children living in the same city due to job mobility. As such, family and household size are getting smaller. The traditional *partrilocal* family where parents and married sons share co-residence is now giving way to the *neolocal* family where young adults are residing in separate housing units. Consequently, compared to previous generations, older people in China today are more likely to maintain separate living households from their adult children than in the past (Chen & Silverstein, 2000). Interestingly, Treas and Wang (1993) found that 79% of men and 65% of women aged 60 and older in metropolitan Shanghai favored a separate residence. Education and resources were related to their preference for a separate residence. Unger (1993) revealed that older people with a pension or work income were more likely to live separately from their adult children. Similarly, Hu and Ye (1991) found that higher-educated elderly were also more inclined to have their own housing units. Though in a separate residence, they also preferred living in the vicinity of at least one of their adult children. Some researchers have dubbed the term *networked family* to describe the intergenerational linkages to provide support when needed (Pan & Ruan, 1995; Xu, 1995). Chinese families have long been described as a corporate kin group that cared for the welfare of all family members and were bound by common goals and interests (Tu et al., 1993). Through the networked family, the norm of reciprocity between the elderly and their adult children is often observed. For example, studies have shown that over half of all elderly helped their adult children with housework and child care (Hu & Ye, 1991).

On the other side of the care spectrum, Yang (1996) stated that in the traditional Chinese family, support for elders was not uniform, but rather varied by gender. Sons were usually expected to support their parents financially. In Gui's study (1988), he found in rural China that sons provided the most in medical care, then spouses, and daughters last.

Likewise, in other places in China, of those legally responsible for the elder, 30% were oldest sons, 10% oldest daughters, and 31% other children (Chinese Population Information and Research Center, 1990). Zhan and Montgomery (2003) investigated the changing dynamics of caregiving in urban China against the backdrop of economic reforms and cultural emphasis of *xiao* (filial piety). Their study showed "a decline in the patrilocal tradition of caregiving." Taking care of the elderly was shifting from sons' responsibility to daughters' responsibility. However, the authors were concerned that those female caregivers today with fewer children, who were more financially dependent and more likely to live longer, faced challenges in future elder care for themselves.

The notion of having daughters as the caregivers is undergoing changes. With the one-child-per-family policy, parents in urban China were willing to invest in their only child's education, be it a boy or girl. Tsui and Rich (2002) revealed that parents held similar expectations and put forth a similar investment for boys and girls from only-child families. Therefore, there is no guarantee that girls would be available to take care of their aging parents, because the education opportunity granted to them today would allow them to have better job opportunities and to move away from their parents. This is consistent with Chen and Silverstein's (2000) study that revealed that the number of children and the gender of children were not significantly related to elder support, rather, having at least one proximate child increased the likelihood of receiving support.

As a result of changes at the family and state levels, researchers cautioned that the family may not remain the panacea for elder care in current China. In fact, the increasing number of older people in China necessitated involvement not only from the family level but also from the state level in elder care. Pei and Pillai (1999) concluded from their study that the following factors mattered at the family level: the number of living adult children; having sons in the family; and the amount of monetary support from adult children. Whereas, at the state level, the following variables were important: a pension; state financial subsidies; and the availability of medical services. Geographic locations mattered as well. In the same study, rural elderly received more financial aid from their adult children than their urban counterparts, while urban elderly received more pension income than rural elderly.

Meanwhile, young adults' attitudes towards elder care are changing. They express less commitment to elder care if there is conflict between employment and caregiving (Zhan, 2004a). Living in a three-generation household does not help improve the attitude either. Zhan (2004b) found that living arrangement impacted today's Chinese young adult's attitudes toward filial responsibility in a negative manner. Young adults from three-generation households were reported to be less committed to their sense of obligation to elder care.

Overall, intergenerational relationships in China are undergoing some changes. The traditional *patrilocal* family is gradually replaced by the *neolocal* family as a result of an increase in housing construction, a decrease in family size, people's attitudes towards co-residence, and job mobility among youths. Meanwhile, because of a lack of a national pension system for elderly at the moment, and the deeply-rooted traditional belief in filial piety (*xiao*), family remains the cornerstone of major support for young children and elders alike, though the role of the state is becoming more paramount and critical.

CONCLUSION

The socioeconomic developments of recent decades have put Chinese families at the crossroads of traditional and modern values. They have challenged many traditional practices, such as the change of residential patterns from patrilocal to neolocal. The last decade also witnessed an increased divorce rate in many parts of China. Chinese urban youths have adopted more liberal attitudes toward marriage and family. For instance, more youths today favor childfree marriages than before, and they are more accepting of cohabitation and premarital sex.

However, the inevitable changes in family dynamics will not eradicate family roles and functions. Chinese families remain the cornerstone of support. Though family size is getting smaller, researchers have coined a new term–networked families–to describe the fact that families maintain in close proximity toward each other and reciprocity is still a recurring theme. Marriage and family strengths identified by Chinese include harmony, affection, the ability to adapt to changes, equity in marriage, mutual trust, compatibility, and family support. The majority of couples report a satisfactory relationship. In terms of support, with the high female labor force participation rate, families are still responsible for child care and child socialization. Without a universal social security system, they are also responsible for elder care. Chinese culture, being collective in nature, still emphasizes that family needs take precedence over individual needs.

Meanwhile, challenges have surfaced as a result of economic growth and development. Major issues facing urban families include the division of household chores, only children's education and socialization, financial issues, and in-laws issues; whereas, issues facing less advantaged rural families are money and the division of household labor. There is also concern that the only-child generation may not have the wherewithal to take care of their older generation, and therefore, it is necessary for the development of state-level programs to implement support at the family level.

REFERENCES

Breault, K. D., & Kposowa, A. J. (1987). Explaining divorce in the United States: A study of 3,111 counties, 1980. *Journal of Marriage and the Family, 49*, 549-558.

Chen, X., & Silverstein, M. (2000). Intergenerational social support and the psychological well-being of older parents in China. *Research on Aging, 22*, 43-65.

Chinese Population Information and Research Center (1990). Beijing: Beijing Institute of Economics Press.

Chow, N. (1999). Diminishing filial piety and the changing role and status of the elders in Hong Kong. *International Journal of Aging, 1*, 67-77.

Chui, F. (1994). Married women's attitudes toward marriage and spouse selection. *Population and Economy, 3*, 30-37.

Ding, S. (1992). Trends in current Shanghai families. *Social Sciences, 3*, 42-46.

Dong, X. P. (2001). DINC families: Contemporary youths' attitudes towards childbirth. *Contemporary Youth Study, 6*, 39-42.

Du, J. M. (1992). The traditional family. In D. Liu (Ed.), *New perspectives on Chinese culture*. Beijing: ShangLing Publishing.

Falbo, T. (1982). The one-child family in the United States: Research issues and results. *Studies in Family Planning, 13*, 212-215.

Falbo, T., & Poston, D. L. (1993). The academic, personality, and physical outcomes of only children in China. *Child Development, 64*, 18-35.

Falbo, T., Poston, D. L., Ji, G., Jiao, S., Jing, Q., Wang, S., Gu, Q., Yin, H., & Liu, Y. (1989). Physical achievement and personality characteristics of Chinese children. *Journal of Biosocial Science, 21*, 483-495.

Fei, X. D., & Xie, S. (1995). *The Shanghai suburban women in recent decades.* Shanghai: Shanghai Academy of Social Sciences.

Fei, X. D. (1983). The issue of elder care amid the change of family structure. *Beijing University News, 3*, 6-15.

Fei, X. D. (1982). On changes of Chinese family structure. *Tienjing Social Sciences, 3*, 2-6.

Fong, V. (2005). *Only hope: Coming of age under China's one-child policy.* Stanford: CA: Stanford University.

Fu, H. (1988). On unhappy marriages. *Guangzhou Study, 8*, 42-45.

Glenn, N. D., & Supancic, M. (1984). The social and demographic correlates of divorce and separations in the United States: an update and reconsideration. *Journal of Marriage and the Family, 46*, 563-585.

Glenn, N. D., & Shelton, B. A. (1985). Regional difference in divorce in the United States. *Journal of Marriage and the Family, 47*, 641-652.

Gui, S. X. (1988). A report from mainland China: Status and needs of rural elderly in the suburbs of Shanghai. *Journal of Cross-Cultural Gerontology, 3*, 149-167.

Ho, D. Y. F. (1981). Traditional patterns of socialization in Chinese society. *Acta Psychologica Taiwanica, 23*, 81-95.

Hsu, J. (1985). The Chinese family: Relations, problems and therapy. In W. Tseng, & D. Y. H. Wu (Eds.), *Chinese culture and mental health* (pp. 95-112). Orlando, FL: Academic Press.

Hu, R., & Ye, N. (1991). *The nine-city survey on aging in 1988.* Tianjin: Tianjin Educational Press.

Jiao, S., Ji, G., & Jing, Q. (1986). Comparative study of behavioral qualities of only children and sibling children. *Child Development, 57*, 357-361.

Lei, J. (1994). *Changes in rural marriages in recent decades.* Beijing: Beijing University Publisher.

Liu, B. (1996). *Contemporary marriages in Shanghai.* Shanghai: Shanling Publisher.

Li, Y. H. (1989). Research on love. *Social Sciences Study, 12*, 33-42.

Li, Y. H. (Fall, 1996). The investigation and study of marriage quality in Beijing. *China Social Sciences Quarterly*, 63-66.

Li, G., & Xu, A. Q. (2004). *Youth's mate selection in the marriage market.* Shanghai: Shanghai Academy of Social Sciences.

Liu, C., Munakat, T., Fujiyama, H., & Usuba, M. (2003). Mental health and psycho-social factors with single child high school students in a city of China. *Nippon Koshu Eisei Zasshi, 50*, 15-26.

Lo, P., & Fen, Y. (2001). On college students' marriage attitudes: A gendered perspective. *Wuhan University Press, 5*, 631-635.

Lu, S. H. (1997). Data analysis of marriage attitudes and changes. *Social Sciences Study, 2*, 37-47.

Pan, S., & Jen, J. (2000). *Chinese college students' sexual attitudes and behaviors.* Beijing: Business Publisher.

Pan, S. (1995). *Sex in China.* Beijing: Guangmin Daily Publisher.

Pan, Y. K. (1987). *Marriages and families in urban China.* Shangdong: Shangdong People's Publisher.

Pan, Y. K., & Ruan, D. Q. (1995). Chinese urban family networks. *Zhejiang Academic Journal, 3,* 66-71.

Pan, Y. K., Roger, J., Bien, F., Bien, Y., Guan, Y., & Lu, H. L. (1997). Housing and family structure in urban China. *Social Sciences Study, 6,* 69-79.

Pei, X., & Pillai, V. (1999). Old age support in China: The role of the state and the family. *International Journal of Aging and Human Development, 49,* 197-212.

Polit, D. F., & Falbo, T. (1987). Only children and personality development: A quantitative review. *Journal of Marriage and Family, 49,* 309-325.

Poston, D. L., & Falbo, T. (1990). Academic performance and personality traits of Chinese children: "Onlies" versus others. *American Journal of Sociology, 96,* 433-451.

Research on Sex Education among College Students (2001). An investigation of Chinese college students' sexual behaviors in 2000. *Youth Study, 12,* 31-39.

Sa, J. (1995). *Contemporary Chinese women.* Beijing: Beijing University Press.

Shen, Chen & Gao (2000)

Shen, S., & Yang, S. H. (1995). *Family studies of urban China.* Beijing: Chinese Social Sciences Publisher.

State Statistics Bureau (1990). *Chinese statistics annually.* Beijing: Chinese Statistics Publisher.

State Statistics Bureau (1996). *Chinese statistics annually.* Beijing: Chinese Statistics Publisher.

State Statistics Bureau (2005). *Chinese statistics annually.* Beijing: Chinese Statistics Publisher.

Stinnett, N., & DeFrain, J. (1985). *Secrets of strong families.* Boston: Little, Brown.

Su, S., & Hu, Z. P. (2000). *Together and separate: Chinese youths' value perspective.* Shanghai: Shanghai Academy of Social Sciences.

The Second Investigation of Chinese Women's Social Status (2001). Data report on the second investigation of Chinese women's social status. *Women Studies, 5,* 4-12.

Treas, J., & Wang, W. (1993). Of deeds and contracts: Filial piety perceived in contemporary Shanghai. In V. Bengston, & A. Achenbaum (Eds.), *The changing contract across generations.* New York: Aldine de Gruyter.

Tsui, M., & Rich, L. (2002). The only child and educational opportunity for girls in urban China. *Gender and Society, 16,* 74-92.

Tseng, W., Juotai, T., Hsu, J., Jinghua, C., Lian, Y., & Kameoka, V. (1988). Family planning and child mental health in China: The Nanjing Survey. *America Journal of Psychiatry, 145,* 1396-1403.

Tu, E. J., Freeman, V. A., & Wolf, D. A. (1993). Kinship and family support in Taiwan, *Research on Aging, 15,* 465-86.

Unger, J. (1993). Urban families in the Eighties. In Davis, D., & Hareel, S. (Eds.), *Chinese families in the post-Mao era.* Berkeley: University of California Press.

Wan, C., Fan, C., Lin, G., & Jing, Q. (1994). Comparison of personality traits of only and sibling school children in Beijing. *The Journal of Genetic Psychology, 155,* 377-388.

Wang, W., Du, W., Liu, P., Liu, J., & Wang, Y. (2000). Five-factor personality measures in Chinese university students: Effects of one-child policy. *Psychiatry Research, 109,* 37-44.

164 STRONG FAMILIES AROUND THE WORLD

Wong, M. G. (1998). The Chinese American family. In C.H. Mindel, R. W. Habenstein, & R.Wright (Eds.), *Ethnic families in America*. NJ: Prentice Hall.

Xie, X., Xia, Y., & Zhou, Z. (2004). Strengths and stress in Chinese immigrant families: A qualitative study. *Great Plains Research, 14*, 203-218.

Xie, X., DeFrain, J., Meredith, W., & Combs, R. (1996). Family strengths as by university students and government employees in the People's Republic of China. *International Journal of Sociology of the Family, 26*, 7-27.

Xie, X., Xia, Y., & Zhou, Z. (2004). Strengths and stress in Chinese immigrant families: A qualitative study. *Great Plains Research, 14*, 203-218.

Xu, A. J. (1995). The situation and changes of urban family and social networks. *Shanghai Academy of Social Sciences Academic Journal, 2*, 77-85.

Xu, A. Q. (1997). *Love and marriage among Chinese at the turn of the century*. Beijing: Chinese Social Sciences Publisher.

Xu, A. Q. (2000). Standard of spouse selection: Reasons for changes in the past 50 years. *Social Sciences Study, 6*, 18-30.

Xu, A. Q., & Ye, W. L. (2002). *Research report on Chinese marriages*. Beijing: Chinese Social Sciences Publisher.

Xu, A. Q., & Ye, W. L. (1999). *Chinese marriages*. Beijing: Chinese Social Sciences Publisher.

Xu, A. Q. (1997). *Love and marriage among Chinese at the turn of the century*. Beijing: Chinese Social Sciences Publisher.

Xu, A. Q. (1995). Investigation of Chinese family structures: A sociological and demographic perspective. *Jenjian Study, 1*, 72-76.

Yang, B., Ollendick, T. H., Dong, Q., Xia, Y., & Lin, L. (1995). Only children and children with siblings in the People's Republic of China: Levels of fear, anxiety, and depression. *Child Development, 66*, 1301-1311.

Yang, H. (1996). The distributive norm of monetary support to older parents: A look at a township in China. *Journal of Marriage and the Family, 58*, 404-416.

Zhan, H. J. (2004a). Willingness and expectations: Intergenerational differences in attitudes toward filial responsibility in China. *Marriage & Family Review, 36*, 175-200.

Zhan, H. J. (2004b). Socialization or social structure: Investigating predictors of attitudes toward filial responsibility among Chinese urban youth from one and multiple-child families. *The International Journal of Aging and Human Development, 59*, 105-124.

Zhan, H. J., & Montgomery, R. J. V. (2003). Gender and elder care in China: The influence of filial piety and structural constraints. *Gender and Society, 17*, 209-220.

Zhang, Y., Kohnstamm, G. A., Cheung, P. C., & Lau, S. (2001). A new look at the old "little emperor": Developmental changes in the personality of only children in China. *Social Behavior and Personality, 29*, 725-732.

Zhang, M. J. (1994). Divorce in Jenjian province. *Jenjian Study, 6*, 67-71.

Zhang, Y. J. (2001). Support networks for urban and rural senior citizens. *Social Sciences Study, 4*, 11-21.

Zhen, N., Zhang, S., Li, M. H., Mao, G. Y., & Wang, J. (2000). *Sexuality among contemporary Chinese college students*. Tienjing: Tienjing University Press.

doi:10.1300/J002v41n01_08

Strengths and Challenges in the Indian Family

Nilufer P. Medora

SUMMARY. Beginning with a brief geographical, historical, cultural, and religious overview of India and her people, this article then presents a summary of family life in the contemporary Hindu family. The family strengths that are unique and based on deep-rooted religious, cultural, and social values that have been in existence and integral to the Hindu family for multiple generations are then outlined. The article also summarizes some challenges that families have to contend with in day-to-day living situations. doi:10.1300/J002v41n01_09 *[Article copies available for a fee from The Haworth Document Delivery Service: 1-800-HAWORTH. E-mail address: <docdelivery@haworthpress.com> Website: <http://www.HaworthPress.com> © 2007 by The Haworth Press, Inc. All rights reserved.]*

KEYWORDS. Culture, extended family network, family challenges, family strengths, Hinduism, Indian family

---

Nilufer P. Medora is Professor and Certified Family Life Educator, Department of Family and Consumer Sciences, California State University, 1250 Bellflower Boulevard, Long Beach, CA 90840 (E-mail: Medora@csulb.edu).

The author wants to extend her sincere appreciation and gratitude to Eri Enomoto and Monica Rottermann for their valuable assistance in researching the information and in the preparation of this article.

[Haworth co-indexing entry note]: "Strengths and Challenges in the Indian Family." Medora, Nilufer P. Co-published simultaneously in *Marriage & Family Review* (The Haworth Press, Inc.) Vol. 41, No. 1/2, 2007, pp. 165-193; and: *Strong Families Around the World: Strengths-Based Research and Perspectives* (ed: John DeFrain, and Sylvia M. Asay) The Haworth Press, Inc., 2007, pp. 165-193. Single or multiple copies of this article are available for a fee from The Haworth Document Delivery Service [1-800-HAWORTH, 9:00 a.m. - 5:00 p.m. (EST). E-mail address: docdelivery@haworthpress.com].

Available online at http://mfr.haworthpress.com
© 2007 by The Haworth Press, Inc. All rights reserved.
doi:10.1300/J002v41n01_09

INTRODUCTION

In this article, the concept of family strengths will be defined, and a brief geographical and historical overview of India will be presented. The pluralistic nature of the Indian people will be explained, and the concept of individualism versus collectivism also will be emphasized so that the reader has a better comprehension of why certain cultural phenomena are significant and different in the Indian family as compared to families in the West. Some of the family strengths in the Indian family will be outlined, and some of the challenges that Indian families encounter also will be discussed. Finally, in the conclusion section some of the rapid changes that are occurring in the metropolitan areas which are *modernizing* India and family life in India will be explained.

There are many different definitions of family strengths. For the purpose of this article, family strengths will be defined as qualities that promote satisfying and fulfilling relationships among family members, and contribute to the family's ability to deal effectively with stress and crises. Hill (1973) defined family strengths as, "those traits that facilitate the ability of the family to meet the needs of its members and the demands made upon it by systems outside the family unit" (p. 3). Family strengths are those relationship qualities that contribute to happiness, emotional health, and well-being of the family. Family strengths are unique qualities that keep a family together and give them positive emotional energy and a sense of connection (DeFrain & Stinnett, 2002). Since family life is significantly influenced by cultural norms, practices, and beliefs, it follows that family strengths are likely to be culturally based and tend to vary from culture to culture. Therefore, a family strength that is emphasized in one culture might not be looked upon that positively in another culture.

An Overview on India

The name Indian comes from *Indoi*, a Greek word that stands for the people who lived along and beyond the Indus River (Elst, 2001). India is situated in Southern Asia and is slightly more than one-third of the size of the U.S. It is the seventh largest country in the world comprising of 1,210,700 square miles (3,287,590 sq. km.). India has a population that recently exceeded the 1 billion mark, making it the second most populous country in the world after China. The majestic Himalayan Mountains that separate India from China form the highest range in the world. The southern half of India is a triangular peninsula that stretches southward to the Tropic of Cancer and extends into the Indian Ocean. The Arabian Sea lies to the west of India, and the Bay of Bengal to the east of India. The countries neighboring India are Pakistan to the northwest, China, Nepal and Bhuttan to the north, and Bangladesh and Myanmar (Burma) in the east. India is the second largest country in Asia after China, and the territory also includes the Andaman, Nicobar, and the Lakshadweep Islands.

India is one of the oldest countries in the world, with a *rich* culture, social, and religious history, and heritage. The Indus Valley civilization dates back at least 5,000 years, and was a complete, advanced, and prosperous civilization where excavations reveal a sophisticated urban culture. This civilization was followed, in around 1500 BC, by the arrival of the Aryans from Central Asia, who settled along the Gangetic Plains in northern India. The merger of the earlier local residents and the Aryans created a distinctive culture that continues to be part of ancient and modern Indian tradition. The ancient verses and hymns of the *Rig Veda* that originated at that time are still recited in Hindu temples and households in the 21st century (CIA World Factbook, 2005).

India has been influenced by many different cultures and rulers. The Greeks, Persians, Turks, Mughals, and the Europeans have each added to the uniqueness and diversity, and have collectively enhanced the religious beliefs, traditions, customs, spirituality, and culture of India.

India is ethnically a very diverse, pluralistic, and the largest secular society in the world. Because of the many invasions and conquests, people of India belong to diverse ethnic groups, have significant cultural variations, adhere to a variety of different beliefs and lifestyles, and speak many different languages that few continents, let alone countries possess. India's culture, like its people, is a diverse mosaic whose myriad elements have been born of its ancient history, its foreign influences, urbanization, modernization, and globalization. The culture and antiquity stems from the manner in which the *great* and *little* traditions intertwine, mingle, and are absorbed.

India is made up of 28 states and 7 union territories. There are 18 different languages and 300 dialects spoken by the Indian people. Although Hindi is the national language, most people living in metropolitan areas speak English. This is the language that is used for national, political, economic, and commercial communication. As a matter of fact, Das (2002) remarked that by 2010, "India will become the largest English speaking nation in the world, overtaking the United States" (p. 19). After being colonized by England for almost 300 years, India won its independence on August 15th, 1947. New Delhi in central India is the country's capital.

The weather in India is tropical except for the northern states bordering the Himalayas. These states experience cold winters and heavy snow. Most of the other states experience three seasons–the rainy season, the cold season, and the hot season.

India is the birthplace of four of the major world religions: Hinduism, Buddhism, Jainism, and Sikhism. In addition, India is home to the third largest number of Muslims in the world after Indonesia and Pakistan. Christianity also has ancient roots here because the apostle St. Thomas introduced it in this country about 2,000 years ago. The Zoroastrians fled Persia in the 8th Century to avoid persecution by the Arabs and they, too, have made India their home.

Hinduism is the dominant religion and is practiced by over 80 percent of Indians. Through the centuries, Indians have learned to co-exist with people from other faiths, religions, and beliefs. A majority (81%) of Indians are Hindu, 13.4% are Muslims, 8% are Buddhists, 4% are Jains, 2.3% are Christians, 2% are Sikhs, and about 0.6% are Bahai, Jews, and Zoroastrians (Census of India, 2001).

There is a tremendous difference in the way people live in urban and rural areas. A majority of Indians live in their native villages in rural areas. According to the Census of India 2001, 72% of residents lived in rural areas and 28% lived in urban communities. The larger metropolitan cities in India continue to have a large influx of residents from the rural areas. They migrate for better job opportunities, medical facilities, and more amenities in life for themselves and for their children. The level of literacy among Indians has increased but still more efforts are needed to reach residents living in the rural communities. As can be expected, urban residents are more literate (73%) as compared to residents living in rural areas (44%). In general, males have a higher literacy rate (76%) compared to females (54%) (CIA World Factbook, 2005).

During the last 3 decades, life expectancy has increased for Indian men and women. In 2001, life expectancy was 61.9 years for men and 63.1 years for women. The infant mortality rate declined from 151 per 1000 births in 1965 to 88 per 1000 births in 1995. In 2001, the infant mortality rate was 61.47 per 1000 births (Census of India, 2001, CIA World Factbook, 2005).

Since India is a secular and ethnically-diverse society, there are religious, regional, cultural, social, and educational variations in structural and functional patterns of family life. It is, therefore, difficult to generalize values, behaviors, practices, attitudes, norms, traditions, and beliefs about family life from one community to all Indian communities. Because the large majority of Indians are Hindus, this chapter will focus primarily on the strengths and challenges experienced by Hindu families.

Religion and Religious Beliefs

Religion and the observance of rituals pervade almost every aspect of life in India. Indians identify themselves with a particular religion but also affiliate themselves with a specific geographical region or state in India. Religion specifies the form of worship and guides their daily behavior, while the specific region generally identifies the language one speaks, the literature, art, music one prefers, the clothes one wears, and the food one eats (Medora, 2003).

The Hindus believe in a multitude of gods and goddesses that are an integral aspect of Hindu mythology. They believe that the three manifestations of God are: Brahma–the creator of the universe, Vishnu–the protector, and Shiva–the destroyer. Hinduism is a major world religion, has approximately 800 million followers, and is the third most widely followed religion in the world. It has influenced many other religions during its history that dates back to 1500 BC. Hindus believe that a person's life is actually the journey of the soul. A person goes through a series of reincarnations that eventually leads to salvation which is the freeing of the body from the cycle of rebirth (this occurs after reaching spiritual salvation). The Hindus follow the scriptures and teaching that are outlined in the Vedas (a collection of religious and philosophical poems and hymns), Upanishads, Bhagavad Gita, the Mahabharata, and Ramayana. These scriptures stress the importance of work, knowledge, sacrifice, respect, devotion, service to others and the renunciation of worldly and material goods in later life (Chekki, 1996; Damani & Damani, 2004; Mullatti, 1995).

Hinduism is not viewed as an organized religion like Western religions but rather a way of life (Almeida, 1996). According to the Hindu beliefs, a person goes through four stages in life that correspond with the human life cycle stages. The first stage is the Brahamacharya ashram (apprenticeship), the period of discipline and education. The second stage is the Grihastha ashram (household duties and time spent with family), the period dedicated to marriage, parenthood, family, and the establishment of a household. Vanaprastha ashram (gradual retreat) is the third stage, and is characterized by a gradual disengagement and loosening of social, emotional, and material bonds. Finally, the goal of the fourth and final stage, the Sanyasa ashram (renouncement), is to seek solitude, indulge in meditation, prepare for death, and strive for salvation and wisdom (Chekki, 1996; Jayapalan, 2001; Medora, 2003; Seymour, 1999).

Most Indians incorporate rituals and ceremonies in everyday life. Gods are not remote and distant figures, but part of every household and street corner. Worship can range from silent meditation, to the chanting of *slokas* (verses), to the staging of large, colorful processions on religious and festive days. Most Hindu households have a prayer platform or room that is considered the most sacred place in the home. Most devoted Hindus are vegetarians and they believe in non-violence. They pray, fast, sing hymns, light incense, adorn the platform with fresh flowers, and worship their deity at least once a day. As part of the religious activities, Hindus take regular morning baths, recite and chant certain mantras from the scriptures, prepare specific food items, offer flowers to deities, and worship ancestors (Medora, 2003).

The Caste System

In many ways, India is similar to other Eastern societies, yet it is different because of the ubiquitous caste system. The caste system has religious elements and is interwoven into the Hindu faith and daily livelihood. Caste is an exclusive phenomenon highly characteristic of Indian society (Katti & Saroja, 1989). Each caste is bound together by a common occupation, common customs, religious beliefs, and rituals. Each member of the Hindu community belongs to one of the many castes and sub-castes (Vohra, 1997). This rigid caste system has been in existence for more than 2,000 years.

The caste system is seen as a form of institutionalized inequality, an instrument of social assimilation, an extension of the joint family, and a system of graded relationships (Laungani, 2005). The caste system puts people into endogamous groups and different social strata. Persons belonging to the highest social caste are the Brahmins (the priestly class, the educated elite, and guardians of the Vedas–the religious Hindu books), followed by the Kshatriyas (the warriors and farmers), the Vaishyas (the merchants, traders, businessmen, merchants, and money lenders), and the Shudras (the servants, workers, and laborers) who are considered the lowest caste. Below the Shudras, are the people considered to be the *untouchables*. These individuals are regarded as impure and unholy (Medora, 2003; Seymour, 1999). They encounter prejudice and discrimination in everyday life.

For non-Indians, it is difficult to comprehend that the social position of each person is determined by heredity, not by personal accomplishments, qualifications, or spiritual deeds. Membership in a caste is decided by birth in a family which further dictates one's occupation, religious beliefs, alliances, and friendship circles (Mullatti, 1992). The caste system bonds people of the same caste together but at the same time the caste system splits society up into sub-groups in which people socialize, work, conduct business, live, and marry within their own caste. Although the caste system was officially abolished by the Indian government in 1950, it continues to play a crucial role and is unchangeable in most of its essential features (Mullatti, 1995). The caste hierarchy among Hindus still continues to be an influential force in everyday life situations, where discrimination continues to persist (Global Action for Dalits, 2005). Unfortunately, as remarked by Laungani (2005), "it is clear that one's caste origins are so strongly ingrained in the Hindu psyche that it is difficult for most to renounce such appalling practices" (p. 93).

The law of *karma* is an important feature of Hinduism and has been integral to the religion over the centuries. Most Hindus generally believe and have faith in the law of karma. Karma means that all human actions and behaviors have consequences. It is believed that each person receives the results of their actions in their current life or in future reincarnations. Jayapalan (2001) stressed that the very basis of the Hindu social organization is the doctrine of karma. It is one of the social values stressing individual responsibility for one's action. Karma is supposed to offer explanations for pain, suffering, misfortune, pleasure, happiness, luck, and success. Hindus tend to be fatalistic in their beliefs and also tend to be deterministic. This implies that one's present life is a consequence of and shaped by actions and deeds accomplished in one's past life. This belief allows Indians to accept misfortunes and successes that they experience in their life cycle. A belief in determinism allows Indians to accept things in life as they come. It often leads to a sense of fatalism, existential despair, and moral resignation, compounded by a state of inertia.

Laungani (2005) noted that, "A belief in the unending cycle of birth and rebirth, a belief that one's life does not end at death but leads to a new beginning, and that one's moral actions in one's present life or past life will lead to consequences in one's future life, may create in the

Hindu psyche a set of psychological protective mechanisms in the face of death. "A belief in an afterlife helps to reduce the terror of death and the fear of extinction" (p. 96).

Individualism versus Collectivism

Some cultures in the world tend to emphasize individualism, while others tend to emphasize collectivism. Triandis and his colleagues (Triandis, 1990; Triandis, Bontempo, Villareal, Asai, & Lucca, 1988) have examined the concepts of individualism and collectivism across various cultures and concluded that individualism is correlated with personal initiative, personal autonomy, self-reliance, and personal freedom. India is definitely a collectivistic society. Despite the fact that Indian society has passed through significant cultural, economic, and social transformations, the family continues to be the most important institution that has survived through the ages. India, like most other developing, and less industrialized, traditional, eastern societies, is a collectivistic society that stresses family unity, family togetherness, family integrity, and family cohesiveness. Collectivism is defined as, "a sense of harmony, interdependence, and concern for others" (Hui & Triandis, 1986, p. 244). More specifically, collectivism is reflected in a greater willingness to work together, emphasis on cooperation, joint decision-making, and most importantly putting the family views, needs, goals, and priorities above individual needs. Social norms and duty are defined and prescribed by cultural and familial needs. The beliefs a person has are those that are similar to and shared by family rather than those that distinguish the person from his or her family (Triandis, 1983; Verma, 1989).

Collectivistic cultures assume that any person through birth belongs to a family, an extended family, or a clan that takes interest in the person's well-being, and looks after their needs, interests, and goals. The individual in turn is expected to be faithful, loyal, grateful, and dedicated. Collectivism manifests itself in the beliefs and practices that reflect the individual's embeddedness in his or her family and the influence of the extended family on the individual in all aspects of life, including mate selection, marriage, choice of occupation, career, place of residence, and submission to head of the household (Medora, 2003; Verma, 1989).

FAMILY STRENGTHS AND SIGNIFICANCE
OF FAMILY IN INDIA

Structure and Family, Family Values, and Family Life

The family has always been the most salient institution and an integral part of Indian culture. It is the cornerstone and foundation of the Indian community and society. For centuries, the ideal and desirable family form in India has been the joint family or the extended family. For many lay people and professionals as well, the term *Indian family* is synonymous with the term *joint or extended family*. A joint family includes elderly parents and their children's families often living under one roof. It includes kinsmen of two or three generations, including uncles, aunts, nieces, nephews, and grandparents living together in the same household. The joint family is generally composed of a number of family units living in separate rooms of the same house. These members eat the food cooked at one hearth, share a common income, share common property, are related to one another through kinship ties, and worship the same idols. The family supports and takes care of the elderly, widows, never-married adults, and the disabled; assists during periods of unemployment; and provides security and a sense of support and togetherness (Chekki, 1996; Sethi, 1989). It has been stated that most Indians at some point in their lives have participated in joint family living (Nandan & Eames, 1980; Carson & Chowdhury, 2000).

The Indian family acts as a socializing agent and provides children and adolescents with varying life experiences within the confines and boundaries of the family. Srivastava (1995) remarked that the Indian family is a transmission belt for the diffusion of cultural standards to the next generation, a psychological agent of society, a shock absorber, and an institution of many enhancing and valuable qualities. Karve's definition of joint family has probably been the most popular and accepted definition. The traditional joint family has been defined as "a group of people who generally live under one roof, who eat food cooked in one kitchen, who hold property in common, participate in certain family worship, and are related to one another as some type of kindred" (Karve, 1965, p. 8).

Growing individualism and mobility have had adverse effects on the joint family system. In contemporary India, the joint family is the exception rather than the rule in most urban households (Shangle, 1995). Kumar and Reddy (2002) remarked that the joint family system is disappearing from society and giving way to the nuclearization of the family. Kapadia (1990) believed that this transformation has occurred primarily because of an emphasis on individualism and the changing status of women. Some researchers (Carson, & Chowdhury, 2000; Roopnarine & Hossain, 1992; Shangle, 1995) have commented that the Indian family is in transition and that the *modified extended family* has become the predominant family form in metropolitan India.

The *modified extended family* is defined as a social unit in which parents, children, and other relatives do not necessarily live under one roof. The family keeps in contact with relatives and kin and receives practical assistance with a variety of tasks, from child rearing, baby sitting, arranging marriages, to buying a house (Rao, 2002). This modified version of the family does not have the geographical proximity, shared hearth, or occupational involvement (Carson & Chowdhury, 2000; Laungani, 2005, Mullati, 1995; Nandan & Eames, 1980; Shangle, 1995) but continues to perform many of the previous functions. Frequent visits, financial assistance, aid and support in child care, household chores, and attendance and participation at life cycle events such as births, marriages, deaths, and festival celebrations continue to be obligations and are integral components of the modified extended family (Gupta, 1994).

The family still continues to be the fundamental unit of Indian society. Despite the social, cultural, educational, technological and global influences, and the adaptations to a pseudo-Western culture, a majority of families in India operate within the extended family network. It is believed that even in contemporary times, if conditions prevent members from residing together, it is incumbent on the members to participate in joyous and tragic family life cycle events. Indians go to great lengths to ensure that family and kin are all present and participate when a family member gets married, when children are born, in times of sickness and crises, when a family member dies, and when holy festivals and holidays are celebrated.

It is difficult and challenging to specifically identify family strengths in the Indian family when the cultural milieu and all of one's life events occur within the context of the family environment. The family adheres to well-defined rules, roles, and sentiments that bind family members together. The welfare of the family is always considered more important than that of the individual. Members share feelings of a *sense of duty, obligation*, and *solidarity* to their family of origin and they strive hard to uphold family dignity and status in society.

A high premium is placed on family unity and cohesiveness, which are necessary for family stability and survival. The Indian family emphasizes social bonds, facilitates group goals, encourages and promotes family solidarity by promoting sharing, cooperation, and interdependence. Any behavior that threatens this cooperative and familial spirit and unity is discouraged. This is achieved and maintained through a hierarchically organized authority structure in which individual needs, desires, goals, and aspirations are ignored to a great extent and group (family) goals are ranked above individual goals and given top priority (Misra, 1995). Sharing and mutual dependence occur at all stages of the family life cycle, thus contributing to and emphasizing a sense of safety and security in the family. In addition, elaborate family functions, life cycle events, and rituals, foster feelings of security and belongingness and convey the message that family bonds are immutable, dependable, and lifelong (Bharat, 1997; Carson & Chowdhury, 2000; Mullati, 1995). When Medora, Larson, and Dave (2000) surveyed 218 undergraduate students in Western India and asked them to identify their major family strengths in their family of origin, the three most popular answers were: (1) a sense of harmony, (2) a feeling of respect and support, and (3) a feeling of cooperation and dependability.

Indians take pride in the centrality of marriage and family life (Mullatti, 1995). As indicated earlier in this chapter, the extended family provides and satisfies the physical, psychological, and economic needs of all family members (Bharat, 1997; Misra, 1995; Mullatti, 1995; Sethi 1989). Children are given a special place in the family, community, and society, and interdependence, support, and nurturing across the generations are valued in the Indian family system (Madan, 1990). Living in an extended family is supposed to be particularly beneficial and advantageous for children, and it could also act as a buffer against the stresses associated with urban living (Chase-Lansdale, Brooks-Gunn, & Zansky, 1994). Hackett and Hackett (1993) stated that residing in an extended family promoted the psychological well-being in children and benefited the overall development of children. The family acted as a socializing agent with cultural values, traditions, norms, and mores that were transmitted to the next generation through family members and kin. The extended family members even today, continue to be the primary socializing agents of children. Family members and kin continue to regulate and maintain ties and connections even when geographical distances separate them (Shukla, 1994).

In the traditional joint family, individuals looked to the family for help and shelter in times of stress and crises. Members of the joint family took the responsibility to nurse the sick, the ailing, and the needy (Shangle, 1995). Even today, many of these elements are still present.

Single unmarried siblings, divorced and/or widowed mothers, elderly members, orphans, and children with special needs are generally cared for by other extended family members (Bhat & Dhruvarajan, 2001).

There is an unwritten and unspoken guarantee that all members in the family clan will be cared for. No member will be made to feel alone, or made to feel as though they were a burden to the family, community, and society. Some experts (Laungani, 2005; Medora, 2003) argue that in contemporary times, although things are gradually changing and some individuals are putting their needs and priorities above the welfare of the family because of the deep-rooted cultural values, that neighbors, friends, and kin are still willing to provide assistance in day-to-day living and in time of need.

The modified extended family structure provides a range of caretakers to look after children. They are likely to be influenced by a variety of role models and influences. Children are less prone to loneliness, rejection, and role confusion during childhood and adolescence because siblings and cousins serve as constant companions, playmates, and role models. As a matter of fact, in many affluent Indian homes, there are many faithful and long-term servants who provide assistance with child care and socialization from the time a child is very young (Laungani, 2005). Despite the fact that children are exposed to multiple care givers, the role played by the mother in rearing the children is of crucial importance, particularly the relationship that she has with her son(s)–a very close bond and relationship that develops between the two of them and is sustained for as long as they live.

Women's Changing Roles

During the last three to four decades, significant changes have taken place with regard to the position of women in Indian society. Women's employment is becoming increasingly more common and a financial necessity for the well-being of the family. The multiple options open to women have increased more than ever before. Married women today hold educational and occupational positions that are pursued outside the home. Child care centers and crèches (family day care centers) are some institutions that are trying to meet the growing needs of dual-career families. Even though these are available, employed women prefer not to use them. Instead they place trust and confidence in extended family members and kin to take care of their children in their absence (Rao, 2002).

Although gradual changes are occurring with regard to the status of women in Indian society, as a rule, women do not have the same rights and privileges as men do, especially in the decision-making process. Typically, in many homes, the mother-in-law dominates the daughters-in-law. The relationship between the daughter-in-law and the mother-in-law is often strained and distant. Researchers have commented that daughters-in-law are often downtrodden by their mothers-in-law (Amato, 1994; Derné 2000; Singh, 2005). This is a significant and ongoing challenge that many young women have to contend with and overcome. Many Indian women cope with this by drawing support from their sisters-in-law and other female relatives. Some researchers argued that the Indian women exert their power and influence indirectly and covertly. They often use passive techniques to exercise their voice and power in their home and get what they want (Sethi, 1989; Derné 2000). One observer argued that many Hindu women use sex as a means to have children, as a way to influence their husbands in their favor, and as an effective weapon to earn security and respect in their husband's home (Derné, 2000). Indian women still have a long way to go before the rules and regulations that oppress and suppress them will change. When Medora, Larson, and Dave (2000) asked college students in India to identify advantages of living in a joint family, the three most popular answers were: (1) a sense of unity and togetherness, (2) division of labor, (3) constant companionship and lack of loneliness.

CHALLENGES ENCOUNTERED BY THE INDIAN FAMILY

Preference for Male Children

A preference for male children in India is similar to that in other Asian cultures. There is a definite preference for sons over daughters. India has always been a patriarchal, patrilineal, and patrilocal society, and has a pronounced preference for sons (Arnold, 2001; Clark, 2000; Gupta, 1994; Philip & Bagchi, 1995). In a male-dominant society like India, girls do not get a place equal to that of boys. Traditional beliefs, customs, and religious practices reflect differences between the two sexes (Mukherjee, 2002). Sons are preferred to daughters because it is through male children that the inheritance, succession, and lineage continue. Essentially, it is believed that male children continue the family lineage, while female children are raised for the families of others; sons are raised to marry and bring women into the family, have children and broaden and extend the family line. Economically, sons are desired because they are expected to provide support for their parents in old age. Also, the Hindus believe that sons are needed to perform the funereal rites and light the funereal pyre, to ensure the safe passage of the soul.

The birth of a daughter is treated with ambivalent feelings and even some misgivings. Daughters are considered a burden to the family because when they get married, the parents of the Hindu bride are expected to give a dowry to the groom's family and after marriage, her responsibilities and obligations are transferred to her husband's family (Banerjee, 1998; Dube, 1997).

Since male children are desired more than female children, they are treated with more respect and given special privileges. Male children are raised to be independent, assertive, domineering, self-reliant, demanding, and as a rule more educated (Kumar & Rohatgi, 1987; Pothen, 1993). They are indulged, pampered, protected, and denied very little. A male child's wishes, desires, and wants take precedence over the needs of female children (Laungani, 2005). While male children are pampered and accorded many privileges, girls are often raised in a very strict and rigid way. Female children are socialized to be good housewives and fit into the family in which they marry. From an early age they are taught to be self-sacrificing, docile, accommodating, nurturing, altruistic, tolerant, religious, and value family above all (Kumar & Rohatgi, 1987; Mullati, 1995). Laungani (2005) remarked that Hindu women are raised to be obedient (initially to their parents and then to the husband and the husband's family), doing one's duty, praying, and ensuring the health and satisfying the needs of the husband and family. The Hindu woman is trained from an early age in the necessary culinary and other domestic skills so that neither she nor her parents are criticized. She is raised to be an ideal wife, a dutiful and faithful daughter-in-law, a compliant sister-in-law, a loving and caring mother, and an indulgent grandmother.

In modern India, there is some evidence that childlessness or bearing only daughters is grounds for abuse. The wife is abused by the husband or the mother-in-law, and sometimes desertion or divorce has also been documented (Gupta, 1991; Shivurkar, 1991; Unisa, 1999). Until recently, some couples were opting to do amniocenteses to determine the gender of the child and if the embryo was not male, the couples aborted the child. Since coming to the attention of the Indian government, conducting amniocenteses to determine the gender of the child has been outlawed and the doctors found guilty have been prosecuted.

Belief in Karma

The belief in the law of *karma* and the belief that one should be passive and accepting of difficulties in life in order to be rewarded in the next life are contrary to beliefs in most other cultures. This belief often encourages individuals to be passive and acceptant of problems. Family life cycle transitions can sometimes be stressful and problematic when they collide with values of passivity, obedience, and sacrifice. The belief that one should be accepting of misfortunes and *taqdeer* (difficulties) that befall us in order to be rewarded in the next life is contrary to the Western beliefs and notions that each person *makes* his or her own destiny and that we are responsible for our own actions. Moreover, Hindus have always believed in and incorporated astrology in their everyday life. They do this, because they believe that a person's destiny is determined by the alignment of the stars, sun, planet, and earth at the time a person is born. Consequently, they believe that their lives are predestined, their faith is predetermined, and thus they are helpless and powerless as far as they are concerned because they must succumb to the celestial factors in the universe. When young people grow up with this belief and ideology, they lack the initiative to take control of their lives, and do not make a conscious effort or take an active role in rectifying situations when crises occur in their life.

Sex and Sexuality Issues

Sex and sexuality are topics that are not openly discussed in the Indian society. Sexuality during adolescence is not experienced as a liberating force that allows them to begin establishing a sense of their own identity and independence outside of family relationships. Instead, reaching adolescence is associated with even more responsibilities, obligations and greater family enmeshments. Almeida (1996) remarked that free expression of sexuality is viewed as incongruent with spirituality. Boys are not permitted to masturbate but rather they are encouraged to channel their energies into more constructive endeavors like focusing on their studies and helping out with the housework. Almeida also commented that girls are seen as requiring more protection after they begin menstruating. Consequently, more restrictions are placed on them, they are told to dress modestly, more curfews are imposed, and they are told to have minimal interactions with the opposite sex. Sexuality is not acknowledged, sex education is not readily available, and premarital sex is severely frowned upon (Segal, 1998).

There is much secrecy attached to sex and sexuality and it is a taboo to discuss these topics in the home environment. This is particularly challenging because adolescents are bombarded with sexual innuendos through the media, billboards, the Internet, and peer relationships. Indian parents are not comfortable discussing sex and sexuality issues with their children because they feel inept and uncomfortable doing so. When the parents were teenagers, their parents never discussed these topics with them so why should they do so with their children? Consequently, adolescents are forced to rely on peers and books to get this information.

Jejeebhoy (1996) remarked that approximately 20 to 30% of all males and 10% of females are sexually active during adolescence. Since sexual topics are not discussed, sexual awareness is largely superficial. A double standard exists whereby unmarried males are far more likely than females to be sexually active; males are also more likely to approve of premarital sexual relations for themselves and are more likely to have opportunities to engage in premarital sexual activity.

Many Indian youth desire to emulate Western youth in many aspects of life. Literature suggests that adolescents generally conform to their peer culture in lieu of parental norms (Segal, 1998). These issues, along with a lack of emphasis on individualism/self-reliance and a lack of involvement/consultation on the part of parents, are major challenges, and points of contention and conflict between Indian parents and their children. When Medora, Larson, and Dave (2000) asked 218 undergraduate students to identify the changes that they desired in their family, the youth stated that they wanted their parents to be more broad-minded, consultative, and desired more freedom and fewer restrictions in their day-to-day living.

Almeida (1996) argued that the life cycle stage of *adolescence* and the *launching years* do not exist in the Indian culture. She stated that a culture that prescribes marriage, childbearing, and economic responsibilities to the extended family leaves little or no room for self-exploration and self-determination. Young adults are less likely to acquire independence, leave home, find their own residence, experiment in finding a dating partner, or for that matter explore their sexual orientation, or decide on a choice of career. It is also important to mention that many Indian youth probably experience challenges including identity confusion if they are gay or lesbian, because in the Indian culture homosexuality is not culturally sanctioned or accepted. Gay youth probably cope with their sexual orientation by not admitting and accepting their homosexuality, by not discussing this issue with family members and kin. For the sake of social appearances, they consent to getting married, and having children. They do this, so that the family is not shamed and ostracized in the community.

Need for Privacy

In most Western societies, having *one's own space* and the need for privacy are highly valued. Living as people do, in an extended Indian family network, there are no clear defining boundaries between *mine* and *ours*. In the rural areas and in metropolitan areas as well, most families live in confined and restricted areas. Most day-to-day activities are shared and done together as the need for psychological and physical space and privacy is not as important to Indians (Laungani, 2005). Thus, the notion of privacy, the need to desire it, to value it, and the thought of intruding on another person's privacy is not understood by most Indian people (Laungani, 2005). Larson and Medora (1992) compared the preferences for privacy between Americans and Indians and concluded that Indians had a lower need for privacy than Americans.

The Significance of Marriage and Marital Customs

Hindus believe that marriage is a sacred and sacramental union. Hence, Hindus view marriage as an indispensable part of life:

> Fulfillment of *dharma* (religious duties) and *praja'* (progeny) has traditionally been the primary functions of marriage. Since marriage in a Hindu society is generally desired for the fulfillment of religious duties and procreation, mutual conjugal fidelity, affection, and respect have been highly emphasized and earnestly solicited. Marriages, as a result, have predominately been monogamous in nature. (Shangle, 1995, p. 426)

Marriages in India even today are arranged by the parents and extended family members. Marriage in the Hindu society is considered to be a union and an alliance between two families and not two individuals (Mullatti, 1995). In arranging a marriage, emphasis is placed on the compatibility and fit of the two families. Arranged marriages tend to be endogamous, and the parents select mates from their own caste and sub-caste, and from families which have higher or equal economic, political, social, and cultural clout and standing. In many families, parents consult an astrologer before the marriage is finalized. The astrologer matches the bride and groom's horoscopes and verifies compatibility to ensure a long and happy married life, good health, economic success, and children. In India, love and romance are not considered to be prerequisites to getting married, nor is courtship a necessary prelude for testing the relationship.

Even in contemporary times, the above-mentioned practices continue to exist. The use of matrimonial advertisements is increasing and is an integral part of the mate-selection process (Mullatti, 1995). Advertisements like the ones that appear below are placed in major national and international newspapers that are likely to attract wide readership. If many people apply, screening is done on the basis of photographs. During contemporary times, after the photographs are sent and a few potential persons appear to fit the specified criteria, the men and women correspond via the Internet to learn more about each other. They exchange information about priorities, goals, expectations, etc., before they actually meet (Medora, 2003). Many Hindus still regard marriage as a social, religious, and cultural duty and obligation. Marriage is not viewed as a means of attaining personal happiness, or a means of sharing one's life with a person one loves. Instead, family unity, family togetherness, and common family goals are of primary importance, and personal considerations are only secondary. It is not considered important whether the groom and bride share common goals or have, similar interests, so long as the family line and family traditions can be maintained (Medora, 2003).

GROOMS WANTED

SEEKING TALL AND PROFESSIONALLY WELL-POSITIONED partner for an attractive South Indian girl who is slim, well-educated and is 5 feet 4 inches in height. She has completed her BCOM, MCOM and is 25 years old. She is professionally employed and comes from a respectable family in Kerala. Girl has east/west values, is good natured and well-trained in home skills and entertainment. Hobbies include music, dance, cooking, and reading. Correspond with photo and bio-data to <matesearch 39@hotmail.com>.

BRIDES WANTED

ALLIANCE INVITED from a good looking professional Indian girl with eastern values for handsome Jat-Sikh male, 31, 6'1" clean shaven, software engineer, salary six figures, from well settled, well connected, good family and green card holder. Correspond with bio-data and returnable photograph to P.O. Box A -7144 c/o India-West or correspond with uncle, Mr. Ashok Singh <asingh59@yahoo.com>.

One of the most salient challenges that Indian families are experiencing today is that many modern youth want to break away from the custom of having their marriages arranged. They want to select their own partner for life. The custom and tradition of arranged marriages has caused acute tensions and turmoil in Hindu families between parents and children. Young Indian men and women want more of a say in whom they marry, when they marry, and the type of family in which they marry. Many youth are dating without their parents' knowledge and behind their backs. Others have fallen in love with, and are in a committed long-term relationship with a person of the opposite sex who belongs to another religion, caste, or sub-caste. These young adults conceal their dating relationship from their parents because they are afraid that if the parents find out, their sense of trust will be betrayed. They are apprehensive that the parents will proceed to arrange a marriage for them which they will not be able to refuse because of family pressure, tradition, and family honor. Most importantly, they will probably never see the person that they are in love with again. This is illustrated in an interview with Bina, a 23-year Gujarati university student majoring in child development and family studies at a major university in Western India. She had been dating in committed relationship with another Gujarati boy from a different sub-caste. She was hoping to tell her parents about her desire to marry this man after she completed her degree. Bina stated:

> One day my boyfriend and I were leaving a theatre after watching a movie. We were seen together by an uncle who is a distant relative. I did not know that my uncle had seen us. Within the same week, my father came to the dormitory and summoned me home saying that my mother was not keeping too well and needed my assistance at home. Unsuspectingly, I immediately left with him. Once I went home, I realized that my father had conjured up a story to get me to go home. My parents confronted me and told me

that they had been informed that I had been seen with a man. First, I denied the allegation, but then I confessed that I was in love with Naveen and would like to marry him. They were absolutely shocked and flabbergasted and forbade me to ever see Naveen again or for that matter, they informed me that since I had dishonored the family, I would not be allowed to return to the university to complete my education. I begged with them but they would not budge. They even refused to speak to me.

Within the next one month, they proceeded to arrange my marriage to another Gujarati man, Vinod, who was from the same sub-caste. I pleaded with them and told them that I could not marry a man I did not know and did not love. My mother told me that she did not even see my father before she married him and she was happy and I, too, will be if I gave the marriage a chance. They and other family members put so much pressure on me and forced me to marry Vinod. I gave in to them and married Vinod. (B. Patel, personal communication, January 15, 2005)

Studies have been conducted to determine the success or failure of arranged marriages. Vijaylaxmi, Saroja, and Katarki (1992) found that couples in love marriages were more educated, had higher incomes, and had more prestigious jobs than couples in arranged marriages. Interestingly, these researchers also found that marriages lasted for a longer duration if the couples had arranged marriages. Marital satisfaction was higher for couples that had arranged marriages than it was for those in a love marriage (Gupta & Singh, 1982; Shangle, 1995). Also, for couples in love marriages, marital satisfaction tended to decrease with the duration of marriage, while it increased over time for those in arranged marriages.

Marriage Dissolution and Divorce

Marriage is viewed as a sacred and religious event in which the couple is expected to stay together, "till death do them part." Divorce was not even a remote possibility or even thought of until recent times. In India, there is a cultural, religious, and social stigma associated with divorce. Familial and community disapproval is stronger for divorced women than it is for divorced men (Lessinger, 2002). In many instances, the wife is economically and socially dependent on her husband, his family members, and their network of relations. She is not in a position to even contest a divorce, let alone take any steps in achieving it (Laungani,

2005). A woman suffers serious consequences, e.g., homelessness, the threat of poverty, probable loss of custody of her children, loss of friends, and the danger of being referred to as a loose woman or a tart. As a matter of fact, a large proportion of divorced women report problems with sexual harassment in their work environment and on the social scene (Amato, 1994; Pothen, 1989). The pressures to stay married are so immense that many women, even under the most adverse conditions (maltreatment, emotional, verbal, and physical abuse, lack of independence, and subjugation at home), believe that it is their moral duty to stay with their husband and elect to stay within the confines of a tyrannical family as a silent sufferer rather than break away (Laungani, 2005). It is important to point out that if a woman gets divorced regardless of whether she or her husband initiated the divorce, it reflects poorly on her, her parents, and her extended family. People are likely to gossip and point fingers at her family and imply that she was too pampered, spoiled, and was not taught to be a giving, tolerant, and accommodating wife.

Meera is a 32-year-old divorced woman who was raised in an urban area in an upper-class family. She had an arranged marriage to an Ashok who was a medical doctor with a thriving medical practice. She had been married to him for eight years and had two children with him. Ashok was an alcoholic and a womanizer. After being unhappy and facing humiliation for eight years, Meera decided to divorce him. In her words:

> When I told my parents that I had decided to leave Ashok, they were both devastated. My mother started crying and said that I was a fool to leave him. She went on to say that after all the material comforts that he provided, how could I do this to him? She accused me and said that if I had been a good wife, he would not be drinking. Men sometimes fool around, but they always come back to their wife and that I needed to be more patient and understanding. If I divorced him, there would be no place for me and my children in their home. They would not provide for me financially either. I would have to make it on my own. My place was with Ashok, and it was up to me to make things work . . . I should try harder. (M. Maolankar, personal communication, January 10, 2005)

Stories like Meera's are common throughout India. Although divorce today is more acceptable than it was a decade ago, divorced women continue to encounter numerous challenges.

The Dowry System

The dowry system has been in existence in India for centuries. It was initially instituted to provide for the physical security of a girl in the event of unexpected circumstances, an emergency, or in case of adversity after marriage. The dowry is given by the girl's parents to their daughter (consequently to the groom's father). The parents generally gave whatever they could financially and materially.

In recent times, this custom has deteriorated to a point whereby some grooms and their families have become very materialistic and greedy. They make tremendous demands, which if not met, result in *dowry deaths*–burning brides alive if the dowry is insufficient, so that the boy can remarry another girl for a higher or better dowry (Mullatti, 1995). The more assets a man has (e.g., good looks, education, political and social status, job prospects, income, potential to settle abroad), the more the expectation for the dowry increases. This expectation limits the pool of potential partners for girls whose parents are unable to pay the dowry. Also, if the daughters are highly educated, it is difficult for the parents to arrange a marriage because as a rule, girls are expected to have more educated husbands (Seymour, 1999).

The Status of Singles

Another challenge that Indians have to contend with is to deal with singlehood. Since the Hindu culture strongly endorses marriage *vivaha*, an individual who remains single and never marries does feel out of place socially and culturally. Traditionally, single family members were supposed to be the responsibility of the extended family. With the significant changes occurring in Indian society, many singles continue to experience a feeling of rejection, and not being *good* enough to be able to find a suitable partner. They experience a sense of not belonging. Remaining single and *not marrying* is considered more acceptable for men than it is for women. When a woman is not married, the community members generally assume that she is difficult to get along with, something is wrong with her, she is uncompromising, and therefore she is single. The thought of her not wanting to marry is absent from people's minds. Single women are not allowed to participate in religious activities and other family life cycle occasions like marriage celebrations, because their presence is considered unlucky, unholy, and inauspicious. Single women rarely live on their own. Most of the time, they end up living in the extended family household or with siblings. Some families might resent this and consider it to be a burden to them. Since there are relatively few single men and women in India, they receive minimal social support and hence many of them experience loneliness and alienation (Medora, 2003).

Coping with Mental Illness

One of the most significant challenges that Indian families encounter is dealing with a family member that has a mental or emotional illness. Indian families face a wide variety of every day problems, including the stresses and strains of rearing children, conflicts with in-laws, difficulties associated with chronic illness, and mental illness encountered by children and family members. In India, the attitude towards mental health is complex, with tradition and modernity thriving side-by-side in a confusing but intimate relationship (Sharma & Chadd, 1990). Many individuals with mental and/or emotional problems go to faith healers, herbal doctors, shamans, and gurus more often than they do to trained professionals. Training of mental health professionals and the acceptance of mental and emotional disorders are minimal and lacking, despite existing national policy guidelines (Carson & Chowdhury, 2000).

Laungani (2005) commented that if a child or family member suffers from a mental disorder, attempts are made to conceal this dysfunction from relatives, friends, and community members because of the fear of social stigma and ostracism befalling the entire family. She also remarked that the fear of social stigma related to mental disorders often leads to secrecy.

> Many parents have been known to keep a severely disturbed member of the family "in hiding," concealed from the outside world, confined to a room. In such situations, the family will go to great lengths to conceal a problem to prevent it being discovered and leading to social censure, which may have an adverse effect on the marital prospects of the girls in the family. (Laungani, 2005, p. 95)

The extended family network is likely to be a breeding ground for problems relating to mental health because of the constant tension and friction between the mother-in-law and the daughter-in-laws. Sometimes there are intrusions of the extended family members that fuel marital tension and conflict between the husband and wife (Chowdhury & Barnal, 1999; Das, 1999; Mullatti, 1995).

Sonuga-Barke and Mistry (2005) investigated mental health problems among grandmothers, mothers, and the children residing in a nuclear
versus extended family. They found that children and grandmothers
tended to be better adjusted in the extended family than in the nuclear
family. In contrast, the mothers in nuclear families were more adjusted
and had better mental health. The researchers concluded that there appears to be a link between residing in an extended family and higher
incidence of mental distress, especially for women.

The Plight of the Elderly

A definite challenge in modern India is the plight of the elderly. In
traditional Indian society, family and kin were guaranteed to look after
all the needs of elderly family members. Family values and traditions
were so strong and ingrained in them that they provided security and care
to all its members, especially elderly members. At that time, with their
ascribed status, elderly persons had more authority, wisdom, maturity,
prestige, and power. Social security in all aspects of life was assured to
the elderly under the institution of the joint family system. In contemporary times, dynamic changes have replaced traditional family values and
priorities. The newly *achieved* status of the young has generally replaced
the *ascribed* status of the elderly. The market economy has improved
significantly and monetary value has taken over the traditional familial
values of caring for elderly family members (Kumar & Reddy, 2001).

CONCLUSION

In conclusion, it would be fallacious to assume that a diverse and traditional society such as India has remained unchanged over time. During the past few decades, dynamic and significant changes have altered
family functioning, cultural values, priorities, mores, and parenting
practices in Indian families. These changes have occurred as a result of
industrialization, urbanization, globalization, a revolution in information
technology, mobility, women's changing roles, foreign investments, and
Western influences. The joint family system, which prevailed for centuries, is disappearing. The number of nuclear families has been increasing.
Family life, especially in urban India is undergoing a transformation.
Western influences are impinging on and altering some of the traditional ways of life, values, beliefs, and familial obligations. One of the

consequences of these changes includes the disintegration of the joint family and the ushering in of the modified extended family.

Indian society has demonstrated a strength and tenacity to withstand and survive foreign invasions through the centuries. It is, therefore, debatable if technology and globalization can completely transform the ancient values and intrinsic beliefs of the Indian culture and society. The Indian family is different from families in the West. The family is unique, resilient, and has many strengths but living in such a closed, hierarchical, and structured society can also be quite challenging and stifling. In this chapter, some of these strengths and challenges have been examined.

India has been, is, and will probably always be a collectivistic society in which the family's needs, interests, and goals will supersede those of the individual. Indian families are strong, defined, resilient, and enduring (see Box 1).

BOX 1. Important Family Strengths of the Hindu Family

Some of the salient family strengths of Hindu families include the following characteristics:

- The welfare of the family is considered to be far more important than that of the individual.
- Cooperation and sharing are strongly encouraged values and competition and individual achievement are discouraged qualities.
- The joint/extended family provides for the physical, psychological, and economic needs of all family members, i.e., the elderly, unemployed, sick, disabled, widowed, and single siblings.
- The joint/extended family provides "built in" playmates for all the children in the family.
- The structure of the joint/extended family ensures that there are "built-in" baby sitters and tutors for children at all times.
- Due to the structure of the joint family system and because so many members live in close physical proximity, coping with crises is sometimes easier because an empathetic listener is generally available. Some family dysfunctions i.e. juvenile delinquency, teen-age pregnancy, substance abuse, child abuse and spouse abuse are less likely to occur because children and adolescents, and adults are closely monitored.
- There is built-in family support for all members at all times including young couples who are starting married life.
- The Hindu religion imparts strong personal discipline on the individual, and stresses a high regard for knowledge and wisdom. Education and literacy are highly regarded and valued among the middle and upper class families and are gaining importance and recognition among lower class families because they realize that education is their way out of poverty and unemployment.
- The Indian culture believes that the elderly are reservoirs of knowledge and wisdom. Because of this belief, the elderly are respected, revered, and obeyed.
- There is a role hierarchy that exists for gender and age so roles are clearly defined and delineated. With so many family members living under one roof, there is a definite division of labor.
- The Hindu and Jain religions stress a respect and love for all organic life. Thus, most Hindus believe in non-violence; they believe that human and animal life is sacred and most of them are vegetarians.
- During times of festivities and celebrations or during times of illness and bereavement, there is support that is readily available from the extended family kin and close relatives.

REFERENCES

Almeida, R. (1996). Hindu, Christian and Muslim families. In M. McGoldrick & J. Giordane (Eds.), *Ethnicity and family therapy* (pp. 395-423). New York: Guilford.

Amato, P. (1994). The impact of divorce on men and women in India and the United States. *Journal of Comparative Family Studies, 25,* 208-221.

Arnold, F. (2001). Son preference in South Asia. In Z. A. Sathar & J. F. Phillips (Eds.), *Fertility transition in South Asia* (pp. 281-299). Oxford, UK: Oxford University Press.

Banerjee, N. (1998). Household dynamics and women in a changing economy. In M. Krishnaraj, R. M. Sudarshan, & A. Shariff (Eds.), *Gender, population, and development* (pp. 245-263). New Delhi, India: Oxford University Press.

Bharat, S. (1997). Family socialization of the Indian child. *Trends in Social Science research, 4*(1), 201-216.

Bhat, A. K., & Dhruvarajan, R. (2001). Ageing in India: Drifting intergenerational relations, challenges and options. *Aging and Society, 21,* 621-640.

Carson, D. K. & Chowdhury, A. (2000). Family therapy in India: A new profession in an ancient land. *Contemporary Family Therapy, 22*(4), 387-406.

Census of India. (2001). *The Religion.* Retrieved February 15, 2005, from http://www.censusindia.net/religiondata/presentation_on_religion.pdf.

Chase-Lansdale, P.L., Brooks-Gunn, J., & Zamsky, E.S. (1994). Young African-American multigenerational families in poverty: Quality of mothering and grand-mothering. *Child Development, 65,* 373-393.

Chekki, D. A. (1996). Family values and family change. *Journal of Comparative Family Studies, 27,* 409-413.

Chowdhury, A., & Baral, S. (1999). A study of vulnerable families. In J. K. Baral & A. Chowdhury (Eds.), *Family in transition: Power and development* (pp.131-138). New Delhi: Northern Book Center.

CIA World Factbook. (2005). *The World Factbook–India.* Retrieved February 14, 2005, from http://www.cia.gov/cia/publications/factbook/geos/in.html

Clark, S. (2000). Son preference and sex composition of children: Evidence from India. *Demography, 37,* 95-108.

Damani, Gaurang D. & Damani, Jayshree G. (2004). *Hinduism.* Retrieved February, 28, 2005, from http://www.diehardindian.com/demogrph/moredemo/hindu.htm

Das, G. (2002). The *elephant paradigm: India wrestles with change.* New Delhi: Penguin Books.

Das, R. C. (1999). Marriage in transition: A bio-social approach. In J. K. Baral & A. Chowdhury (Eds.), *Family in transition: Power and development* (pp. 139-147). New Delhi: Northern Book Center.

DeFrain, J., & Stinnett, N. (2002). Family strengths. In J. J. Ponzetti et al. (Eds.), *International encyclopedia of marriage and family* (2nd ed.) (pp. 637-642). New York: Macmillan Reference Group.

Derné, S. (2000). Culture, family structure, and psyche in Hindu India: The "fit" and the "inconsistencies." *International Journal of Group Tensions, 29,* 323-348.

Derné, S. (1994). Violating the Hindu norm of husband-wife avoidance. *Journal of Comparative Family Studies, 25,* 249-267.

Dube, L. (1997). *Women and kinship: Comparative perspectives on gender in South and South-East Asia.* New York: United Nations University Press.

Elst, K. (2001). *Who is a Hindu? Hindu revivalist views of Animism, Buddhism, Sikhism, and other offshoots of Hinduism, 2.* Retrieved February 15, 2005, from http://voi.org/books/wiah/ch2.htm

Global Action for Dalits. (2005). *India caste system discriminates.* Retrieved December 8, 2005, from http://www.imadr.org/project/dalit/wcar1.html

Gupta, B. (1994). Modernity and the Hindu joint family system: A problematic interaction. *International Journal on World Peace,* 11, 37-60.

Gupta, K. (1991). Research on marital disruption in India: Some theoretical formulations. In M. Desai (Ed.), *Research on families with problems in India, 2* (pp. 374-382). Bombay, India: Tata Institute of Social Sciences.

Gupta, U., & Singh, P. (1982). An exploratory study of love and liking and type of marriages. *Indian Journal of Applied Psychology, 19,* 92-97.

Hackett, L. & Hackett, R. (1993). Parental ideas of normal and deviant child behavior: A comparison of two ethnic groups. *British Journal of Psychiatry, 32,* 851-856.

Hill, R. (1973). *Strengths of black families.* New York: National Urban League.

Hui, C. H., & Triandis, H. C. (1986). Individualism-Collectivism: A study of cross-cultural researchers. *Journal of Cross-Cultural Psychology, 17,* 222-248.

Jayapalan, N. (2001). *Indian society and social institutions. Volume 1.* New Delhi: Atlantic Publishers and Distributors.

Jejeebhoy, S. J. (1996). *Adolescent sexual and reproductive behavior: A review of the evidence from India.* Washington, DC: International Center for Research on Women.

Kapadia, K. (1990). *Marriage and family life in India.* Calcutta: Oxford University Press.

Katti, M., & Saroja, K. (1989). Parents' opinion towards intercaste marriage and their preference in mate selection for their children. *Indian Journal of Behavior, 13,* 28-34.

Karve, I. (1965). *Kinship organization in India.* Bombay: Asia Publishing House.

Kumar, P., & Rohatgi, K. (1987). Value patterns as related with high and low adjustment in marriage. *Indian Journal of Current Psychological Research, 2,* 98-102.

Kumar, S. V., & Reddy, V. N. (2002). Social security for the elderly in India: Present status and future challenges. In P. S. Reddy & V. Gangadhar (Eds.), *Indian society: Continuity, change and development* (pp. 256-269). New Delhi: Commonwealth Publishers.

Larson, J. H., & Medora, N. P. (1992). Privacy preferences: A cross-cultural comparison of Americans and Asian-Indians. *International Journal of Sociology of the Family, 22,* 55-66.

Laungani, P. (2005). Families in global perspective. In J. L. Roopnarine & U. P. Gielen (Eds.), *Changing patterns of family life in India* (pp. 85-103). Boston, MA: Pearson Education, Inc.

Lessinger, J. (2002). Asian Indian marriage: Arranged, semi-arranged, or based on love? In N. V. Benokraitis (Ed.), Contemporary ethnic families in the United States: Characteristics, variations, and dynamics (pp. 101-104). Englewood Cliffs, NJ: Prentice Hall.

Madan, G. R. (1990). *Social welfare and security.* New Delhi: Vivek Prakashan.

Medora, N. P. (2003). India. In J. J. Ponzetti, Jr (Ed.), *International Encyclopedia of Marriage and Family* (pp. 876-883). New York: Macmillan Reference USA.

Medora, N. P., Larson, J. H., & Dave, P. B. (2000). Attitudes of East-Indian college students toward family strengths. *Journal of Comparative Family Studies, 31*, 407-425.

Misra, G. (1995). Reflection on continuity and change in the Indian family system. *Trends in Social Science Research, 2*, 27-30.

Mukherjee B. M. (2002). Intergeneration integration: A possible remedy and prospect for the girl child. In P. S. Reddy & V. Gangadhar (Eds.), *Indian Society: Continuity, change and development* (pp. 112-115). New Delhi: Commonwealth Publishers.

Mullatti, L. (1992). Changing profile of the Indian family. In UNESCO (Ed.), *The changing family in Asia: Bangladesh, India, Japan, Philippines, and Thailand.* Bangkok: Principal Regional Office for Asia and the Pacific.

Mullatti, L. (1995). Families in India: Beliefs and realities. *Journal of Comparative Family Studies, 26*, 11-25.

Nandan, Y., & Eames, E. (1980). Arranging a marriage in India. In J. K. Norton (Ed.), *India and South Asia* (pp. 113-116). Guilford, Connecticut: Brown & Benchmark Publishers.

Phillip, M., & Bagchi, K. S. (1995). The *endangered half.* New Delhi: Upalabdhi, Trust for Development Initiatives.

Pothen, S. (1989). Divorce in Hindu society. *Journal of Comparative Family Studies, 20*, 377-391.

Rao, M. H. (2002). Employed women and the extended family. In P. S. Reddy & V. Gangadhar (Eds.), *Indian society: Continuity, change and development* (pp. 116-122). New Delhi: Commonwealth Publishers.

Roopnarine, J. L., & Hossain, Z. (1992). Parent-child interactions in urban Indian families: Are they changing? In J. L. Roopnarine & D. B. Carter (Eds.), *Parent-child socialization in diverse cultures* (pp. 1-16). Norwood, NJ: Ablex.

Segal, U. A. (1998). The Asian-Indian family. In C.H. Mindel, R. W. Habenstein, & R. Wright (Eds.), *Ethnic families in America: Patterns and variations.* New Jersey: Prentice Hall.

Sethi, B. B. (1989). Family as a potent therapeutic force. *Indian Journal of Psychiatry, 31*(1), 22-30.

Seymour, S. C. (1999*). Women, family, and child care in India: A world in transition.* New York: Cambridge University Press.

Shangle, S. C. (1995). A view into the family and social life of India. *Family Perspective, 29*, 423-446.

Sharma, S., & Chadd, R. K. (1990). *Mental hospitals in India: Current status and role in mental health care.* Delhi: Institute of Human Behavior and Allied Sciences.

Shivurkar, N. (1991). Deserted women: A grave social problem. In M. Desai (Ed.), *Research on families with problems in India* (Volume, II, pp. 439-448). Bombay, India: Tata Institute of Social Sciences.

Shukla, M. (1994). India. In K. Hurrelmann (Ed.), *International handbook of adolescence* (pp. 191-206). Westport, CT: Greenwood Press.

Singh, J. P. (2005). The contemporary Indian family. In B. N. Adams & J. Trost (Eds.), *Handbook of world families.* (pp. 129-166). California: Sage Publications.

Sonuga-Barke, E. J. S., & Mistry, M. (2000). The effect of extended family living on the mental health of three generations within two Asian communities. *British Journal of Clinical Psychology, 39*, 129-141.

Srivastava, S. (1995). Family, deviance, and delinquency. *Trends in Social Science Research, 2*, 95-96.

Triandis, H. C. (1983). *Collectivism vs. individualism.* Champaign-Urbana: University of Illinois Press.

Triandis, H. C. (1990). Cross-cultural studies of individualism and collectivism. In J. Berman (Ed.), *Nebraska Symposium on Motivation* (pp. 41-133). Lincoln: University of Nebraska Press.

Triandis, H. C., Bontempo, R., Villareal, M. J., Asai, M., & Lucca, N. (1988). Individualism and collectivism: Cross-cultural perspective on self in group relationship. *Journal of Personality and Social Psychology, 19*, 323-338.

Unisa, S. (1999). Childlessness in Andhra Pradesh, India: Treatment-seeking and consequences. *Reproductive Health Matters, 7*, 54-64.

Verma, J. (1989). Marriage opinion survey and collectivism. *Psychological Studies, 34*, 141-150.

Vijaylaxmi, A. H., Saroja, K., & Katarki, P. A. (1992). A comparison of socio-economic profiles of mixed married and intracaste married working women. *Indian Journal of Behavior, 16*, 1-7.

Vohra, R. (1997). *The making of India a historical survey.* Armonk, NY: M.E. Sharpe.

doi:10.1300/J002v41n01_09

How Strong Families Encounter
Social Challenges in the Republic of Korea

Young Ju Yoo
Insoo Lee
Gyesook Yoo

SUMMARY. Research on family strengths began in Korea in the 1990s. With increasing academic and social interest in the study of family strengths, a number of investigations have been conducted. Western measurements do not properly reflect unique features of Korean familism and culture. *Pursuit of coexistence* and *we-ness* are unique Korean qualities of family strengths that represent the solidarity of members and familism. However, these qualities are sometimes called obstacles to the adjustment of Korean people to changing norms in a rapidly individualizing society today. In this context, it is time to reexamine the concepts of family strengths in Korea. doi:10.1300/J002v41n01_10

Young Ju Yoo is Professor Emeritus, College of Human Ecology, Kyung Hee University, and President of the Institute of Korean Family Strengths, # 372-1, Seokyo-dong, Mapo-gu, Sam-Yeon Bldg. 501, Seoul 121-210, Korea (E-mail: yjy@khu.ac.kr). Insoo Lee is Co-Director, Korean Family Welfare Counseling and Education Institute, # 501 Suktop Bldg., Changchun-Dong 114-9, Seodaemoon-Gu, Seoul 120-835, Korea (E-mail: einsoo@hanmail.net). Gyesook Yoo is Assistant Professor, College of Human Ecology, Kyung Hee University, # 1 Hoegi-dong, Dongdaemun-gu, Seoul, 130-701, Korea (E-mail: dongrazi@khu.ac.kr).

Address correspondence to: Young Ju Yoo.

[Haworth co-indexing entry note]: "How Strong Families Encounter Social Challenges in the Republic of Korea." Yoo, Young Ju, Insoo Lee, and Gyesook Yoo. Co-published simultaneously in *Marriage & Family Review* (The Haworth Press, Inc.) Vol. 41, No. 1/2, 2007, pp. 195-216; and: *Strong Families Around the World: Strengths-Based Research and Perspectives* (ed: John DeFrain, and Sylvia M. Asay) The Haworth Press, Inc., 2007, pp. 195-216. Single or multiple copies of this article are available for a fee from The Haworth Document Delivery Service [1-800-HAWORTH, 9:00 a.m. - 5:00 p.m. (EST). E-mail address: docdelivery@haworthpress.com].

Available online at http://mfr.haworthpress.com
© 2007 by The Haworth Press, Inc. All rights reserved.
doi:10.1300/J002v41n01_10

[Article copies available for a fee from The Haworth Document Delivery Service: 1-800-HAWORTH. E-mail address: <docdelivery@haworthpress.com> Website: <http://www.HaworthPress.com> © 2007 by The Haworth Press, Inc. All rights reserved.]

KEYWORDS. Family strengths, Korean family, qualities of strong families, Republic of Korea

GEOGRAPHIC AND DEMOGRAPHIC CHARACTERISTICS

Korea lies adjacent to China and Japan. Because of its unique geographical location, Chinese culture filtered into Japan through Korea. The west coast of the Korean Peninsula is bounded by the Korean Bay to the north and the West Sea to the south; the east coast faces the East Sea. The Korean Peninsula extends about 1,000 kilometers southward from the northeast Asian continental landmass. The peninsula and all of its associated islands lie between 33° N and 43° N parallels and 124° E and 131° E meridians. The latitudinal location of Korea is similar to that of the Iberian Peninsula and Greece. The land area of the peninsula is 220,000 km² and is divided into two parts–South Korea and North Korea.

The Korean Peninsula is divided into three distinct regions: Central, South and North. These macro regions are divided into three separate geographical spheres, each of which shows particular economic, cultural and physical distinctiveness. In the Central region are the Seoul metropolitan area, Chungcheong and Gangwon provinces; in the South, Gyeongsang, Jeolla and Jeju provinces.

The climate of the nation is temperate, under the influence of a continental dry winter and a moist maritime monsoonal summer. With four distinct seasons, it shows a vast difference in temperature between winter and summer. Rainfall averages 1,200 mm per year. From June through August, the monsoonal summer climate brings 50-60 percent of the total yearly rainfall. During the winter, from December through February, the climate is cold and dry with some snowfall.

Population. The population of the Republic of Korea as of 2005 was 48.3 million. The population density of the country is among the highest in the world, with approximately 490 persons per square kilometer. As of 2002 the population of North Korea was 22.2 million. Fast population growth was once a serious social problem in the Republic, as in most other developing nations. Due to successful family planning campaigns and changing attitudes, however, population growth has been curbed re-markably in recent years. As a result of a lengthened life expectancy and the sustained implementation of birth control, the annual rate of popula-tion growth was 0.44 percent in 2005 (Korean National Statistical Office, 2006).

A notable trend in the population structure is that it is getting increas-ingly older. The 2005 population estimate revealed that 9.1% of the total population was 65 years old or over. The number of people in the age of 15-64 years accounted for 71.8%.

In the 1960s, Korea's population distribution formed a pyramid shape, with a high birth rate and relatively short life expectancy. However, the structure is now shaped more like a bell with a low birth rate and extended life expectancy. Youth (under the age of 15 years) will make up a de-creasing portion of the total, while senior citizens (65 years or older) will account for some 20.8% of the total by the year 2026.

Language. All Koreans speak and write the same language, which has been a decisive factor in forging their strong national identity. The Korean alphabet, *Hangeul*, is another source of pride for Koreans. Kore-ans have developed several different dialects in addition to the standard used in Seoul. However, the dialects, except for that of Jeju-do province, are similar enough for native speakers to understand each other without any difficulties.

The *Hangeul* was created by King Sejong the Great during the 15th century. *Hangeul*, which consists of 10 vowels and 14 consonants, can be combined to form numerous syllabic groupings. It is simple, yet systematic and comprehensive, and is considered one of the most scientific writing systems in the world. *Hangeul* is easy to learn and write, which has greatly contributed to Korea's high literacy rate and advanced publication industry.

A Changing Picture: Demographic Trends in Korea

Income. Korea had remained a predominantly agricultural society until the first half of the twentieth century. Korea was able to join the leading group among developing countries, despite its poor natural re-sources and thanks largely to the five government-led five-year economic development plans implemented since the early 1960s.

As of 2002, per capita Gross National Income (GNI) of Korea is $14,162 and the amount of trade is $3,146 (IMF, 2002), making Korea the 13th largest trading country in the world. The government of Korea has pressed for the development of heavy and chemical industries, high technology and expansion of exports (see Table 1).

Employment. The employment structure of Korea has undergone a noticeable transformation since the dawn of industrialization in the early 1960s. In 1960 workers engaged in the agricultural, forestry and fishery sectors accounted for 63% of the total labor force. However, this figure dropped to a mere 8.1% by 2005. By contrast, the weight of the tertiary industry (service sectors) has gone up from 28.3% of the total labor force in 1960 to 73.3% in 2005 (Korean National Statistical Office, 2006).

In the latter half of the 1970s, the Korean labor market went through a series of major changes. Korea emerged as a competitive country in the global market with its labor-intensive industry such as textiles and footwear. And the stabilization of supply and demand in the Korean labor market enabled workers to demand their rights, which resulted in the organization of an increasing number of trade unions and collective action. The wages of Korean workers has sharply increased since then.

As Korea faced the economic crisis of 1997-98, a national consensus has been established on the need for a flexible labor market. In March 1998, the government introduced a law which permits companies to lay off employees if there is no other feasible alternative. The law has been in effect since June 1998. As of 1998 women's participation in economic activities decreased from a year earlier by 2.5% to 47.0% due to the economic crisis that placed Korea under the IMF supervision since the end of 1997. In 2005, employed women accounted for 50.2 % of the total labor force. The average age of employed women is on a steady rise.

Family life. The vast changes that have swept Asia and the rest of the world in the latter half of the 20th century have naturally been felt in the day-to-day lives of every Korean. Traditional customs and beliefs have undergone a great deal of change due to the rapid modernization of society. Despite these changes, however, Korea is still one of the most

TABLE 1. Gross national income (GNI) index.

Sectors	1990	1995	1998	2000	2002	2004
Growth rate(%)	8.7	8.1	−6.9	8.5	7.0	4.6
Per capita GNI (US $)	5,886	10,823	7,355	10,841	11,499	14,162

Source: The Bank of Korea (2006).

Confucian nations in the world. The traditional ways of the past and the long-cherished customs continue to influence Koreans' newly acquired modern ways.

Confucianism posits the family as the fundamental unit of society, incorporating the economic functions of production and consumption as well as social functions of education and socialization, guided by moral and ethical principles (Lee, 1997). The values and traditional family system of Confucianism were given new impetus during the late Joseon dynasty, although the origins of that belief system date back to the historical and social conditions of two millennia before (Park & Cho, 1995).

In the past, three or four generations often lived together, and people believed many children were desirable for the stability and security of the family. Traditionally, the eldest male of a family was regarded as the source of supreme authority. All family members were expected to do what was ordered or desired by him. Strict instructions were to be obeyed without protest. It would have been unthinkable for children or grandchildren to place themselves in opposition to the wishes of their elders. Obedience to one's superior was deemed natural; in addition, filial piety in particular was viewed as the most important of all Confucian virtues. On the other hand, it was understood that the patriarch of the family would be fair in all matters relating to the discipline of family members.

Under the patriarchal system, the man has traditionally been given the responsibility of representing, supporting and protecting his family. Order at home is maintained through the principle of hierarchy in which children must obey parents, the wife the husband, the servants the master. Reverence and respect for one's elders is a long-held social tradition in Korea (Choi, 1989).

There are many monuments throughout Korea commemorating loyal subjects, filial sons and faithful women. These monuments were erected as a way of honoring such people as models for society. Community service and spirit were also nurtured and promoted by the social recognition given to those who adhered to family values, the social order, family loyalty, filial piety and fidelity.

The rapid industrialization and urbanization of the country in the 1960s and 1970s were accompanied by an effective birth control drive, and the average number of children in a family has been dramatically decreased from 2.8 in 1980 to 1.08 in 2005.

Having a long Confucian tradition under which the eldest son takes over as head of the family, a preference for sons was prevalent in Korea. To deal with the problem of male preference, the government has completely rewritten family-related laws in a way that ensures equality for sons and daughters in terms of inheritance.

Industrialization of the country has made life more hectic and complicated. Young married couples have begun to separate from their extended families and start their own homes. Now almost all families are couple-centered nuclear families.

CHANGES AND CONTINUITY
IN MARRIAGE AND THE FAMILY

In Korea current trends include fewer marriages, a later age of marriage, fewer children, more divorce, more blended families, and more working mothers throughout the last 40 years. These changes in the concept of family are having a dramatic effect on the traditional concept of family values and on sexual consciousness, which results in the weakening of the solidarity between different generations, the appearance of individualism, the influx of values concerning gender equality among family members and so forth, thus causing dramatic changes in current family values (Byun, Baek, & Kim, 2000).

Trends in Marriage

Marriage and the family have survived over time despite all the predictions of their imminent collapse. In Korea, although marriage is the most popular institution in our society, there are several changes in marriage, which are not necessarily lasting (Korean National Statistical Office, 2006).

*   The total number of marriages recorded in 2005 was 316,375 cases (couples), down from 434,911 cases in 1996. The crude marriage rate (number of first marriages per 1,000 persons) stood at 6.5 cases in 2005, which dropped by 2.9 from 9.4 cases in 1996 and edged up by 0.2 from 6.3 cases in 2003.
*   As for males, the average age of the first marriage recorded was 30.9 years in 2005, which rose by 0.3 of a year from 2004 and by 2.5 years from 1996. As for females, the average age of first marriage was 27.7 years in 2005, which climbed by 0.2 a year from 2004 and by 2.2 years from 1996.
*   In 2005 there were 233,714 marriages between people marrying for the first time, an increase of 585 from 233,129 cases in 2004.

Meanwhile, remarriages totaled 66,666 cases in 2005, up 3,111 from 63,555 cases in 2004.

- Factors such as a rapid decline in fertility rate (from 4.53 in 1970 to 1.08 in 2005), late marriages and a rise in life expectancy have brought about changes in women's family life cycle. As of 1997, Korean women got married for the first time at the age of 25.9 on average, up 1.4 years from a decade ago. This trend toward later marriage can again be seen in the fact that the proportion of single women aged 30 rose by 2.7 times from 3.4% in 1975 to 9.2% in 1995.
- Although Korea has had a dominant cultural identity as a single ethnic group for a long time, Korea today is one of the culturally diverse nations. The international marriages between Korean men and women who have an ethnicity such as Chinese, Ethnic Korean Chinese, Japanese, Vietnamese, Russian and others are rapidly increasing. There were 35,447 marriages between different ethnic groups in 2004, which rose by 30,737 cases from 1990.

Trends in Divorce and Remarriage

Let us now look at trends in divorce and discuss why so many couples divorce in Korea:

- The number of divorces in Korea is on the rise, from 45,694 in 1990 to 128,468 in 2005. The crude divorce rate (number of divorces per 1,000 persons) was 2.6 in 2005, a considerable increase from 1.1 cases in 1990.
- In 2004, the average age of divorced males was 41.8 years, which had climbed by 0.5 a year from 2003 and by 3.7 years from 1994. The average age of divorced females was 38.3 years, which inched up by 0.4 year from 2003 and by 4.1 years from 1994.
- As for the length of marriage before divorce, the percentage of divorced couples that had lived together four years and less decreased to 25.8% in 2005 from 33.7% in 1994. At the other end of the spectrum, the percentage of divorced couples who had lived together 20 years and more jumped to 18.7% in 2005 from 7.2% in 1994, increasing more than twofold.
- The main reason for divorce in 2005 was dissimilarities in personality between spouses (49.1%), followed by economic problems (14.9%), trouble issues among family members (9.5%), spousal infidelity (7.6%), mental and physical abuse (4.4%) and others

(13.8%). The percentage of couples divorcing due to economic problems increased, while the percentage of couples divorcing because of dissimilarities in personality decreased, compared to the percentage in 2004 (see Table 2).

Trends in Family Structure

Significant changes have occurred in Korean family structure in recent years, including the transformation from a patriarchal system of family members arranged in a hierarchical order to a nuclear family based on a married couple; from a single-income family to a dual-income couple family structure; and increases in the number of weekend couples and DINKs (Dual Income No Kids) (Byun et al., 2000).

The following trends illustrate the changes in family structure in Korea:

* Double-income families, divorced families, single-mother families, and the aged living alone are all increasing, while a growing number of women are seeking a job to be economically active as they are now less burdened by the responsibility for household work and the care of children.
* As of 2000, over 70 percent of all Korean households (12.96 million) were two-generation families. Three-generation extended families accounted for 13.8 percent; one-generation families were 10 percent; and single households were 12.7 percent. Households headed

TABLE 2. The main reason for divorce.

	2000	2001	2002	2003	2004	2005
Total	100.0	100.0	100.0	100.0	100.0	100.0
Spousal infidelity	8.1	8.7	8.6	7.3	7.0	7.6
Mental and physical abuse	4.3	4.7	4.8	4.3	4.2	4.4
Trouble among family members	21.9	17.6	14.4	13.0	10.0	9.5
Economic problem	10.7	11.6	13.6	16.4	14.7	14.9
Dissimilarity in personality	40.1	43.0	44.7	45.3	49.4	49.2
Health problem	0.9	0.7	0.6	0.6	0.6	0.6
Others*	14.0	13.7	13.3	13.1	14.1	13.8

Source: Korean National Statistical Office. Annual Report on the Vital Statistics. 2000-2005.

by women numbered 2.15 million (or 16.6 percent of the total), an increase of 650,000 since 1985.

Changes in the Role of Women in the Family

The role of women in the family has undergone considerable change since the liberation of Korea from Japan in 1945. For centuries Koreans lived in extended families. It was not uncommon for one household to include three generations or more, including younger male siblings and their wives and children. However, this situation changed dramatically during the 1960s and 1970s when Korea experienced rapid economic growth and people began to populate the cities in great numbers.

- Women's economic participation started in the early 1960s with the industrialization of Korea, and the participation rate increased continuously and peaked in the late 1980s. However, women's economic participation rate currently shows an M-curve, which is characterized by highest rates for ages in 20s and 40s but lowest in childbirth age. This curve represents severance of working experience due to marriage and childbirth. The women's advancement to management and high-income position is compromised by such disconnect in job experiences.
- In addition to these changes, more and more older people are living away from their grown children. One out of five women (or 19 percent) 65 years or older now live alone. Due to the formation of "nuclear" and one-person households, the size of the average family has been decreasing steadily.
- The number of elderly women aged 65 and over was 4.9% of the total population in 1980. This percentage reached 11.3% in 2000. As of 1995, 19% of elderly women aged 65 and over lived alone, perhaps indicating difficult conditions in the lives of some elderly women.
- The average life expectancy for Korean women was 66.7 years compared to 59.8 years for men in 1970. In 2003, these figures have increased to 80.8 years and 73.9 years, respectively. On average, women live 7 years longer than men.
- Ninety percent of Korean women get married in their 20s, although the average age of first-time brides has been steadily rising over the years. Today's women are getting married significantly later than their grandmothers. In 1950, the average age of marriage

was 20.4 years; in 1960, 21.6 years; in 1985, 24.8 years and in 2005, 27.7 years, respectively. Until the 1960s, the ideal number of children was thought to be four; however, today's women believe that two children are enough.

- As a result of all these changes, the relationship between married couples has also undergone a significant transformation, with more values being placed on mutual cooperation and affinity between husband and wife than ever before.
- Traditionally, it was the man of the house who made all the significant monetary decisions. However, recent surveys show that seven out of 10 Korean couples now make joint decisions when they buy a house, a piece of land and other big-ticket items. More and more wives are making the final decision on matters concerning children's education and childcare.
- Today's women are very different from their mothers and grandmothers. Today's wife is an equal partner of her husband. She is a capable person, constantly trying to expand her role and realize her potential both in the home and the society in which she belongs.

FAMILY STRENGTHS AND CHALLENGES IN KOREA

Individuals have the desire to understand their own strengths, characteristics and resources, and such an internal desire is increased when people face considerable stress and changes in life (Giblin, 1996). While individuals are responsible for themselves and control their own fate, the development of individual identity is influenced by the family, the primary environment in which people live. Thus, the more that people emphasize the establishment of individual identity and a focus on individual needs and desires, the more essential a peaceful and healthy family becomes.

Most research on the family in the Western societies in the 20th century concentrated on the problems in the lives of families, focusing on the question, "Why did the family fail?" and pathological phenomena. However, studies of the strengths of families and positive aspects of life together began in the 1960s and 1970s, asking the question, "How does the family lead a successful life?" (DeFrain, 2002; DeFrain et al., 2006; Olson, 1993; Otto, 1962; Stinnett & DeFrain, 1985; Stinnett & Sauer, 1977; Stinnett, Sanders, & DeFrain, 1981).

The family strengths perspective, a conceptual framework for thinking about families, has a positive and optimistic attitude toward life and includes the following propositions: All families have strengths and the capability to meet challenges and the potential for growth. If a family focuses only on problems and not strengths, the family will only see problems. If a family tries to see its strengths or merits, the family will discover its merits. The merits can be developed and become the foundation for the positive growth and change in the future. Furthermore, when a person has grown up in a strong family, he or she can more easily build the strong family in the future (DeFrain et al., 2006).

Strong families need to be cultivated in our society, because they produce truly well-rounded individuals, developed through positive emotional and relational processes in the family. The dysfunctional family causes family problems and transmits family violence, chronic anxiety, stress, family misunderstandings and counter-productive values from generation to generation. Preventing family problems in advance requires less effort and fewer resources than to repair the damage done by families already suffering misfortune and restoring them to happiness after considerable injury has already been inflicted. It is very urgent to change the unhealthy family to a strong family under the current situation in which the divorce rate, family violence, alienation of the aged and the deviation and misconduct of youth have all been increasing. These family-focused changes are more valuable for a country in the long run than economic and political development, the increase in family dissolution and dysfunction have resulted in increasing social welfare costs, as well as devastation of the quality of life in families, putting the country in a downward spiral. Thus, it is urgent that solutions are found and that we begin to empower and strengthen our families.

Research on Strong Families

Research on strong families was initiated in Korea in the 1990s. Yoo (1994) was the first to suggest an academic definition for the term *strong family* in the Korean context. Since then, with increasing academic and social interest in strong families, a number of studies have been conducted Choi, Yoon, Han, Cho, & Lee, 1999; Eo & Yoo, 1995, 1997; Heo, 1998; Yang, 2001). However, most of the studies modified and edited the means used in other countries to measure the family strengths. The Western scales reflected Western culture and perspectives on family life. Thus, such scales raised the problems that they couldn't properly reflect Korean cultures and unique features of Korean families. Eo and Yoo

(1995) corrected these problems with the existing scales and developed family strengths scales reflecting Korean values. Their studies indicated that patriarchal consciousness still remained in Korea, because the major characteristics of a strong family were seen to be peace and harmony, respect, and prescribed roles for family members in Korea, while the characteristics of the strong family in the US had more individual aspects, such as love, respect, sharing time and commitment (Stinnett Sanders, & DeFrain, 1981). According to a recent pilot survey by Yoo (2001) related to Korean perspectives on family strengths, it was found that the individualistic tendency had increased in Korea, as the elements of a strong family were love, affection, positive communication, respect and the self-confidence of individuals in the family.

As we can see from the research discussed above, the family has been continuously changing along with the changes in Korean society. The times in which we live impact many aspects of our lives in families. Therefore, it is essential that researchers continuously study the family. Research on the concepts and elements of strong families need to be renewed and restructured to reflect changes in our society.

Further, as the strong family has been recently highlighted more than ever throughout the world, family researchers globally, including the US, have been conducting comparative cultural studies of strong families in many countries, and this work has been enhanced by international conferences and joint research and program development projects uniting researchers and practitioners from diverse cultures.

Accordingly, a national empirical study of Korean family strengths was necessary. A fundamental survey of Korean families with the ultimate aim of helping to strengthen families in our society was designed with ideas and concepts drawn from global efforts. Korean family strengths scales needed to be developed that were sensitive to Korean social and cultural values and customs. We will now turn to a discussion of the qualities of strong families in Korea, as delineated by the survey using the Korean Family Strengths Scales (Yoo, 2004).

Qualities of Strong Families as Delineated by Korean Researchers

The term of *strong family* is a compound of the words *strong* and *family*. The definition of the word *strong* is more suitable and familiar in the realm of physical health. The term *strong* suggests the absence of disease and the presence of physical health. The World Health Organization (WHO) defines *health* as not only being without diseases but also a state of physical and mental wellbeing. *Physical health* implies a state in which the individual can perform appropriate activities without a sense of inconvenience or helplessness, and *mental health* means that the individual feels happy, optimistic, and has a vigorous approach to life. Mental health also implies that the individual is relatively free of anxiety and physically abnormal conditions. A number of studies have found significant correlations between physical health and mental health (Ross, Mirrowsky, & Goldstein, 1991).

Herbert Otto (1962, 1963), an early pioneer in family strengths research, designed a conceptual system for thinking about the strong family and family strengths after a pilot study. He considered family strengths as the ultimate product of consistently changing elements that interrelate with each other through the family life cycle. Some researchers have more recently contended that a sense of spiritual well-being should be included in definitions of a strong family (Lee, 2000; Stinnett & Sauer, 1977; Stinnett & DeFrain, 1985).

The concept of *family* has been defined by a number of theoreticians and researchers. The definition of *modern family* today does not focus so much on family structure as it did in the past, emphasizing kinship patterns and other structural issues. The focus, instead, is more on the internal dynamics of the group and what actually goes on in the life of the family. Researchers are likely to focus on internal functioning, on how family members behave toward each other. Investigators are likely to conduct research on feelings toward each other in families, on love, boundary awareness, paradigms and rules, day-to-day activities, communication and conflict resolution, decision-making, resource management, family relationships, and so forth. The predominant interest of researchers has shifted from studies focusing on family structure to studies focusing on family functioning.

Family researchers, family therapists and other clinical practitioners and educators are influenced by findings in many allied fields, such as sociology, psychology, education and cultural anthropology. However, professionals in family studies are likely to focus on the family system and close relationships within the family (Burr, Day, & Bahr, 1993). Thus, the strong family is a system that promotes the healthy development of each family member, shares important values as a group through the positive interaction among family members (communication, decision-making processes, and effective solutions for stress management) and interacts successfully with other social systems. The following table outlines the qualities of strong families as uncovered by Korean scholars (see Table 3).

TABLE 3. Qualities of strong families as delineated by Korean researchers.

Year	Researchers		Qualities of Strong Families
1995	Eo, Eun-Ju & Yoo, Young-Ju		A bond with each other Communication Ability to solve problems A shared value system
1996	Heo, Bong-Ryeol		Love Rules Generosity Adaptability Positive communication
1998	Jee, Young-Sook & Lee, Young-Ho		A sound family environment Parent-children relationship Couple relationship Economic activity Community life Kinship and brothers' and sisters' relationship
1999	Choi, Sun-Hee	Family strengths evaluation (Professional group)	Communication Affection/love Autonomy Confidence/support Economic stability Physical health Problem-solving ability Resilience/value system
		Family strengths of a broad sample of families	Affection/love Confidence/support Communication Autonomy Role performance Resilience Problem solving ability Others
2000	Yoo, Young-Ju		Appreciation Love, respect, support Interest in each other and responsibility Communication Respect for individuality Sharing time Shared goals for life, ethical values Financial management Positive thoughts and cooperation in case of family risks and problems Close relationship with society
2001	Yang, Soon-Mi		Communication, coping to problems, and family identity Decision making and family bond Resilience and social recognition Creation of family customs

Year	Researchers	Qualities of Strong Families
2004	Yoo, Young-Ju	Respect Commitment Appreciation/affection Positive communication Sharing values and goals Role performance Ability to solve problems Economic stability Connectedness with the social system
2004	Yoo, Gye-Sook	Pursuit of coexistence Positive interaction Spiritual strengths

Qualities of Strong Families as Delineated by Korean Family Members

Young Ju Yoo (2004) examined the qualities of strong families as perceived by urban Korean family members. *The Family Strengths Concept Scale* was administered to 806 adults living in Seoul. This scale is a self-report questionnaire, consisting of 26 items on a 5-point Likert scale. The scale was influenced by earlier research on strong families by DeFrain, Stinnett and their colleagues (DeFrain & Stinnett, 1999; University of Nebraska-Lincoln for Families, 2006) and Olson and his colleagues (Olson & DeFrain, 2006). The scale items are listed in Table 4. Higher scores indicate higher levels of perceived strengths on various items. The reliability of the scale, computed using Cronbach's alpha was .95 for the sample.

Table 4 indicates that *trust* was regarded as the most important quality of strong families in Korea, followed by *honesty, caring for each other, friendship*, and *respect for individuality*. Relatively less important family strengths were *faith, compassion, shared ethical values*, and *enjoying each other's company* (see Table 4).

To identify the qualities of strong families, a principal component analysis with varimax rotations was conducted on adults' responses to the 26 family-strength items. As seen in Table 5, three factors of adults' concepts of the qualities of family strengths were yielded as follows: *pursuit of coexistence, positive interaction*, and *spiritual strengths. Pursuit of coexistence* represents those qualities such as *the ability to cope with stress* and *time together. Positive interaction* consists of the qualities such as *commitment, positive communication* and *appreciation and affection*. And *Spiritual strengths* represent the qualities of *faith* and *ethical and moral values*. Among these three factors, *Spiritual strengths*

TABLE 4. Means and standard deviations of perceived qualities of family strengths ($N = 806$).

Family Strengths	M	SD
Trust	4.66	.63
Honesty	4.57	.64
Caring for each other	4.52	.67
Friendship	4.50	.67
Respect for individuality	4.50	.67
Faithfulness	4.49	.67
Sharing feelings	4.44	.70
Giving compliments	4.38	.72
Dependability	4.37	.74
Sharing fun times	4.36	.71
Being able to compromise	4.35	.69
Agreeing to disagree	4.32	.77
Resilience	4.30	.77
Oneness with humankind	4.30	.80
Avoiding blame	4.25	.83
Growing through crises together	4.15	.83
Simple good times	4.14	.76
Openness to change	4.07	.85
Quality time in great quantity	4.07	.78
Adaptability	4.06	.81
Playfulness & humor	4.05	.80
Good things take time	4.05	.79
Shared ethical values	3.95	.93
Enjoying each other's company	3.95	.82
Compassion	3.80	.96
Faith	3.67	1.18

supports the International Family Strengths Model (DeFrain & Olson, 2004), implying that this factor is a universal quality of family strengths. On the contrary, the other two factors, *Pursuit of coexistence* and *Positive interaction*, could be interpreted as the Korean specific qualities of family strengths that represent solidarity of family members and familism.

Gyesook Yoo (2004) examined the perceptions of family strengths among married men and women in Korea. The subjects of this study were a total of 1,675 men (854) and women (821) in Seoul and 5 provinces. All of them selected "*Yes*" on the question, "Do you think your family is healthy?"

This study used *The Korean Family Strengths Scale* (Yoo, 2004). Each factor is explained in detail below. The *Respect* factor contains the

TABLE 5. Principal component analysis on adults' perceptions of qualities of family strengths (*N* = 806).

Qualities of family strengths	Factor Loadings			
	factor I pursuit of coexistence	factor II positive interactrion	factor III spiritual strengths	h^2
Adaptability	.78	.20	.25	.71
Simple good times	.75	.24	.18	.65
Growing through crises together	.73	.25	.17	.63
Openness to change	.73	.28	.24	.66
Quality time in great quantity	.71	.27	.28	.66
Good things take time	.70	.25	.27	.62
Sharing fun times	.69	.31	.06	.57
Resilience	.68	.33	.16	.60
Enjoying each other's company	.66	.17	.32	.57
Playfulness & humor	.65	.25	.31	.58
Agreeing to disagree	.45	.43	.24	.44
Honesty	.19	.79	.11	.67
Trust	.17	.79	−.04	.65
Faithfulness	.23	.71	.25	.61
Friendship	.31	.68	.21	.60
Dependability	.15	.66	.15	.48
Caring for each other	.31	.63	.20	.54
Respect for individuality	.45	.59	.10	.56
Giving compliments	.30	.58	.37	.57
Sharing feelings	.39	.57	.26	.54
Being able to compromise	.39	.52	.35	.54
Avoiding blame	.25	.46	.46	.49
Compassion	.30	.15	.80	.76
Shared ethical values	.30	.29	.72	.70
Faith	.19	.08	.72	.56
Oneness with humankind	.35	.44	.52	.58
Cronbach's α	.93	.92	.82	
Eigenvalue	12.25	1.93	1.33	Σh^2
Total Variance (%)	47.11	7.40	5.13	
Cumulative Variance (%)	47.11	54.51	59.64	15.54

questions related to the respect for individuality, acceptance of each other, interest in each other, positive expectations of each other, confidence, trust, consideration, and encouraging growth in each other. The "We-ness" factor measures the bond, cooperation and harmony, pride for family tradition, sharing good times together, family history (past time) and sharing leisure and hobbies together. The *Appreciation and affection* factor measures the expression of affection (love) and affinity, expression of positive feelings and gratitude, and the awareness of the family as a psychological nest. The *Positive communication* factor comprises the questions focusing on approaches to positive communication, communicating with an open mind, reflective listening, and warm and attentive communication with each other. The *Sharing values and goals* factor measures how closely family members' views of life agree with each other, respect for elders in the family, keeping family traditions, consensus on issues regarding what is right and wrong, compliance with family rules, sharing common interests, and positive thoughts and attitudes toward life. The *Role performance* factor examines devotion to family roles, equity in role sharing, devotion to each individual's role, responsibility to these roles, and awareness of each role. The *Ability to solve problems* factor includes questions on the family's ability to manage risk, their ability to cope with difficulties, and the positive meanings they apply to difficult situations.

The qualities of strong families that participants described are suggested in Table 6. According to the comparison on the mean scores of family strengths by sub-factor, the highest mean scores were *respect for family members* and *a bond* (M = 3.71) followed by the *affection and appreciation* and *positive communication* in that order. The factors *sharing value and goals, the ability to solve problems,* and *role performance* were on the same rank with the mean score of 3.53 (see Table 7).

CONCLUSION

We-ness in the Korean family is both an advantage as well as a disadvantage. The current post-modern society in which we live is dominated by rapid change through periods of industrialization and post-industrialization. Personal abilities, personal identities and personal confidence and values are required if an individual is to successfully navigate in the world today. However, members of many Korean families are often faced with the ideal of extreme *We-ness* that could lead to

TABLE 6. Qualities of strong families as delineated by Korean people.

Qualities of strong families	Descriptions	Response frequency*
Respect	- Respect for individuality - Accept and understand others - Admit each other - Support, encouragement and help for growth - Confidence and reliability - Generosity, consideration and practice of virtue	344
We-ness	- Sharing joys and sorrows with family members - A sense of unity, a bond, affiliation - Harmony - Solidarity, cooperation - Pride for family tradition and the clan - Keeping the bond through meeting with brothers, sisters and relatives - Sharing the story of the family history (past story) - Sharing the entertainment activities with family members and hobbies	306
Appreciation/ Affection	- Share affection and love - Express closeness - Give emotional and sentimental stability support - Express appreciation - Psychological and emotional refuge	261
Positive Communication	- Positive communication methods - Open conversation - Reflective listening (carefully listening to others) - No cynical or ignorant expressions toward each other - Enjoy discussion on various issues - Enjoy the conversation - Jokes	256
Sharing Values and Goals	- Share the view of life - Respect for the elderly - Unique traditions - Family rules, customs and etiquette - Sound thoughts - Right values - Religious beliefs - Positive thoughts on life	224
Role Performance	- Faithful to roles - Equity of role sharing - Faithful to roles of each other - Responsibility for duties - Admit the roles of other members	193
Abilities to Solve Problems	- Ability to manage risks - Ability to cope with hardship - Problem solving ability	173

*The response frequency includes the overlapped responses.

TABLE 7. Means, standard deviations, and ranks of sub-factors on the family strengths scales ($N = 1,675$).

Rank	Factors	M	SD
1	respect	3.71	0.59
2	we-ness	3.71	0.66
3	appreciation and affection	3.61	0.66
4	positive communication	3.60	0.60
5	sharing values and goals	3.53	0.62
6	role performance	3.53	0.59
7	ability to solve problems	3.53	0.63

enmeshed relationships, in which there is very little individual right to decide one's own lifestyle and values. The self-differentiation that Bowenian theory describes is not a reality for many Korean family members. Thus, the individual's experience in society can cause substantial conflicts and challenges for families. *Family comes first*, the traditional concept, works well when the family is in harmony and everything is going smoothly. However, when women or the elderly need to sacrifice themselves or unconditionally obey the patriarch for the harmony of family, the ideal of personal achievement or individual development and independence cannot be realized in many cases.

Rapid social change in Korean society and *We-ness* in the Korean family can cause significant problems. In this context, the *Strong Family Movement* in Korea will be no more than a simple motto. It is time to reexamine the true meaning of the term *strong family*, and develop a viable vision for Korean families in the future.

Some observers assert that individuals are free to control their own fate, and should be allowed to grow and change in ways they themselves determine. Other observers are more likely to focus on social continuity, noting that our cultural and family backgrounds give us a solid foundation and purpose for living while shielding us from the difficulties life inevitably brings (Jang, Je, &, Kim, 2000, p. 15). This on-going discussion over the value of continuity and the value of change in society and in families is a healthy interchange, for it focuses on two great needs in life: the need for roots and the need for wings.

The development of self-identity is heavily influenced by the family of origin into which we are born, and by the institutional family groups, such as child care centers, schools, and care centers for the elderly where we spend a significant amount of our time in life. Positive self-identity is formed by the strong and healthy families in which we live (Stinnett, Sanders, & DeFrain, 1981). The quality of family life is a critical influence on who we are, who we will become, our emotional security, happiness, and mental health.

REFERENCES

Burr, W., Day, R., & Bahr, K. (1993). *Family science.* Pacific Grove, Brooks/Cole.

Byun, W., & Cho, E. (2004). Study of changes in family structure and the prospective goals for family laws. KWDI research report. Seoul: Korean Women Development Institute.

Byun, W., Baek, K., & Kim, H. (2000). A study of the changes in the Korean family and the role and status of females. KWDI research report. Seoul: Korean Women Development Institute.

Choi, J. (1989). *Korean family study.* Seoul: Illjogak.

Choi, S. J., Yoon, H. G., Han, D. W., Cho, G. H., & Lee, S. W. (1999). *Oriental psychology.* Seoul: Jisik Saneop.

DeFrain, J. (2002). Global perspectives on strong families. Paper presented at the Chinese International Building Family Strengths Conference, sponsored by the Shanghai Academy of Social Sciences, June 12-14. Shanghai, People's Republic of China.

DeFrain, J., et al. (2006). Family treasures: Creating strong families. Lincoln, NE, USA: University of Nebraska Extension. Website: unlforfamilies.unl.edu

DeFrain, J. & Olson, D. H. (1999). Contemporary family patterns and relationships. In M. Sussman, S. Steinmetz, & G. W. Peterson (Eds.), *Handbook of marriage and the family.* NY: Plenum.

DeFrain, J., & Olson, D. H. (2004). Family and couple challenges and strengths in the USA. Paper presented at the Korean International Family Strengths Conference, June 10. Seoul, Korea.

DeFrain, J. & Stinnett, N. (2002). Family strengths. In J. J. Ponzetti et al. (Eds.), *International encyclopedia of marriage and family* (2nd Ed.). NY: Macmillan Reference Group, pp. 637-642.

DeFrain, J., & Stinnett, N. (2006). American family strengths inventory. Lincoln, Nebraska, USA: University of Nebraska-Lincoln. Website: www.ianrpubs.unl.edu/epublic/live/nf498/build/nf498.pdf

Geggie, J., DeFrain, J., Hitchcock, S., & Silberberg, S. (2000). Family strengths research project: Final report to the Australian Commonwealth Government Ministry of Family and Community Services, Canberra, A.C.T. Callaghan, N.S.W., Australia: Family Action Centre, University of Newcastle.

Giblin, P. (1996). Family strengths. *Family Journal, 4,* 339-347. LA, CA: Sage.

Jang, H., Je, S., & Kim, J. (2000). *Family therapy*. Seoul: Jungang Jeoks Publishing.
Korean National Statistical Office (2006). Annual Report on the Vital Statistics. Seoul: KNSO Publishing.
Korean National Statistical Office (2006). Korea Social Index, 2005. Seoul: KNSO Publishing.
Korean Research Institute of Population & Health (1985). *A study on the current state of Korean aged people's life*. Seoul: Korean Research Institute of Population & Health.
Lee, I. (2000). *Modern marriages and families: Social changes and Korean family.* Seoul: Singwang Publishing.
Lee, J. (2005). The change of the public/private spheres and family policies beyond "the family." *The Women's Studies, 68*, 137-164.
Lee, K. (1997). *Korean family and kinship*. Seoul: Jipmoondang.
Lee, S. (2000). *Health and the elderly*. Seoul: Daeyoung Publishing Co.
Olson, D. H. (1993). Circumplex model of marital and family systems: Assessing family functioning. In F. Walsh (Ed.), *Normal family processes* (2nd ed.) (pp. 104-137). NY: Guilford Press.
Olson, D. H., & DeFrain, J. (2006). *Marriages and families: Intimacy, diversity, and strengths* (5th Ed.). New York: McGraw-Hill Higher Education.
Otto, H. A. (1962). What is a strong family? *Marriage and Family Living, 24*, 77-81.
Park, I., & Cho, L. J. (1995). Confucianism and the Korean family. *Journal of Comparative Family Studies, 26*, 117-129.
Stinnett, N., & DeFrain, J. (1985). *Secrets of strong families*. Boston: Little, Brown.
Stinnett, N., Sanders, G., & DeFrain, J. (1981). A nation-wide study of strong families. In N. Stinnett, J. DeFrain, K. King, P. Knaub, & G. Rowe (Eds.), *Family strengths 3: The roots of well-being*. Lincoln, NE: University of Nebraska Press.
Stinnett, N., & Sauer, K. (1977). Relationship characteristics of strong families. *Family Perspective, 1*, 3-11.
University of Nebraska-Lincoln for Families. (2006). Building strong families. Website: unlforfamilies.unl.edu.
Yoo, G. (2004). A survey of the elements of strong families: Focusing on family systems and family strengths. *Journal of Korean Family Relations, 9*, 25-42.
Yoo, Y. (2000). Healthy family created by 10 precepts. Seoul: Kyung Hee Family Counseling and Education Center.
Yoo, Y. (2004). A study on Korean Family Strength Scale development for family enhancement. *Journal of Korean Family Relations, 9*, 119-151.

doi:10.1300/J002v41n01_10

OCEANIA

The Shaping of Strengths
and Challenges of Australian Families:
Implications for Policy and Practice

Judi Geggie
Ruth Weston
Alan Hayes
Simone Silberberg

SUMMARY. This article traces some of the key historical events that have combined with Australia's geography, climate and patterns of immigration in shaping characteristics of Australian families–characteristics

Judi Geggie is Director, Family Action Centre, University of Newcastle, Callaghan Campus, Faculty of Health, CALLAGHAN NSW 2308 Australia (E-mail: Judi.Geggie@ newcastle.edu.au). Ruth Weston is General Manager–Research, Australian Institute of Family Studies, 485 La Trobe Street, Melbourne Vic. 3000, Australia (E-mail: ruth. weston@aifs.gov.au). Alan Hayes is Director, Australian Institute of Family Studies, 485 La Trobe Street, Melbourne Vic. 3000, Australia (E-mail: Alan.Hayes@aifs.gov.au). Simone Silberberg is Community Consultant, AWE Consultancy, P.O. Box 1191, Mullumbimby NSW 2482 (E-mail: Simone.Silberberg@portstephens.nsw.gov.au).
Address correspondence to: Judi Geggie.

[Haworth co-indexing entry note]: "The Shaping of Strengths and Challenges of Australian Families: Implications for Policy and Practice." Geggie, Judi et al. Co-published simultaneously in *Marriage & Family Review* (The Haworth Press, Inc.) Vol. 41, No. 3/4, 2007, pp. 217-239; and: *Strong Families Around the World: Strengths-Based Research and Perspectives* (ed: John DeFrain, and Sylvia M. Asay) The Haworth Press, Inc., 2007, pp. 217-239. Single or multiple copies of this article are available for a fee from The Haworth Document Delivery Service [1-800-HAWORTH, 9:00 a.m. - 5:00 p.m. (EST). E-mail address: docdelivery@haworthpress.com].

Available online at http://mfr.haworthpress.com
© 2007 by The Haworth Press, Inc. All rights reserved.
doi:10.1300/J002v41n03_01

that are remarkable for their diversity on many fronts. These factors, along with changing patterns of family formation, stability and structure, evolving parenting roles, and the ever-increasing spatial concentration of families, have all contributed to diverse strengths, vulnerabilities and lifestyles of families. Policies directed towards helping families identify and draw on their own strengths and those of their community have gained momentum since the late 1990s. The article outlines some of these policies, along with a project on family strengths that has helped shape interventions. doi:10.1300/J002v41n03_01 *[Article copies available for a fee from The Haworth Document Delivery Service: 1-800-HAWORTH. E-mail address: <docdelivery@haworthpress.com> Website: <http://www. HaworthPress.com>* © *2007 by The Haworth Press, Inc. All rights reserved.]*

KEYWORDS. Family challenges, family formation, family strengths, government policies, historical events

THE AUSTRALIAN FAMILY

What is the iconic picture of an Australian family? Is it a father throwing "a shrimp on the barbie," with the beer in one hand and surrounded by mates, while his wife and children are well in the background, or is it a family of parents working long hours, children in childcare, and not a shrimp nor a barbie in sight? Is it a farming family living in the rural backblocks or an urban family living on a quarter acre block? Is it a newly arrived Vietnamese or Sri Lankan family, or a family of mixed Italian, Greek, British or Irish descent? Is it a lone-parent family, stepfamily, or so-called "intact family," or an Indigenous family, defined by blood relationships that differ markedly from other families?

Whichever image springs to mind, it will be challenged by others, for Australian families are distinguished by a striking diversity that has its roots in many interacting factors. These include Australia's history of immigration policies, vast thirsty landscape and geographic position relative to other countries, along with a highly concentrated population distribution, and changing fortunes in rural areas. Behind some of these factors are others that cannot be dealt with here, for example, the social, economic and political forces in other countries that have encouraged emigration to Australia, and structural change in industry, job markets and globalisation of the economy. Indeed, Australia's dynamic social and economic context has partly resulted from, as well as contributed to, the patterns that are outlined below.

This article explores five issues: (a) key historical events and features of Australia that contribute to the diverse characteristics of Australian families; (b) the extent and ways in which the roles of men and women in Australian families have changed; (c) some of the challenges facing Australian family life today; (d) the strengths on which families rely to meet these challenges; and (e) the influence of family strengths and resilience research on family practice and policy.

Non-Indigenous Settlement

The arrival in 1788 of convicts from the British Isles should be seen as a defining moment in Australia's (white) (and black) history. These convicts, their officers and military personnel arrived in a vast brown land that had been inhabited for probably well over 40,000 years by Aboriginal and Torres Strait Islanders. Indigenous Australian families inhabited most of Australia and, while sharing a fundamental connection with the natural environment, their cultural traditions, languages and lifestyles varied across the regions. For these original Australians, the First Fleet marked the beginnings of death, disease, dispossession and dislocation, along with the disappearance of most of their numerous distinct languages. For Australia in general, it marked the beginning of an overarching British culture whose legal framework is the Westminster system of government. By 1836, around 100,000 convicts had arrived, of whom only 13,000 were female. As the demand for labour increased, convicts were sent out more frequently, with the numbers peaking in 1833. While the transportation of convicts continued until 1868, free immigrants arrived from the early 1790s, and became the main source of population growth from the 1830s. Rapid population growth continued with the gold rush and the expanding wool industry during the 1850s.

Life was extremely harsh for the early generations of settlers, including the large numbers of convicts and free settlers from Ireland whose resentment of British oppression continued on Australian shores. This resentment may well have contributed to Australian society's disparagement of "tall poppies" (i.e., those whose success appears to have resulted in a sense of superiority) and emphasis on egalitarianism and a "fair go."

Between 1860 and 1900, 95% of the one million people who migrated to Australia were English, Irish or Scots (Australian Government Department of Immigration and Multicultural and Indigenous Affairs [DIMIA], 2001). Others to arrive in Australia during the 19th Century included Germans, many of whom settled in South Australia, and Italians who worked in the cane fields in Queensland. The gold rush attracted large groups of Chinese immigrants whose industriousness, different appearance and unique customs generated considerable antagonism amongst other miners and service providers, leading to riots, violence towards them, and pressure on governments to limit their intake. This experience of racial unrest played a major role in the development of the "White Australia Policy"–a policy that lasted more than 70 years. The associated legislation was the first major change to be handled upon the establishment of the Commonwealth of Australia and is a central reason behind the strong British-Celtic culture in Australia today.

Federation and the "White Australia Policy"

The Commonwealth of Australia was formed in 1901 through the passing of an Act in the British Parliament, which united six British colonies (or Australia states) under a single constitution. Most of the 3.8 million non-Indigenous population were of Anglo-Celtic descent, and almost half lived on rural properties or in small rural towns of less than 3,000 people. Men outnumbered women (115 men for every 100 women) and primary industries predominated.

Soon after federation, the Immigration Restrictions Act (1901) was introduced to retain the Anglo-Celtic profile and thereby limit any disharmony linked with racial or cultural intolerance. British immigration was particularly encouraged. Although rules on the immigration of non-Europeans were gradually relaxed, it was not until the early 1970s that the "White Australia Policy" was formally abolished.

After World War II, concerns that Australia would be incapable of defending its borders from attack and the need for unskilled labor gave rise to the slogan "populate or perish," and led the Government to actively encourage immigration from Britain and Europe. To further preserve cultural homogeneity, policies were introduced to encourage non-Anglo immigrants to assimilate to mainstream Anglo culture. This emphasis on cultural homogeneity for harmony eventually switched to recognition of the dynamism generated by diversity. Australia is now one of the most ethnically diverse countries in the world, although the proportion of Australians who were born overseas was virtually the same in 1901 and 2001 (23% and 22% respectively). People born in the United Kingdom represented 58% of all overseas born people in 1901 and only 20% in 2001 (DIMIA, 2001; ABS, 2002a).

The number of people recorded as Indigenous Australians has also increased in recent decades (from nearly 161,000 in 1976 to more than

427,000 in 2001, representing an increase from 1.2% to 2.2% of the total population) (ABS, 1994, 1998, 2003). This trend can be attributed not only to natural increase, but also to improved census coverage of this population and a greater inclination for people to identify as an Australian. Estimates of the size of the Indigenous population at the time of European settlement vary from 300,000 to more than one million (ABS, 2000).

Although multicultural diversity is diluted by intermarriage and the socialisation of children within an overarching culture that still carries strong British overtones, each successive wave of migration has made its mark on the ways Australian families live their lives, including the foods they eat, the sports they play, the religion (if any) they follow, and the languages they speak at home. However, another important influence on families is Australia's vast, "sunburnt country (with its) land of sweeping plains" (a quotation, which captures the essence of outback Australia, from a much-loved poem by Dorothea MacKellar 1904, entitled "My Country").

Spatial Concentration of Australian Families

In Australia, there are six states, two major mainland territories, and several minor territories. The states are New South Wales, Queensland, South Australia, Tasmania, Victoria and Western Australia and the two major mainland territories are the Northern Territory and the Australian Capital Territory. Each state and territory has its own governmental control, but the Commonwealth Parliament can override any legislation of the individual parliaments.

Where families live dictates fundamental aspects of their lifestyles, including their economic wellbeing. In terms of the number of people per kilometre, Australia is one of the most sparsely populated countries (fewer than three people per km) (ABS, 2000), but also has one of the most spatially concentrated populations. Most people live on the east and southwest coastlines, with 85% living within 50 km of the coast (ABS, 2001a). While Australians are often portrayed as "Battlers" roughing it in the "bush" (i.e., rural Australia), most Australians live in the suburban sprawl that surrounds its large cities. Government policies have attempted to contain this "sprawl" by encouraging medium density housing. The "bush" image, however, is historically accurate. Over the 20th century, the rural population fell from about 40% to less than 15%, with a concomitant fall in the proportion of workers in agriculture–from around 33% to less than 5% (Hugo, 2001).

In 2001, close to 40% of Australia's population (of more than 19 million) lived in Melbourne and Sydney and around 24% lived in the other five capital cities. People from overseas are particularly likely to settle in capital cities (81%, compared with 64% of the total population), especially Sydney and Melbourne (ABS, 2001).

The Structure of Australian Families

While at the beginning of the 20th Century, families often lived with other relatives and unrelated people including boarders, nuclear families increasingly predominated during the post-World War II period (ABS, 2001). Young women rejected life as domestic servants as opportunities opened up in manufacturing, retailing and non-domestic service industries, thereby requiring families that employed servants to reshape their lifestyles. This adjustment contributed to the increasing number of women across all social classes who became "housewives" (Gilding, 2001). As Gilding noted, the gradual introduction of government social security measures also meant that many families no longer needed to house vulnerable members of their kin, including the aged and disabled (see Figure 1 for details).

Although the most common family type is still a couple with dependent children, "couple only" (comprising parents whose children have left home and couples who have not (yet) had children) have almost caught up. In 1976, couples with dependent children represented nearly half (48%) of all families, while over one quarter (28%) were couple only families. In 2001, however, these types of families represented 39% and 36% of all families respectively. Families containing one parent have also increased (from 7% to 11% between 1976 and 2001). While one-parent family households have always existed, death of a parent was the primary reason for these cases in the early 20th century. By contrast, most of today's children who live in one-parent family households have a parent living elsewhere.

Likewise, stepfamilies have always existed, but were mostly formed by a widowed parent remarrying some 100 years ago. Under these circumstances, the children and their stepparent typically lived in the same household. Today, on the other hand, stepfamilies mostly result from parental separation following relationship breakdown. As a result, some children have a co-resident stepparent, some have a non-resident stepparent, and others have both. Of all couple family households with children under 18 years old in 2003, 5% were "co-resident step-families,"

FIGURE 1. Australia's Evolving Social Protection for Families

1900	Social Security System	None. Individuals and families in need had to rely on extended family networks or voluntary organizations. These organizations sometimes received assistance in the form of government grants
1909	Means-tested age pension	First forms of social security introduced at a national level
1910	Pensions for invalids	Introduced at a national level
1912	Maternity allowance	Introduced at the national level
1912	Social Security Benefit	Not payable as a lump sum-means tested
1914	War Widow's Pension	Introduced at the national level
1945	Unemployment & Sickness	Introduced at the national level
Benefits Currently Available:		
	Maternity Payment	Lump sum payment to the primary caretaker of each new baby, adopted child or child in foster care in the family born on or after 1 July 2004
	Parenting Payment	Income support payment for low-income families with caring responsibilities for a child under 16 years of age
	Parenting Payment (single)	Paid to single parents with no or low income
	Parenting Payment (partnered)	Paid (subject to income and assets tests) to the primary caretaker in a couple family where both parents have no income or a low income
	Maternity Immunization Allowance	Payment for children aged 18-24 months who are fully immunized or have an approved exemption from immunization
	Double Orphan Pension	Payment for children (under 16 or a full-time student) whose parents are dead or one is dead and the other cannot care for the child and, under certain circumstances, for refugee children
	Family Tax Benefit Part A	Paid (at three different rates) to low and middle income families with dependent children under 21 and/or dependent full-time students aged 21 to 24 years
	Family Tax Benefit Part B	A non-means tested payment providing additional assistance to single-income families, including single parents, with a child under 16 or a child aged 16 to 18 years studying full-time

and 4% were "blended" families (containing at least one natural child of the couple and one stepchild of one parent) (ABS, 2004).

The socio-economic circumstances of all these different families vary markedly. One-parent families, in particular, tend to be financially disadvantaged–a situation that has continued for decades despite the introduction of a scheme directed towards ensuring that separated parents support their children according to their capacity to do so. In fact, it has long been noted that the only way for many resident single mothers and their children to escape financial disadvantage is for the mother to repartner (Weston, 1986; Smyth and Weston, 2000; Kelly and Harding, 2005).

In contrast to the increasing diversity of family types and cultures, families have become less diverse in relation to the number of children born. Two-child families have become increasingly dominant, while families with four or more children have become unusual. Of women aged 40–44 years, the proportions who gave birth to two children increased from 29% in 1981 to 40% in 2001, while the proportion who had four or more children nearly halved (from 28% to 15%) and the proportion who remained childless increased (from 9% to 13%). Women giving birth when at least 30 years old are increasingly likely to be first-time mothers (38% of all first births in 2001 were to women of this age, compared with 28% in 1993) (ABS, 2002b). As a result, women are progressively shortening their total potential childbearing period, lowering their chance of having as many children as they might prefer and increasing their chance of childlessness. An exception to this would be Indigenous women, who have a fertility rate of 5.8, twice that of all Australian women (ABS, 2001b).

Changing Role of Parents

One of the most dramatic changes in family life has been the shift away from the male breadwinner: female homemaker model to one where couple parents increasingly shared the breadwinning role. This trend is linked with girls' increased participation in education. Until the mid-1970s, girls tended to leave school earlier than boys. This was consistent with the notion that they were destined to become full-time homemakers and that they were inherently suited for a narrow range of routine occupations. Indeed, it was not until 1966 that the Commonwealth Public Service permitted married women to be appointed or remain as permanent officers in the Commonwealth Service and to return to their jobs after the birth of their children. Increasing numbers of women maintained some attachment to the labour force upon having children. In 2005, dual employment applied to 58% of couple families with dependent children in the home. Of these families, 42% of mothers were working full-time and 58% were working part-time (ABS, 2005a).

A combination of "push and pull" factors have contributed to this major shift in parenting roles, including increases in housing costs, the prolonged financial dependency of children, the increased availability of part-time and casual work as well as formal child care services, the opportunity costs of not working, and various changes in legislation and national policies that have improved women's education and employment opportunities, and wages.

As the importance of mothers' breadwinning role increased, fathers have been called upon to play a more active role in domestic life. While the average amount of time fathers devote exclusively to their children has increased, mothers still take on most of the responsibilities for home making and nurturing the children (Bittman, Craig & Folbré, 2004).

Relationship Breakdown

Another clear way in which family functioning has changed is reflected in the above-noted increase in families with separated parents. It is now more than 30 years since the Family Law Act 1975 was introduced. The Act allowed a divorce based on only one ground–"irretrievable breakdown,"as measured by at least 12 months of separation.This led to a spectacular rise in the divorce rate, and the ABS estimates that around one third of marriages are likely to end in divorce (ABS, 2002c).

However, the divorce rate has become a poor indicator of relationship breakdown, given that many couples (especially young couples) cohabit rather than marry. While the vast majority of men and women under 25 years old do not have partners, those who have partners are more likely to be cohabiting than married (82% vs. 18% of partnered individuals under 20 years old, and 61% vs. 39% of partnered individuals aged 20-24 years). For older age groups, marriage increasingly dominates (ABS, 2001). However, cohabitation tends to be short-lived (lasting no more than five years) and the chances of the relationship converting to separation or marriage are now almost the same (Weston, Qu & de Vaus, 2003).

Implications of Partnership Trends for the Other Transitions

The increasing trend towards starting partnerships with cohabitation has been accompanied by an increase in unwed births (from 9% in 1971 to 32% in 2003). Little is known about the relationship trajectories of these families, although it appears that a pregnancy or first birth amongst cohabiting couples increases the likelihood that cohabiting couples will marry (Weston, Qu & de Vaus, 2005). Secondly, while most children spend all of their childhood with both natural parents, an increasing proportion of children spend some or all of their childhood apart from one natural parent. By age 18, 30% of children who were born 1976-1983 had experience some period of their life without one natural parent (de Vaus & Gray, 2003).

FUTURE CHALLENGES FOR AUSTRALIAN FAMILY LIEE

The trends outlined above have resulted in a number of challenges facing Australia. For example, the fall in fertility rates and the significant improvement in life expectancy have inevitably resulted in an "aging" of the population both in absolute and relative terms. According to the Australian Bureau of Statistics (2005b) projections, the representation of children under 15 years in the total population will fall from 20% in 2004 to around 15% by 2051, while that of people aged 65 years and over will increase from 13% to 26-28% of the population. The proportion of the population of the traditional working age (15-64 years) is projected to fall from 67% in 2004 to around 60% between 2031-2041.

Various repercussions of these trends have been suggested, including a higher tax burden for the working population given the greater costs of elderly people than children; potential growing resentment between the generations as a result of this tax burden; changing demand for services such as housing, health care, leisure, and education, with those for families with dependent children being "fewer and far between"; an aging workforce reinforced by policies encouraging later retirement and relative loss of young adults whose age-related talents often produce important technological advancements; and possibly a society that becomes progressively less "child-friendly." In addition, while there is considerable evidence that families are the most significant sources of support for the elderly, increasing rates of childlessness coupled with family breakdown and children pursuing jobs overseas, will mean that many elderly parents have no children to provide support (see Weston, Qu, Parker & Alexander, 2004). Such social and economic implications of aging populations are clearly pressing matters for South Australia and Tasmania, given that these states have the highest concentration of elderly people are projected to be the first states to experience natural decline (an increase in births over deaths).

The process of urbanization continues to have different effects for different localities, with many of the country towns that exhibit the greatest growth being located within or just beyond commuting distance of major cities, while those experiencing static or declining populations being in less accessible areas, with out-migration from these areas being dominated by young people who have recently left high school. These less accessible areas tend to be the most socially disadvantaged (Hugo, 2002) and their declining in populations and services have intensified (Collits, 2001).

Although ageing of the population is inevitable in the next few decades, a key challenge for Australia is to prevent further falls in fertility and therefore ensure that those who would like to have a first or additional child can achieve their ambition. While surveys suggest that less than 10% of childless men and women do not want any children, various projections suggest that up to one quarter of young women today will not have children (see Weston et al., 2004).

The fragility of couple relationships also continues to represent a challenge for Australia. In some cases this leads to dashed hopes about having children, and in others, it leads to considerable financial disadvantage and disruption for children. The increase in the proportion of children who experience parental separation has important implications, given that such children have an increased risk of experiencing immediate and long-term adverse outcomes, with multiple transitions being more problematic than a single transition (see de Vaus and Gray, 2003). Furthermore, around one million children aged under 18 years old live have a parent living elsewhere, and around 26% of children have little or no contact with one of their parents (ABS, 2004). On 1 July 2006, the Australian Government introduced a new family law system which has several aims, including: helping to prevent separation and build strong, healthy family relationships; and, in the event of separation, encouraging the involvement of both parents in their children's lives (where it is safe to do so); protecting children from violence; encouraging parents to reach agreements outside the court; and ensuring that any parenting proceedings in the court are child-focused. By July 2008, there will be 65 Family Relationship Centres across Australia, which will provide three hours of free dispute resolution to help parents reach agreement about arrangements for their children after separation and make appropriate referrals to other services. Many other relationship support services for families facing difficulties are also being expanded.

Women's participation in the workforce continues to increase and has called for many adjustments in the home, workplace and community to help couples have and raise healthy and well-adjusted children, care for elderly relatives, and have the time to nurture their own relationship and enjoy family life. The adjustments required relate particularly to workplace flexibility, fathers' contributions on the home front, and the nature and hours of operation of services for children, parents and extended families.

Finally, there will always be families facing multiple disadvantages. Many Indigenous families are a case in point, given their higher risk of exposure to complex, interacting problems including unemployment (13% compared to 5% for non-Indigenous), poverty (four times more likely than the non-Indigenous to have financial stress), family violence (double the victimization rate of the non-Indigenous population) and alcohol abuse (more likely than non-Indigenous to drink excessively). In addition, many Indigenous families live in remote areas of Australia, where access to employment and services such as healthcare, communications, and community services are very limited (ABS, 2005c).

AUSTRALIAN FAMILY STRENGTHS

The Family Action Centre (FAC) (Faculty of Health, University of Newcastle) conducted the Australian Family Strengths Research Project (Geggie, 2000) in 1999, with funding from the Australian Government Department of Families, Community Services and Indigenous Affairs. A national advertising campaign enlisted over 600 parents who considered their families to be "strong" to participate in a survey designed to ascertain (a) the characteristics of their families that they consider to be their strengths and (b) the language they use to describe these strengths. This was the first study of its kind in Australia and involved the use of a list of 85 positive statements about family life, developed for the project by DeFrain (2000), and 14 open-ended questions on family structure, strengths, challenges, stress, commitment, communication, affection, spirituality, family time, and role division.

One theme that emerged from the respondents' perceptions of their families in the research captures the essence of being strong–*resilience*. Walsh (1998) previously described resilience as the ability to withstand and rebound from crises and diversity. Indeed, around half the respondents in the Australian family Strengths Research Project, indicated that they became aware of their family's strengths when their family was faced with serious challenges. Seven other themes emerged that may be seen as important means by which such resilience is achieved. These were: (i) open, positive and honest *communication* (with some families mentioning humor as a strength in their communication);

(ii) *togetherness*– the "invisible glue" linked with the sharing of values, beliefs and morals that bonds the families and provides them with a sense of belonging; (iii) *sharing activities*, such as sports and hobbies, camping, games, reading stories, socializing, holidays; (iv) regular expressions of *affection* (i.e., love, care, concern and interest for each other) through hugs, cuddles, kisses and thoughtfulness; (v) regular expressions of *support*, such as assisting, encouraging, reassuring and "looking out for each other"; (vi) regular expressions of *acceptance*, as reflected inrespect, appreciation and understanding of each other's individuality and therefore tolerance of differences; and (vii) readily apparent signs of *commitment*, for example, showing dedication and loyalty toward the family as a whole and to the co-parental relationship, parent-child relationships, sibling relationships, the extended family and/or community. Although these outcomes are based on stories from families who considered themselves as strong, it is important to recognise that all families have their strengths. It is these strengths and the ability to identify these strengths that assist families in challenging times.

The Nature and Influence of Family Strengths Research on Practice and Policy

By the end of the 20th century the strengths perspective to family issues gained momentum and was widely accepted as an empowering approach to deal with entrenched and chronic issues. Australian practitioners have extended on the frameworks within the strengths perspective that were initially developed by Jody Kretzmann and John McKnight, and brief solution-focused therapy (White & Epston, 1990). These approaches focus on what is working well rather than on what is missing in a family's life. They acknowledge and recognise the ability of many families to endure extreme hardship and survive seemingly insurmountable challenges (Silberberg, 2001). These approaches encourage practitioners to listen differently–to listen in awe of the family's resilience. Families who are in the thick of their struggle often lose sight of their strengths and their previous successes to overcome challenges.

The strengths perspective views the family as the expert of their family life and therefore the best persons to consult on the pathway of change (Clay & Silberberg, 2004). It views professional workers as facilitators who walk alongside family members, supporting them to set their own agenda for change, rather than leading them along paths that the workers deem appropriate. Workers facilitate the process of change by hearing the weight of the family's problems, highlighting their strengths, including skills and resources, and helping them draw upon these to achieve their vision of change. Such an approach appears to be particularly effective for practitioners who are dealing with families whose health and wellbeing outcomes are minimised by contextual forces.

Government Policies

At state and federal levels in Australia, there has been an increasing move up the public political agenda of the importance of early childhood development and the community's role in creating the conditions that support the healthy development of young Australians. This interest in the first few years of a child's life, is based on neuroscientific research suggesting that nutrition, care and nurturing directly affect the wiring of the brain's pathways in the first three years of life, thereby influencing children's learning, behaviour and health throughout life (DHS, 2001). In response, an array of programs for families with very young children have been implemented worldwide, involving home visits, parent education, preschools, and community programs. Virtually all these initiatives are strength-focused and promote service delivery models that empower the individual and the community by embracing sustainability, self-reliance, resilience and self-determination. The family services that have become available within the community in recent times have extended the support families can access to beyond that of the family unit, with Uncle Arthur's story (see Figure 2) highlighting this development.

At a national level, strength-focused initiatives include the *National Stronger Families and Community Strategy*, an important policy framework of the Australian Government's Department of Community Services and Indigenous Affairs. The current second four-year phase focuses on early intervention projects developed at a local community level (for details, see: http://www.facsia.gov.au).

Most State and Territory Governments have developed comprehensive plans targeting the developmental needs of young children with a strong focus on early intervention, family support and overcoming disadvantage. Examples include: (a) the *Australian Capital Territory Children's Plan* (2004-14), a plan entailing several principles including strength-focus and inclusiveness, that will guide decisions by government and non-government sectors about policies, programs and services for children up to 2 years of age (ACT, 2004); (b) the *New South Wales: Families First–a better start for children in New South Wales*,

FIGURE 2. Uncle Arthur's Story

An insight from my own family's history gives an opportunity to reflect on families, with an eye both to the present and the future. This personal anecdote reflects the key importance of families for children's development, illustrates the strengths they bring to facing and overcoming challenges, and highlights the difference in the supports available to families then and now (Hayes, 1996).

My Uncle's birth, on the eve of the First World War, was not an entirely positive event. Uncle Arthur, my Mother's youngest brother, was born with Down's Syndrome. The prognosis was bleak. For his cohort of children with Down's Syndrome, the survival age was less than ten years. Within the family, the mythology was that he did not have Down's Syndrome, or Mongolism as it was then labelled, but had suffered brain injury as a result of a complicated birth to an elderly mother. His first year was marked by repeated illnesses. One evening, in exasperation at yet another late night call out, the community nurse finally told my Grandmother that it was better to "let him go."

My Grandmother chose to ignore that advice. She sat up nursing him and administering brandy from a teaspoon. Against the odds, he survived, and the earliest photo that I can remember of him is as a nine or ten year old, with a wicked grin in his eye, preparing to take a pot shot with a slingshot at a cameraman who was endeavouring to take a very formal 1920s family photograph. Space precludes a full history of Uncle Arthur and his place in our family, but suffice it to say that with the ongoing commitment of my Grandparents and his siblings, against the odds, Uncle Arthur lived to the age of 64. He had quite a full life, with some home schooling and occasional part-time employment. Uncle Arthur was a much-loved member of our family, and was generally well accepted by his community. The love of his family, and the strength of their commitment to him, was keys to the quality of his life. As were the informal supports of friends and neighbours and the opportunity to live within his family and their community.

There is, however, an interesting postscript to the story. He was probably not my Grandmother's child, but the offspring of one of her unmarried daughters. Acceptance and tolerance had their limits then, as they do now. Of course, now, for children with disabilities, life in the community is taken for granted, and occurs against the backdrop of very sophisticated family services and supports for children's development, health and wellbeing. I cannot imagine what Uncle Arthur's life would be like were he to have been born now. While disability was less visible then, systematic supports for persons with disabilities and their families were simply not available.

Today, many organizations and agencies provide the comprehensive and extensive supports that my family lacked as they strove to give Uncle Arthur a good start in life, and the opportunities to develop despite his disability. The world has indeed changed for families, and families have changed in ways, and at a pace, that has been truly remarkable.

Alan Hayes

a strengths-based initiative introduced in 1998 to provide a support network to all families with children from 0-8 years, involving locally developed community programs such as family worker services, supported playgroups, volunteer home visiting services, schools as community centres (New South Wales Government (NSWG, 2001); (c) *Victoria: Best Start*, a prevention and early intervention project that aims to improve the health, development, learning and wellbeing of Victorian children, through such measures as the establishment of partnerships and linkages within and across communities, including linkages between existing services (DSH, 2002); (d) *Queensland: Families–Future Directions,* which primarily focuses on prevention and early intervention services for young people whose families are in crisis, or lack the means to ensure their children advance at school and beyond (QG, 2002); (e) *Western Australia: Early Years Strategy,* which was launched in 2003 and was subsequently expanded and incorporated into the *Children First Strategy*–a program designed to achieve several outcomes including helping families and communities to identify their priorities and develop appropriate plans, coordinating policies and programs across departments and organizations, establishing working groups to focus on priority areas, and developing creative ways for reaching children and families who are in most need of services (WAG, 2003); (f) *South Australia: Department for Families and Communities*–a department created in mid-2004 that will involve all its agencies working together to provide integrated services to protect the wellbeing of children, young people, families and communities (GoSA, 2004); and (g) *Tasmania: Our Kids Action Plan,* which was launched in 2003 with the aim of enhancing the resilience of children and families (DoHHS, 2004).

The Service Provider's Perspective

Many service organizations in Australia use a strength-based approach in service delivery. One example, St. Lukes Anglicare, Bendigo is well known throughout Australia for its innovative, whole-of-agency incorporation of a strengths-based philosophy. In the late 1980s St Lukes pioneered its then radical model for delivering family services. It also spawned *Innovative Resources*–a unique publishing and training venture that has equipped countless family workers and other human service workers around the world with practical, hands-on material for identifying and mobilising client strengths.

Another example is the Family Action Centre, one organization that has been on the forefront of promoting strengths-based practice. The Family Action Centre (FAC) is located at the University of Newcastle and combines community service, research dissemination and advocacy on issues relating to family support and building community capacity. It adopts a strength-based approach in all its programs and has developed many related resources to assist practitioners across Australia. Two specific examples of this approach are outlined below.

Boys in School. In Australia, a growing concern over the poor academic performance, (ACER, 2002; 2003; DETYA, 2000; Rowe & Rowe, 2002) disrespectful behaviours and apparent lack of direction of many boys sparked an inquiry in 2002 by the Australian Government into the education of boys (Department of Education, Science and Training [DEST], 2002). Research points to differences between boys and girls in reading comprehension (up from 3% in 1975 to 8% in 1995) and school retention rates (up from 0% difference before 1976 to 11.6% difference in 1990). In addition, 80% of those suspended from school are boys as suspensions increase as boys move into the upper grade levels (*Boys: Getting It Right*, October, 2002). Governments and schools in the last five years have invested resources into developing strategies and programs that best tackle boys' education. Schools that are having success in improving both the social and academic outcomes for boys are adopting strategies that could be characterised as strength-based. The *Boys in Schools Program* at the Family Action Centre has assisted many schools across Australia in this process. The Boys in School program offers a range of services for schools and educational bodies that include workshops and seminars, postgraduate courses in boys' education, and books and teaching resources.

A strength-based approach begins with identifying what is already going really well in a school (Hartman, 2006). Schools identify the strengths of the boys and of the teachers, schools and the community. Without being naively "sweet" about boys or dismissive of the difficulties that some boys present, there is an acknowledgement that every boy, no matter how "difficult," has strengths that can be used and extended. The schools analyse a broad range of school-based data to give them clues about where they are, and are not, progressing well with the boys and use this information to identify priority concerns and shape their intervention. Through this approach, resources have been developed to assist schools to improve the boys' self-images, promote positive images of boys to teachers, and to provide teachers with approach, reward and appraisal systems. As a result, after one program was conducted, the violence and behavior referrals have decreased and suspensions were down by 50% despite a 30% growth of the school population (Hartman, 2006). In 2005, the program was implemented in over 20 schools in Victoria, New South Wales and Queensland. Of most satisfaction was with three schools in particular (one in each state) that have conducted in-depth and long-term action learning projects. Results from these schools, while still in the preliminary stages, indicate greater student engagement and motivation indicated by better attendance, decreases in behaviour problems and increases in academic results. Teachers also reported improved job satisfaction.

Engaging Fathers Project. Social changes cause ripple effects requiring other adjustments to be made, yet responses can be slow to evolve. A key example of this lagged effect relates to the increased participation of mothers in paid work that has called for adjustments in the home, workplace and community. Research indicates that children do better educationally and academically when their fathers are involved in the education. Children learn more, exhibit healthier behavior, and have increased self-esteem when their fathers play an active role in their learning (Ortiz, 2001). Although there is some evidence that fathers are more actively engaged in their children's lives (McBride, Rane & Bay, 2000; Ortiz & Stile, 2000), a recent study of family-related services in the Hunter Region of NSW indicated that only 5% of users were men (Fletcher, Silberberg & Baxter, 2001). It seems likely that a low level of usage applies across Australian communities.

Another issue of concern is for non-custodial fathers. Around one million children under 18 live with one parent. For 88% of these children, the parent is their mother. Approximately one in three of these one million children have little if any contact with their father (Smyth & Weston, 2003). The role that fathers play in the family is a national concern. In 2005, a significant focus on father's engagement at the national level led to the Father's Inclusive Practice Forum for the Commonwealth Government and the result was A Framework for Father Inclusive Practices for Family Service Providers. The Australian Institute of Family Studies, a source of research expertise to the government of Australia, recently set out their research plan for 2006-2008 that included the impact of fathers on the long-term wellbeing of children (Families through Life, 2006).

The Engaging Fathers Project, funded by the Bernard van Leer Foundation, aimed to increase the number of fathers or father-figures who access ante and postnatal services, parent education courses, schools, and other family support services). The project team found that many practitioners (who are predominantly female in family services) believed that men were either not interested or not available to attend their service. The team therefore worked with services to develop strategies to attract fathers to their service. The strength-based approach has proven to be particularly effective in this endeavour. It sought to identify the skills of the fathers and the means by which the service could engage fathers and use their strengths for the benefit of the service, the father and the children.

For example, teachers in a pre-school in a disadvantaged socioeconomic area developed skills/assets/gifts maps of the children's fathers in order to engage these men who had previously been difficult to engage, even in conversations. Through this approach, one unemployed father who would literally run out the door as quickly as possible when leaving his child at the pre-school, was able to share his hobby of raising birds with all the children attending the centre. Children were able to observe the whole breeding cycle of the pigeons and budgerigars over several months. The father's belief in the importance of his role and what he had to offer his child increased significantly.

The Engaging Fathers Project team has also investigated the service delivery and needs of young Aboriginal fathers in the Hunter Valley region (Hammond, Fletcher, Hester, & Pascoe, 2004). (Indigenous Australians tend to enter parenthood at a much younger age than non-Indigenous Australians.) Their study showed that the young fathers lacked access to positive images of Indigenous fathers engaging with their infants or young children. The team worked with many local Indigenous fathers to produce a series of posters that provide clear, positive messages for the waiting room at the regional hospital's birthing unit. These replaced existing posters that focused on domestic violence. Messages conveyed include: *Our Kids Need Dads Who: Stay Strong, Smile, Take an Interest, Be There and Listen.* An eight-minute video was also produced, conveying images of Indigenous fathers engaged in simple activities with their children–bathing their baby, playing with their children on the swings, playing ball games, wrestling and helping small children with their meals was produced.

CONCLUSION

The above short but effervescent history of Australia has highlighted a range of changes to the stereotypical 'family' unit. The reasons for such changes are varied and the pace of change has gained impetus in the past 30 years. It is therefore more important than ever to identify ways of helping families meet their diverse daily and longer-term challenges.

While Australia's history has created a unique societal composition, the basic needs of the Australian family and community are relevant to all societies. Regardless of religion, ethnicity, gender or family type, all children have a fundamental right to be raised in family environments that meet their physical, emotional, educational, and social needs and thereby help them to mature into well-adjusted and active participants of society in adulthood.

However, "it takes a village to raise a child"–a village that is a source of much strength to families. Families need support that is directed to children, parents (or potential parents) and extended family members to help them draw upon their own strengths and those of their "village" to fulfil their many roles (e.g., parents, partners, adult children, grandparents, workers, friends, and community members). It is the role of the governments, relevant agencies, community groups and broader society to recognise that all families have strengths; to support families to draw on these strengths and to provide them with other resources they need to meet their diverse challenges. Furthermore, all policy directed towards strengthening family and community capacity may need to be in place for several years before outcomes become sustainable.

Perhaps it is best to conclude with a real world experience: how one of the participants in the *Family Strengths Research Project* explains the way in which he and other family members draw in their strengths to withstand setbacks and crises, to adapt to changing circumstances, and to think positively towards the challenges of life. All families need the same potential for success.

> *We just need to calm down, take a deep breath and relax, rethink the situation in a positive light–how and why is this going to make us better people in the future The key to NOT turning that moment into a real bad memory, {but} that we kept a positive, opportunity-based attitude on the experience. (Father in a nuclear family)*

REFERENCES

ABS (1994). *Australian Social Trends*. Catalogue No. 4102.0, Canberra: Australian Bureau of Statistics.

ABS (1998). Australian Demographic Trends 1997. Catalogue No. 3102.0. Canberra: Australian Bureau of Statistics.

ABS (2000). *Australian Social Trends 2000*. Catalogue No. 4102.0. Canberra: Australian Bureau of Statistics.

ABS (2001a). *Census of Population and Housing: Australia in Profile–A Regional Analysis*. Catalogue No. 2032.0. Canberra: Australian Bureau of Statistics.

ABS (2001b). *Statistical Geography*, Volume 1, Australian Standard Geographical Classification (ASGC), 2001, Catalogue No. 1216.0, Canberra: Australian Bureau of Statistics.

ABS (2002a). *Census of Population and Housing: Selected Social and Housing Characteristics, Australia*. Catalogue No. 2015.0. Canberra: Australian Bureau of Statistics.

ABS (2002b). *Births Australia 2001.* Catalogue No. 3301.0. Canberra: Australian Bureau of Statistics.

ABS (2002c). *Marriages and Divorces 2001.* Catalogue No. 3310.0. Canberra: Australian Bureau of Statistics.

ABS (2003). *Australian Social Trends.* Catalogue No. 4102.0. Canberra: Australian Bureau of Statistics.

ABS (2004). *Family Characteristics Australia 2003.* Catalogue No. 4442.0. Canberra: Australian Bureau of Statistics.

ABS (2005a). *Australia: Labour force status and other characteristics of families–* electronic delivery (ST FA5). Catalogue No. 6224.0.55.001. Canberra: Australian Bureau of Statistics.

ABS (2005b). *Population Projections Australia 2004-2101,* Catalogue No. 3222.0, Canberra: Australian Bureau Statistics.

ABS (2005c). *The Health and Welfare of Australia's Aboriginal and Torres Strait Islander Peoples,* Catalogue No. 20054704.0, Canberra: Australian Bureau Statistics.

ACER (2002). *Achievement in literacy and numeracy 1975-98.* Report 29 of the longitudinal survey of Australian youth (LSAY).

ACER (2003). *Gender differences in educational and labour market outcomes,* Report 8 of the longitudinal survey of Australian youth (LSAY).

ACER (2003). *School leavers in Australia: profiles and pathways,* Report 31 of the longitudinal survey of Australian youth (LSAY).

ACT (2004). *ACT Children's Plan,* 2004-2014. Australian Capital Territory, [Online http://www.children.act.gov.au/pdf/childrensplan.pdf#search=%22www.children.act.gov.au%2Fpdf.childrensplan%22]

Bittman, M., Craig, L., & Folbré, N. (2004). Packaging care: What happens when children receive nonparental care? In N. Folbré and M. Bittman (Eds.), *Family Time: The Social Organization of Care* (pp. 133-151), London: Routledge.

Boys: Getting It Right (October, 2002). Report to the House of Representatives Standing Committee on Education and Training, Canberra: The Parliament of the Commonwealth of Australia.

Clay, V., & Silberberg, S. (2004). *Resilience Identification Resources.* Family Action Centre, Faculty of Health, University of Newcastle.

Collits, P. (2001). Small town decline and survival: Trends, causes and policy issues. In M. F. Rogers and Y. M. J. Collins (Eds.) *The Future of Australia's Country Towns,* Bendigo, Centre for Sustainable Regional Communities, La Trobe University.

DeFrain, J. (2000). What is a strong family, anyway? University of Nebraska-Lincoln, For Families website: http://unlforfamilies.unl.edu.

DEST (2002). House of Representatives Standing Committee on Education and Training Inquiry into Vocational Education in Australian Schools. Department of Education, Science and Training of the Australian Government [Online http://www.dest.gov.au]

DETYA (2000). Submission to the House of Representatives Standing Committee on Employment, education and Workplace Relations, Inquiry into the Education of Boys.

DHS (2001). *Best Start: The Evidence Base Underlying Investment in the Early Years (children 0-8 years).* Department of Human Services, State Government of Victoria. [Online http://www.beststart.vic.gov.au/docs/evidence_base_project_1002v1.2.pdf]

DHS (2002). *Best Start.* Department of Human Services, State Government of Victoria. [Online http://www.beststart.vic.gov.au]

DeVaus, D., & Gray, M. (2003). Family transitions among Australia's children. *Family Matters, 65,* 10-17.

DIMIA (2001). *Immigration–Federation to Century's End 1901-2001,* Australian Government Department of Immigration and Multicultural and Indigenous Affairs Department of Immigration and Multicultural and Indigenous Affairs.

DoHHS (2004). *Our Kids Action Plan, Working Towards a holistic Response for Tasmania's Children 2004-2007.* Department·of Health and Human Services Tasmania. [Online http://www.dhhs.tas.gov.au/agency/pro/ourkids/documents/5394_ActionPlan.pdf]

Families Through Life: Diversity, Change and Context. (2006). *Family Matters, 73,* 4-12.

Fletcher, R., Silberberg, S., & Baxter, R. (2001). *Father's Access to Family Related Services.* Report produced for Hunter Families First, NSW Department of Community Services.

Gilding, M. (2001). Changing families in Australia 1901-2001. *Family Matters, 60,* 6-11.

Geggie, J., DeFrain, J., Hitchcock, S., & Silberberg, S. (2000). Family Strengths Project.

Government of South Australia (2004). *Connecting individuals, families and communities* Department for Families and Communities, Government of South Australia [Online http://www.familiesandcommunities.sa.gov.au/]

Hammond, C., Fletcher. R., Hester, J., & Pascoe, S. (2004). *Young Aboriginal Fathers Project.* Research Report produced by the Family Action Centre and Umulliko Centre for the NSW Department of Aboriginal Affairs.

Hartman D. (2006). *Educating Boys–The Good News.* Adelaide: Griffin Press.

Hayes, A. (1996). "Family life in community context." In B. Stratford & P. Gunn (Eds.), *New approaches to Down Syndrome* (pp. 369-404), London: Cassell.

Hugo, G. (2001). "A century of population change in Australia." *In Year Book of Australia 2001.* Catalogue No. 1301.0. Canberra: Australian Bureau of Statistics.

Hugo, G. (2002). *Regional Australian Populations: Diversity Dynamism and Dichotomy.* Paper presented at the Academy of the Social Sciences Session on Rural Communities at the Outlook 2002 Conference, Canberra, 5-7 March.

Kelly, S., & Harding, A. (2005). *Love can hurt, divorce will cost: Financial impact of divorce in Australia,* AMP: NATSEM Income and Wealth Report Issue 10. National Centre for Social and Economic Modelling Pty Ltd, published by AMP. [ONLINE: http://www.natsem.canberra.edu.au/publications.jsp]

McBride, B., Rane, T., & Bay, J. (2000). Intervening with teachers to encourage father/male involvement in early childhood programs, *Early Childhood Research Quarterly, 16,* 77-93.

NSWG (2001). *Families First–a better start for children in New South Wales.* New South Wales Government [Online: http://www.familiesfirst.nsw.gov.au]

QG (2002). *Families–Future Directions.* Queensland Government [Online http://www.thepremier.qld.gov.au/library/pdf/DPC048Families.pdf]

Oritz, R., & Stile, S. (2000). Training Fathers to Develop Reading and Writing Skills in Young Children with Disabilities, paper presented at the Head Start National Research Conference 5th, Washington, DC 28 June-1 July, 2000.

Rowe, K. J., & Rowe, K. S. (2002). *What matters most: Evidence-based findings of key factors affecting the educational experiences and outcomes for girls and boys throughout their primary and secondary schooling*, invited supplementary submission to House of representatives Standing committee on Education and Training Inquiry into the Education of Boys, ACER & Department of General Paediatrics, Royal Children's Hospital, Victoria.

Silberberg, S. (2001). Searching for family resilience. *Family Matters*, *58*, 52-57.

Smyth, B., & Weston, R. (2000). *Financial living standards after divorce: A recent snapshot*, Research Paper No. 23. Australian Institute of Family Studies, Melbourne. [ONLINE: http://www.aifs.gov.au/institute/pubs/smyth.html]

Smyth, B., & Weston, R. (August, 2003). *Researching fathers: Back to basics.* Paper presented to National Strategic Conference on Fatherhood, Parliament House Canberra.

WAG (2003). *Early Years Strategy*. Western Australian Government. [Online http://www.earlyyears.wa.gov.au]

Walsh, F. (1998). *Strengthening Family Resilience*. New York: Guilford Press.

Weston, R. E. (1986). Changes in household income circumstances. In P. McDonald (Ed.) *Settling up: Property and income distribution on divorce in Australia*. Sydney: Australian Institute of Family Studies and Prentice-Hall of Australia.

Weston, R., de Vaus, D., & Qu, L. (2003). Partnership formation and stability, Paper presented at the National Conference, National Council on Family Relations, Vancouver, 19-22 November.

Weston, R., Qu, L., & de Vaus, D. (2005). Pathways from cohabitation. Paper presented at the HILDA Survey Research Conference 2005. University of Melbourne, September.

Weston, R., Qu, L., Parker, R., & Alexander, M. (2004). It's not for lack of wanting kids: A report on the Fertility Decision Making Project, Research Report No.11, Australian Institute of Family Studies. [Online: http://www.aifs.gov.au]

White, M., & Epston, D. (1990). *Narrative means to therapeutic ends*. New York: Norton.

doi:10.1300/J002v41n03_01

New Zealand Families

Richard Cook

SUMMARY. Family life in New Zealand benefits from a bountiful natural environment and a bicultural heritage. As the first people of the land, Maori contribute rich relational attributes that affect people of all cultures who have settled here. Health, education, welfare and economic realities create particular challenges for New Zealand families, especially those at the lower end of the socio-economic spectrum. Labor shortages and the leeching of highly skilled and qualified people offshore in the pursuit of higher incomes places strain on the infrastructure, yet families particularly enjoy time together in the beauty of the land, commitment to the raising of families and the richness of cultural diversity. doi:10.1300/J002v41n03_02 *[Article copies available for a fee from The Haworth Document Delivery Service: 1-800-HAWORTH. E-mail address: <docdelivery@haworthpress.com> Website: <http://www.HaworthPress.com> © 2007 by The Haworth Press, Inc. All rights reserved.]*

KEYWORDS. Challenges, culture, family strengths, New Zealand families

Richard Cook, MCouns, is Senior Lecturer, Bethlehem Tertiary Institute, Private Bag 12015, Tauranga, New Zealand (E-mail: r.cook@bethlehem.ac.nz).
The author would like to acknowledge his wife, Lucelle, for the wonderful family she has partnered in creating and his parents who showed what commitment to family means.

[Haworth co-indexing entry note]: "New Zealand Families." Cook, Richard. Co-published simultaneously in *Marriage & Family Review* (The Haworth Press, Inc.) Vol. 41, No. 3/4, 2007, pp. 241-259; and: *Strong Families Around the World: Strengths-Based Research and Perspectives* (ed: John DeFrain, and Sylvia M. Asay) The Haworth Press, Inc., 2007, pp. 241-259. Single or multiple copies of this article are available for a fee from The Haworth Document Delivery Service [1-800-HAWORTH, 9:00 a.m. - 5:00 p.m. (EST). E-mail address: docdelivery@haworthpress.com].

Available online at http://mfr.haworthpress.com
© 2007 by The Haworth Press, Inc. All rights reserved.
doi:10.1300/J002v41n03_02

INTRODUCTION

About New Zealand

Barry Crump was a famous New Zealander whose rugged "down on the farm" appearance and voice epitomises one picture of New Zealand and her people. His book, *The Half-Dozen, Quarter-Acre, Pavlova Paradise* (Crump, 1972), was a bestseller for many years. From earliest colonial times, having a piece of land has been most families' dream. The quarter-acre section has given New Zealand low-density housing, with towns and cities often nestled into harbours, bays, and inlets around its considerable coastline.

New Zealand is a similar size to Japan and Great Britain in terms of land area–but not in population. It is a young country geologically, with many large mountain ranges, most along fault lines and many with dramatic upwards thrusting land forms. In the far north are isolated towns that have suffered from a prolonged exodus to the cities. Poised on a narrow isthmus is New Zealand's largest city, Auckland. It sprawls along the coastlines, rolls over low hilly terrain, circles a number of extinct volcanic landmarks and spreads up and down the east and west coasts to the shorelines, where millionaire owners enjoy the expansive sea views.

In the middle of the North Island is a large volcanic plateau. The most famous city for tourists is Rotorua, with boiling mud pools and geysers. Farms of various descriptions are the key feature of the landscape and the economy. The rugged hills of the capital Wellington bring the North Island to an abrupt end at Cook Strait. Ferries and planes are needed to cross this sometimes treacherous stretch of water.

Once across, the beauty of the South Island fiords, Alps, and plains captivate visitor and resident alike. While much bigger than the North Island, the population density is noticeably less in the South, and there is a more provincial and conservative atmosphere. A land of contrasts, New Zealand offers outdoor, water sport, ski, and sporting enthusiasts the paradise Barry Crump spoke of. This is a rich resource for families who frequently develop an enthusiasm for an outdoor pursuit and pass that down from generation to generation.

Temperate would describe the New Zealand climate. The long coastline bathes in the warm Pacific currents balanced by the chills of Antarctic wind flows. New Zealanders also tend to be temperate people, known for their "laid-back," informal, and leisurely ways. Immigrants often comment on the laissez-faire approach of Kiwis, as New Zealanders are affectionately called when compared to more formal and structured societies. A well-known Kiwi phrase is "She'll be right, Mate." It signifies a reluctance to get too concerned about an issue, and a belief that events will work out without too much effort needed.

People travelling overseas know that New Zealand is also a very isolated country. A long way from anywhere, it has earned the nick-name "down under" just as it is in Australia, away from those from the Northern Hemisphere. It is this isolation that has produced phrases like "Kiwi ingenuity." This fond New Zealand myth holds that a piece of number eight gauge fencing wire can be used to fix anything that is broken.

The People

New Zealand now has a population of just over four million. 75.8% of these are European and 13.8% are Maori. Many years of immigration have also seen many other cultures settle in the country: 4.5% of New Zealanders are Asian, 5.3% from various Polynesian islands and 0.6% from other places in the world. The multi-cultural nature of New Zealand is an increasingly obvious phenomenon, especially in Auckland where 33% of the city's population were born overseas–especially from the Pacific Islands (Statistics NZ, 2005a). This creates overt racial tensions in some communities, but also a simmering undercurrent of European nationalism across the country. Again, this becomes evident when politicians on the campaign trail touch this sensitive issue.

The ethnocentrism of many *Pakeha* (European) New Zealanders has meant that political parties surge in popular support when they object to the assistance of Maori and recompense for land loss. But this view ignores the fact that Maori family life in New Zealand is plagued by disproportionately high levels of struggle in health, employment, and educational achievement (Statistics NZ, 2005a). Health issues were highlighted in the report *"Progress Towards Closing Social and Economic Gaps Between Màori and Non-Maori,"* which identified that Maori health status levels are considerably lower than those of non-Maori across a range of health indicators. In addition, the official unemployment rate for Maori is 19% as compared to the non-Maori rate of 6%. (Te Puni Kòkiri, 2000).

History shows Maori to be remarkably resourceful. Early in the colonial settlement, Maori had thriving businesses and trade arrangements. They took bold political steps and until overpowered, were a forthright and fierce proponent of their own interests (Orange, 1987). In his book, *Shadow of the Land*, Wards (1968) writes about the accounts of the battles between British soldiers and the Maori. Their resourcefulness in being able to "live off of the land" is one reason why the conflict took so long to resolve.

The History

Knowing the history is vital in order to understand the attitudes of New Zealanders. In the 1300s, Polynesian explorers from the central Pacific travelled in long canoes and landed in New Zealand–a land they call *Aotearoa* (Land of the Long White Cloud). The various canoes and their landing places became the basis of tribal identities. Though many have moved away from traditional practices and places, Maori today still identify themselves and their origins by these tribal affiliations (Orange, 1987).

In 1642, Abel Tasman was the first European to discover New Zealand, and in 1769 Captain James Cook mapped New Zealand and claimed it for Britain (Governor General, 2005). Whalers and sealers were followed by missionaries and traders. The country began to be settled.

A Declaration of Independence by the Maori tribes of *Aotearoa*, New Zealand, in 1835 was recognized by the British crown. This necessitated a treaty if colonization was to occur. The famous and hurriedly written and translated Treaty of Waitangi was signed in 1840. However, not all chiefs agreed to the Treaty, and the English and Maori versions were not exactly the same. The notion of sovereignty was translated into Maori as meaning *just governorship*. Consequently, the principles of the Treaty were not universally understood or applied (Orange, 1987).

Maori considered land a perpetual resource belonging to the extended families of a tribe, not to individuals. When asked to sell it, they understood that to mean *allowing people to steward it for a time*. Europeans understood it to mean *ownership* and bought huge tracts of land for pittances. Other Maori land was confiscated when Maori began to challenge the colonization process, the lack of respect for the principles of the treaty, and the takeover of land areas. Language was suppressed, and although it is said that New Zealand Maori fared much better than first-peoples in other colonised nations, the culture, traditions, and sacred places were gradually whittled away (Orange, 1987).

In 1975, the first acknowledgement of the Treaty of Waitangi led to initial steps at making amends for the land losses of Maori. Language learning and a resurgence of the culture began. The urban migration, the loss of connection to the *marae* (tribal village), and *whānau* (extended family) meant that Maori families were often fragmented. Children were not achieving in the European dominated education system. Adults were disproportionately represented in prison populations and the desire for greater self-determination was frustrated (Orange, 1987).

The Culture

Politics. Proportional representation has meant that New Zealand has moved from a political landscape dominated by two major parties, one to the left and one to the right on the political spectrum, to a nation with a range of parties representing a range of opinion in Parliament. Some of these parties offer overtly family-centred policies. One party reminds New Zealand, with its history of women's suffrage, social welfare, and family support initiatives, that the country has been called "the social laboratory of the world" (NZ First, 1999). For most parties, however, benefits to families are seen as a side-effect of economic direction.

Economics. In terms of economics, New Zealand has long depended on the agricultural sector. Increasingly, the much acclaimed Kiwi ingenuity has produced viable exports such as the horticultural icon, the Kiwi fruit. Selling to markets that are long flights or sea voyages away presents ongoing challenges to a small nation.

Religion. Over two million New Zealanders are Christian. The main denominations are Anglican (17%), Catholic (14%), and Presbyterian (11%) (Statistics NZ, 2005a). Religion has declined in terms of attendance since the 1950s. Nominal attendance at church is no longer expected. Numbers of people in Pentecostal churches are gradually rising in number while numbers in older denominations are still dropping (Statistics NZ, 2005b).

More significant in terms of spirituality in New Zealand, however, is the effect of Maoridom. Traditionally, Maori begin all gatherings with *karakia* (prayer), and there is widespread acceptance of the spiritual in the everyday experience of living. This has kept the spiritual very much in the awareness of New Zealanders. It would be an offence to ignore it in events attended by Maori. They see a spiritual essence in all relationships, institutions and objects. There are no realities that are secular for Maori. Spirituality is integral to their culture, identity and their way of experiencing the world, and this has influenced the wider culture of New Zealand (Te Wahaaiti, McCarthy & Durie, 1997).

Recreation. Better known is the sporting prowess of New Zealand, which has a prominent place in New Zealand family life. Support for the All Black rugby team is synonymous with patriotic pride. But other sports are also increasingly prominent in the media and family activities often centre on the watching or playing of one sport or another. As a country, New Zealand is small, but it has influenced sporting, political, and social ideas and practices throughout the world. Families in New Zealand live with the inspiration these aspects from our history give, but also with the challenges they present.

Challenges for New Zealand Families

Cultural Diversity. New Zealand families face a range of cultural challenges. Contributing to Maori family development is seen as a key challenge by the New Zealand Families Commission (2005). While demands for higher skills in the knowledge-based economy call for higher qualifications, Maori families encounter an education system that uses very few Maori ways of learning. Compulsory education in New Zealand is divided into primary, intermediate and secondary schooling. Maori students comprise around 20 percent of the student population. By 2020, it is estimated that approximately 40 percent of all primary school children and 35 percent of all secondary school children will be of Maori and/or Pasifika descent. A significant proportion of Maori students (15%) are suspended from school further exacerbating the situation (Te Puni Kokiri, 2000). Western cultural values permeate schooling and Maori worldviews are not given a great deal of attention. Maori have answered the challenge to raise education and skill levels by developing a range of language immersion schools from early childhood through to tertiary levels. Maori culture, values, and traditions are modelled and taught alongside their language in these government-funded initiatives.

The notion of biculturalism as a nation is still a vexing issue in New Zealand. Many *Pakeha* (European) parents pass on to their children the view that Maori efforts at self-determination are a threat. "Separate development" is feared, even though it is not promoted in mainstream Maoridom. The challenge of biculturalism is to find ways to express the principles of the founding Treaty of Waitangi commitment–partnership with Maori, protection of their traditional resources, and participation in determining governmental, social, political, legal, and educational practices compatible with their cultural values (Waitangi Tribunal, 2005). The added challenge is attempting this without polarising New Zealanders. *Pakeha* families are often unaware of the painful results of tribal fragmentation and deprivation that Maori families grapple with on a daily basis. The New Zealand Index of Deprivation provides insight into the differences between the two groups, with Maori more likely to live in deprived areas and have a life expectancy eight years less for Maori males than non-Maori, and nine years less for Maori females than non-Maori. The infant mortality rate for Maori is 7.4 per thousand live births, whereas the non-Maori rate is 5.5 per thousand (Statistics NZ, 2006).

While Maori are more qualified than in the past, only 11% of Maori compared with 17% of non-Maori stay in school until age 18 and 10% more non-Maori complete higher education than Maori (Statistics NZ, 2004). The average incomes of Maori are $6000 per person, per annum less than non-Maori consistent through all levels of educational qualification (Statistics NZ, 2001a).

In terms of alcohol consumption, the New Zealand Health Survey in 1997 found that while more Maori report not drinking at all, those who do drink were found to consume more on a drinking occasion than non-Maori and show more hazardous patterns of binge drinking (Ministry of Health, 1997).

Recompense for land loss through the Treaty of Waitangi tribunal is a significant part of reconciliation. It is enabling tribal communities to improve standards of education and health for their people. But this redress requires tax revenue and that means money coming out of the pockets of other families.

Multiculturalism is another challenge for New Zealand. A walk down the main street of any large New Zealand city shows how many cultures now call New Zealand home. The challenge is to create a cohesive society that accommodates diversity. For many European families, their life at home carries on without being affected by the growing diversity. But for immigrant families there is considerable stress living in a culture whose norms of behavior, values, and attitudes are so different. Children of immigrants often have to move between two cultures–their ethnic culture at home and the New Zealand milieu they encounter at school. Many immigrants say they encounter rejection of their values, ways of living, ways of speaking, and even their very presence in the country. Few programs exist to help immigrant families find ways of fitting in to the New Zealand cultural scene (Ministry of Social Development, 2004). Skilling (2005) suggests that there are fundamental differences between the nation's interests (security and prosperity) and values (openness, tolerance and respect for international human rights laws) that come into conflict and make adequate immigration policy in New Zealand so difficult to achieve. Supporting the adjustment and settlement of refugee and migrant families and promoting the social and economic development of Pacific families in particular is a key challenge for New Zealand (Families Commission, 2005).

Diversity is evident in New Zealand in other ways as well. The dominant form of family structure fifty years ago was a mother, father, and children. The proportion of children in single parent and repartnered families has risen sevenfold since 1970 (Dharmalingam, Pool, Sceats, & Mackay, R. (2004). While the stigma that was attached to those family forms has largely disappeared, the challenges have not. Sole parents often experience the stress of parenting alone, financial demands, not being part of the more dominant couple-culture, and loneliness. Ensuring policies and services are responsive to diverse forms of family has been identified as a key challenge (Families Commission, 2005).

Family Structure. Subtle changes in family structure have been noted in the shifts in family formations and marriage patterns. Despite a recent up-turn, marriage rates are only one-third of what they were at the peak in the early 1970s (45.5 marriages per 1000 non-married population age 16 and over). Common law unions (unmarried partners living together) are more common than marriages with young New Zealanders with one in four men and women age 15-44 in partnerships and unmarried. Since the 1990s, divorce rate has risen sharply but appears to be stabilizing at about 10,000 per year or 12.5 per 1000 (Statistics NZ, 2001b). One-fifth of all New Zealand women and children experience life in a blended family (Dharmalingam et al., 2004). Re-partnered families face the challenge of blending two established sets of values and habits together, of developing roles and routines that suit both, of guiding and disciplining, and of giving time to all children without favouritism. While this is demanding work, many such blended families bond and develop harmonious ways of functioning.

Isolation and External Influences. Isolation presents other challenges to New Zealand families. Interaction with the wider world is low until a young person has what is termed their OE (overseas experience). Young people often grow up largely unaware of the implications of many global issues. On the other hand, isolation also means the challenge of finding new and creative ways to function in a global economy. Kiwi ingenuity is passed from parent to child and has produced many profitable inventions for the economy.

While isolation may prevent a young person from being aware of critical global issues, the influences that are brought from the outside world in the form of entertainment presents a different challenge. Many New Zealand parents are concerned with some of the values television programmes present to their children, particularly around sexuality, relationships, status, and wealth. Promoting positive parenting and child development, including the monitoring of television-watching has been identified as another key issue by the New Zealand Families Commission (2005).

Economic Challenges. Economic challenges also affect New Zealand families on several fronts. Low population growth, skills shortages, and restraining financial policies have kept economic growth slightly behind many trading partners for a number of years (Alexander, 2005). The population growth of New Zealand is 0.99% and is higher than the United States and many European countries but is lower than many African and Middle Eastern countries whose growth is well over 2% (Central Intelligence Agency, 2006). While many New Zealanders are content with a slower pace and simpler life, others, particularly those with sought-after skills, leave New Zealand shores in search of higher salaries and more prosperous lifestyles. This is known in New Zealand as the challenge of "the brain-drain."

The move to right-wing, monetarist economic policy since 1990 has meant families have to pay considerably more than their parents of 20 years ago for a range of services: tertiary education, health care, and retirement. At the same time, the aging population is presenting the gradually shrinking workforce with the challenge of higher taxation. Isolation and the high transportation costs feed into higher costs for fuel, freight, and travel. For families this means a significant proportion of income goes to petrol and limits their opportunities to give children a wider perspective of the ideas, opportunities, and wonders of the global village. For industry, this is a significant challenge to their competitiveness as they attempt to get New Zealand products into the global market.

Green Values. Many families are concerned with *green values* in New Zealand. This includes concern for conservation of the iconic clean, green environment, for the perceived threat of genetic engineering, and for the ozone hole that lies over the country each summer, apparently worsened by global warming.

Violence. Police statistics in 2001 show that violence in families results in over half the homicides in New Zealand and a third of the victims are children. New Zealand ranks 24 out of the 27 Organisation for Economic Cooperation and Development countries, in terms of death by child-maltreatment (UNICEF, 2003). Violence is associated with other risk factors such as poverty, and is identified as a key challenge for family research and policy-making (Families Commission, 2005). It has been suggested that the difference between higher rates of offending within the criminal justice system for Maori as opposed to non-Maori can be explained by the disadvantages both socially and economically (Te Puni Kòkiri, 2000).

New Zealand has one of the highest rates of young people taking their own life in the world. The incidence of youth suicide has risen 40% in the last 20 years (Ministry of Health, 2001). Many parents feel the responsibility for noticing and responding supportively to young people at risk of drug abuse (particularly methamphetamine or "P"), alcohol abuse, physical and sexual abuse, and suicide. The rate of suicide was higher for Maori (21.1 for male and 6.4 for female deaths per 100,000) than for non-Maori (15.6 for male and 5.9 female deaths per 100,000) (Ministry of Health, 2006).

A particular challenge for New Zealand is the differences in orientation between Maori and non-Maori in terms of justice. A mix of pioneers and warriors make for a range of approaches to life. The first people of the land, the Maori, are known for their warrior spirit. This is a kind of fierceness that can be frightening to people encountering Maori *haka* (or war dance) for the first time. But Maori are also known for being less concerned with the progress orientation, pace, and structures of many Europeans (or *Pakeha*). The Maori have always had their own beliefs about justice that may not correspond with the justice system established by the Europeans. In Maori justice, expulsion from the group was considered appropriate punishment. To be excluded from the group carried enormous shame and the severance of all ties to the community. It seems illogical that today the severest punishment is jail, whereas the result of banishment in one sense is locking someone out (Ministry of Justice, 2001). This sense of justice may be one explanation for why a higher percentage of *Maori* are sentenced inmates in New Zealand prisons (49% of Maori, 38% European). In addition, there are a higher percentage of high risk offenders from the Maori population (Department of Corrections, 2006).

Access to Health Care. Access to health care and its rising cost places strain on New Zealand families, particular where there is disability (Ministry of Social Development, 2004). Long hospital waiting lists and the high price of private health insurance make this an ongoing worry for many families. New Zealand ranks unfavourably when compared to other OECD countries in terms of support for family living standards. Addressing family poverty has been identified as another key challenge for New Zealand (Families Commission, 2005).

Work and Family Balance. Sustained economic growth is one challenge, but more pressing for families is balancing work, family, and community commitments (Families Commission, 2005). This pressure of *business* is a more insidious challenge. Many New Zealanders talk of the increased pace of life within their lifetime. New Zealand has changed in forty years from a quiet, agricultural-based country, where bars closed at 6:00 p.m. and no shops opened on weekends, to a bustling, seven-day-a-week, urbanized environment. Family members are often also involved in a wide range of sporting and cultural activities.

A lack of secure and reasonably-paid jobs for unskilled or semi-skilled workers, the pressure of non-standard working hours, and the ongoing challenge for women losing their footing on the promotional ladder when they choose to take years out of the workforce are considered related challenges (Ministry of Social Development, 2004). Educational achievement is an ongoing concern for New Zealand families as well as employers. At the early childhood level, the challenge to prepare children for school has been a recent focus of government policy and funding (Ministry of Social Development, 2004).

Concerns over literacy dominate the primary or elementary school level while recent changes to the qualification system have resulted in a competency-based secondary school curriculum with unit-standard assessment. Families struggle to understand the complex system of academic results and join employers in calling for clearer and higher educational outcomes.

The cost of higher education in New Zealand continues to challenge families who now have to pay significant sums for their children to study. A high level of student debt and low salaries compared to other developed nations contribute to the brain drain. Qualified professionals desperately needed in the New Zealand marketplace are moving offshore in significant numbers seeking to repay their student loans more quickly. They form networks overseas and often start a family. This makes their return to New Zealand increasingly unlikely. The shortage of skilled labor is increasingly concerning (Alexander, 2005).

William Doherty uses the analogy of putting a canoe in a river. If you paddle, you may stay where you are. If you don't, you'll certainly be carried out to sea. But if you want to get somewhere, he says you have to have a plan (Doherty, 2000). He calls this period in history the time of the intentional family. Without a plan and the effort to nurture time together against the pressures, the river of busyness can quickly carry the New Zealand family downstream. The next section describes some ways families are paddling against the stream and creating strengths to celebrate.

Strengths of New Zealand Families

Cultural strengths: pioneers and warriors. These large islands in the expanse of the southern Pacific Ocean have always been settler colonies. The Maori settled here. The British settled here. Europeans, Pacific Islanders, Asians, and South African immigrants have all settled here. Settlers face the stressful changes of geography, climate, people, and ways of living. Those who stay and make a life are evidence of family strengths alive and well down under. This section will describe some of the strengths such families exhibit in making New Zealand home. Because very little research has been done on New Zealand families that are working well (Families Commission, 2005), features of New Zealand families will be described using the six-category Family Strengths framework.

The ability to face crises and stress. Early Maori immigrants faced an untamed land in the 1300s. From the early 1800s, European settlers faced a similarly rugged and only partly-tamed landscape. Phrases like "Kiwi ingenuity," "She'll be right," and "All you need is a piece of number eight fencing wire" are signs woven into the New Zealand vocabulary, of families creatively overcoming the challenges and crises faced in this young land.

In the face of rising levels of violence and crime among Maori, elders on some *marae* (ancestral home village) in New Zealand have taken the initiative to face this crisis. "*Marae* justice" provides a way of holding Maori offenders within a supportive community while still providing accountability for their actions. With health issues such as diabetes, obesity, mental illness, and heart disease, Maori communities have developed strategies to provide care and intervention that are culturally relevant and *marae*-based. These initiatives show how the extended Maori family has responded to challenges in culturally-specific ways. It also reinforces the notion that effective projects "address social and economic outcomes by collective rather than individual intervention" (Ministry of Social Development, 2004, p. 97).

In the wider population, New Zealand families respond to crisis in a variety of ways. Many do not thrive, especially where poverty, living conditions, and multiple risk factors are present (Ministry of Social Development, 2004). Families that do bounce back from crisis or stress tend to have family strengths developed prior to the crisis and protective factors commonly identified in resilience literature (Walsh, 1998).

A preliminary study of strengths of New Zealand families found that a sense of being a team inspired positive responses to stressors (Cook & DeFrain, 2005; Cook, 2000). Similar to the notions of teamwork in the ever popular arena of sport in New Zealand, families consistently spoke in terms of being a team, being dedicated to the team, pulling together, one person's strengths making up for the weaknesses of another, each having a part to play, making sacrifices for the good of the team, working hard, and sticking together in the face of tough times. Families also spoke of the need to shut out some influences in order to limit their effects. For example, actively choosing television programs to switch off that would undermine the values giving strength to the family in the face of fragmentation.

Recent immigrants speak of the stress of adjusting to a country whose ways are so different from those of their country of origin. South Africans, for example, often speak of struggling with the relaxed ways of many New Zealanders, and the informality with which relationships are conducted. As a colony, settlers rose to the challenge of creating a new nation by rejecting the more stratified class structure of "mother England." Society and politics tend to revolve around being an egalitarian nation. While creating a level playing field for all and in its extreme, the nation has produced what Kiwis call the *"Tall Poppy Syndrome."* This is the tendency of New Zealanders to speak in derogatory terms about people who excel or stand out in their achievements. The one exception to this is people who excel in the sporting arena. They are praised and made into celebrities. Increasingly though, New Zealanders are rising to the economic, sporting, and cultural challenges and learning to affirm excellence.

Immigrants who do adjust and develop a sense of being at home in New Zealand speak in terms of coming to accept Kiwi ways and at the same time believe they have something to contribute to this growing country.

Commitment. Maori families who have retained or regained connection to their *marae* have a strong commitment to their nuclear and extended family. Valuing this, they actively incorporate their children into *marae* life. The Maori writer Witi Ihimaera has written powerfully of the pull that many Maori feel back to their *marae*–particularly at times of bereavement (Ihimaera, 1973; 1974; 2003). For celebrations, funerals (*tangi*), unveiling of tombstones a year after a person's death, as well as the beginning of new jobs or in times of difficulty, many Maori families will come together from all over the country. Members will take time off work or study to prioritize their commitment to their *whānau* (extended family). As mentioned earlier, the warrior spirit of the Maori also have a fierce commitment that will defend members of the *whānau* when threatened or attacked. This strength is evident in school playgrounds and also in gang culture, even when other strengths may not be evident.

In European families, commitment ranges from the very disparate to the strongly bonded. Divorce rates have reached a plateau after a steady rise over the last 20 years (Statistics NZ, 2005). Families I have interviewed, consistently speak of the fear of family breakdown and their desire to make their relationships work. Divorce is seen by many as failure and carries a sense of dread for many. As one family put it, "We need to stick together and succeed" (Cook, 2000).

The settler mindset tends to galvanise immigrant families. Often cut off from extended family networks, connections between family members and between families of similar nationality tend to be strong. Most cities have clubs based around nationality like the New Zealand Philippine Society and the Dutch Club. This strength of commitment seems to dissipate down through the generations as children find a sense of belonging in friendship networks beyond their family and ethnic associations.

Time together. Many New Zealand families who speak of their strengths cite time together as a significant element (Cook, 2000). The ability to have fun, go places together, and be involved in hobbies together is prominent. The "great outdoors" is valued by many families. This leads to family activities that are often passed down from generation to generation. The number of seaside beaches and the penchant for boats is visible in any town or seaside city. Coastal properties have risen dramatically in price as families buy up land in these coveted areas.

Sport is another way that many Kiwi families spend time together. Saturday morning is the traditional time for initiating young New Zealanders into the love of sport. Parents taxi youngsters all over their region in junior sporting leagues. Saturday afternoon then becomes the time for more senior-level games. Sidelines all over the country are packed with family members cheering, jeering, and joining in both the coaching and refereeing of the game they're watching. Sport is a common topic of conversation in workplaces and social events; a point of connection. In past generations this was particularly the focus for men, but in recent years, women have joined in the following. Sports involving women have also risen in prominence via television coverage and the granting of celebrity status to outstanding sportswomen.

Sense of spiritual well-being. Urban drift in the mid-1900s has meant many Maori have lost connection to their *marae*. The *ahi ka* or link to the home fire, has grown dim or never been lit. Families who re-ignite this fire, or who begin an association with an urban *marae*, reconnect to the spiritual strength to face the challenges of fragmentation (Waitangi Tribunal, 1988).

Maori sense the spiritual in all things. *Mauri* or life-force is acknowledged and nurtured. There is a deep sense of connection to the land and created world. A clear dualism is sustained between things that are *tapu*, or special, sacred or even untouchable, and things that are *noa*, or common, everyday, and useable. This shared spirituality provides a code of honor for people, places, and things. It offers a sense of spiritual well-being when respected.

The spiritual awareness of Maori has meant that spirituality has remained prominent in New Zealand society. Schools, while secular by law, still have aspects of Maori spirituality practised. This means that *karakia* (prayers) and *waiata* (songs) are often participated in by Maori and *Pakeha* (European) alike. Many schools officially close for half an hour a week to allow for religious education. While parents have the option of withdrawing their children from those times, most have no objection and often speak of feeling that it benefits their children with morals, values, and a sense of right and wrong.

The legal provision in New Zealand for Catholic and other Christian private schools to integrate with the state system means they receive funding at much the same level as state schools. Moreover, it has meant that spirituality is widely acknowledged as an important part of life. In spite of church attendance declining to just 10% (Jamieson, 2001), a recent survey found that 35% of New Zealanders believe in a personal God, and a further 40% in some kind of higher power or supernatural force (Webster, 2001).

Strongly religious families and those with strong values commitments are very intentional in shaping the spirituality of their children. For most however, values, commitments, beliefs and spiritual perspectives are caught rather than taught. That is, the family provides an environment in which spirituality is passed on by osmosis (Garland, 2001). For Maori, because spirituality is so integral to their view of the world, most families pass this worldview on as part of their everyday life. So many life events are imbued with a sense of the spiritual. As mentioned earlier, all objects and events are either *tapu* (sacred or special), or *noa* (common or able to be freely used or enjoyed). An object like a table, for example, is *noa*. It can only be touched by parts of the body that are also *noa*. As such, one would not sit on a table because the bottom is considered *tapu*. A sense of well-being follows from complying with this spirituality and a sense of danger and threat spiritually and physically follows from breaking the rules of *tapu* and *noa*. This code is passed on daily in Maori families. At a time when the major European religions are declining, it is especially difficult for the Maori to justify the inclusion of religious values within in the school system.

Affection and appreciation. Maori are generally a very warm and affectionate people. Despite the disproportionate representation of Maori in criminal statistics mentioned earlier, traditional Maori families exude a quality known as *aroha*–or warm love. The origin of aroha is Polynesian and is the equivalent of the Hawaiian word, aloha. Both terms mean friendly, hospitable, and welcoming. Visitors speak of the aroha "spirit" that they feel. Williams and Robinson (2004) describe the aroha feeling as social captial in the Maori home. It quickly enfolds a stranger and hospitality is generous.

European families have changed in terms of affection since the 1960s. The British phenomenon known here as "the stiff upper lip" meant that many parents were not very demonstrative with their children. In recent years there is much more talk about the importance of affection and the need for men to express more affection towards their children (Bay of Plenty Times, September 26, 2006).

The fear of being thought a child abuser has been one factor holding men back from expressing love through touch, particularly toward their daughters (Roger, 1997). Equally, men fear being labelled homosexual if seen touching another man. It is far more acceptable for women to express affection through touch. While this is a common feature of family life, these social messages limit the way affection is expressed particularly in Pakeha families.

The expression of appreciation is not a strong feature in New Zealand interaction. Seminars for business people often teach the skill to managers because it is not common practice. The *Tall Poppy Syndrome* mentioned earlier influences the tendency to criticise and cut people down who stand out rather than praise them. Appreciation tends to be more subtle and the phrase "Good on ya mate" is often used in the workplace and even featured on television ads that epitomise the rugged Kiwi male.

Positive communication. Communication in traditional extended Maori families and on *marae* is characteristically forthright. Formal welcome ceremonies (*powhiri*) are full of respect and inclusion. Speechmaking at the events (*hui*) following the formal welcome is honest and can be full of emotion, passion, and strong reaction. Each is allowed to speak their mind until they have finished. While not always positive, it is nonetheless frank and clear. There is no doubt where people stand, and this is generally respected, although the standpoint is not always agreed with.

Developing positive communication is a frequent need when couples and families present for counselling in New Zealand. Working with existing capabilities often helps these clients to build further strengths. Narrative therapy, developed down under in Australia and New Zealand, has been a considerable influence in family counselling and support in this country. Experience with clients shows this approach helps develop a sense of their existing strengths and to build on these (DeFrain, Cook & Gonzales-Kruger, 2004). Te Aroha Noa, a leading community development agency, has been recognized as exemplary for its impact using this approach in a poorer suburb of Palmerston North city (McKay, September 12, 2006; Awards, September 9, 2006).

Feedback from students learning strengths-based practice at Bethlehem Tertiary Institute in Tauranga, New Zealand, report that when interviewed, families are invariably surprised to find that they possess strengths in their life together. Even though they volunteer for the conversations knowing it is part of a paper focused on strengths, family members most often hold a negative view of their shared life. As a previous study found, the very act of talking about family strengths is strengthening (Cook, 2000). New Zealanders have a reputation for being somewhat pessimistic. They know well the challenges and shortcomings of their family life. Conversations focusing on strengths reveal that the capabilities discussed in this section are more common than first thought. This may explain why so many family agencies in New Zealand are reorienting their work to strengths-based practice. Over time, this may well nurture both an awareness of the strengths already inherent in New Zealand families, as well as further develop strong family life down under.

REFERENCES

Alexander, T. (2005). BNZ weekly overview. Wellington: BNZ.

Awards, (September 9, 2006). Dynamic Community Learning Award Winners. Retrieved on November 1, 2006 from http://adultlearnersweek.org.nz/natlaunch/ natlaunch/natlevents_files/category-3.html.

Bay of Plenty Times, (September 26, 2006). Sometimes kids needs hugs, teacher says. Tauranga: Bay of Plenty Times.

Central Intelligence Agency (2006). The World Factbook. Retrieved October 25, 2006 from https://www.cia.gov/cia/publications/factbook/geos/nz.html

Cook, R. (2000). Discourses inspiring the strengths of a selection of New Zealand families. Unpublished Masters Thesis, University of Waikato, Hamilton, New Zealand.

Cook, R., & DeFrain, J. (2005). Using discourse analysis to explore family strengths: A preliminary study. *Marriage & Family Review, 38*, 3-12.

Crump, B. (1972). *The half-dozen, quarter-acre, pavlova paradise.* Wellington: Whitcombe & Tombs

Dharmalingam, A., Pool, I., Sceats, J., & Mackay, R. (2004). Patterns of family formation and change in New Zealand. Wellington: Centre for Social Research and Evaluation, Ministry of Social Development.

DeFrain, J., Cook, R., & Gonzales-Kruger, G. (2004). Strengthening couple and family relationships. In R. Coombs (Ed.), *Family Therapy Review* (pp. 3-20). Mahwah, New Jersey: Lawrence Erlbaum and Associates.

Department of Corrections (2006). A census of prison inmates and home detainees 2003 retreived October 24, 2006 from http://www.corrections.govt.nz/public/research/census/2003/index.html

Doherty, W. (2000). The intentional family. In K. Gilbert (Ed.), *Marriage and family 00/01.* Guilford: Dushkin/McGraw-Hill.

Families Commission, (2005). Giving families a voice: Statement of intent 2005/6. Wellington: Families Commission.

Garland, D. (2001). The faith dimension of family. Transforming ministry in a time of transition. USA: Wayne Oates Institute. Retreived on January 2, 2002 from: https://64.226.182.156/olc/pub/a0200/transforming_ministry/presentation_index.htm

Governor General, (2005). About New Zealand. Retrieved 9/19/2005 from http://www.gg.govt.nz/aboutnz/

Ihimaera, W. (1973). *Tangi.* Auckland: Heinemann

Ihimaera, W. (1974). *Whānau.* Auckland: Heinemann

Ihimaera, W. (2003). *Whale rider.* Auckland: Reed

Jamieson, A. (2001). The future of the church in New Zealand. *Reality, 43*, 8-13.

McKay, C. (September 12, 2006). Early childhood centre wins award. *Manawatu Standard.*

Ministry of Health, (1997). Taking the pulse: The 1996/7 New Zealand health survey. Retrieved on November 1, 2006 from http://www.moh.govt.nz/moh.nsf/

Ministry of Health, (2001). Suicide prevention. Retrieved on September 9, 2005 from http://www.newhealth.govt.nz/toolkits/suicide/background_2.htm

Ministry of Health. (2006). *Suicide Facts: Provisional 2003 All-Ages Statistics. Monitoring Report No. 1.* Wellington: Ministry of Health.

Ministry of Justice. (2001). He Hinatore ki te Ao Maori: A Glimpse into the Maori World Wellington: Ministry of Justice.

Ministry of Social Development, (2004). New Zealand families today: A briefing for the Families Commission. Wellington: Ministry of Social Development.

NZ First (1999). The women leaders have lost their way. Speech to Grey Power organisation, Kawerau, August 1999. Retrieved September 9, 2005, from http://www.nzfirst.org.nz/content/display_item.php?t=1&i=21

Orange, C. (1987). *The treaty of Waitangi.* Wellington: Allen & Unwin [993.01 ORA]

Roger, W. (1997). The real fear of the 90's man with children. *The Evening Post.* Wellington, 1 Dec 1997.

Skilling, P. (2005). National identity and immigration: Contemporary discourses. *New Zealand Sociology, 20,* 98-121.

Statistics NZ, (2001a). Highest Educational Qualification and Total Personal Income by Ethnic Group and Sex. Retrieved on November 1, 2006 from http://www2.stats.govt. nz/domino/external/web/prod_serv.nsf/htmldocs/Customised+Tables+Repository +-+Womens+Affairs/$file/C12044wg.xls

Statistics NZ (2001b). Marriage and divorce in New Zealand. Retrieved October 25, 2006, from http://www.stats.govt.nz/products-and-services/Articles/marriage-divorce-99.htm?print=Y

Statistics NZ. (2004). Maori education. Retreived on November 1, 2006 from http:// www.stats.govt.nz/analytical-reports/looking-past-20th-century/maori/maori-education.htm

Statistics NZ. (2005a). Census snapshot: Cultural diversity. Retrieved September 9, 2005, from http://www.stats.govt.nz/products-and-services/Articles/census-snpsht-cult-diversity-Mar02.htm

Statistics NZ. (2005b). 2001 census. Retrieved September 9, 2005, from http://www. stats.govt.nz/NR/rdonlyres/937947E3-D4DA-4D75-A9A9-6C4BA594A8DB/0/R SVolume101.pdf

Statistics NZ, (2006). A history of survival in New Zealand. Retrieved on November 1, 2006from http://www.stats.govt.nz/NR/rdonlyres/D2B767FB-6338-4E70-9ECB-41AE48E95520/0/AHistoryofSurvivalinNZreport.pdf

Te Puni Kòkiri. 2000. *Progress Towards Closing Social and Economic Gaps Between Màori and Non-Màori.* Wellington: Te Puni Kòkiri.

Te Wahaaiti, P., McCarthy, M., & Durie, A. (1997). *Mai I Rangiaatea Maori wellbeing and development.* Auckland: Auckland University Press

UNICEF. (2003). A league table of child maltreatment deaths in rich nations. Geneva: UNICEF Innocenti Research Centre.

Waitangi Tribunal, (1988). Report of the Waitangi Tribunal on the Muriwhenua fishing claim. Retrieved November 1, 2006, from http://www.waitangi-tribunal.govt. nz/scripts/reports/reports/22/796C25F5-7F61-4F4F-8C50-EED0218276F3.pdf

Waitangi Tribunal (2005). Principles of the Treaty: National overview. Retrieved September 16, 2005, from http://www.waitangi-tribunal.govt.nz/about/treatyofwaitangi/principles.asp

Walsh, F. (1998). *Strengthening family resilience.* New York: Guilford Press

Wards, I. (1968). *Shadow of the Land–A Study of British Policy and Racial Conflict in New Zealand 1832-1852.* Mystic, CT: Lawrence Verry.

Webster, A. (2001). *Spiral of values.* Hawera: Alpha Publications.

Williams, T., & Robinson, D. (2004). Social capital and philanthropy in Maori society. *International Journal of Not-for-Profit Law, 6*(2), NA

doi:10.1300/J002v41n03_02

NORTH AMERICA

Canada and Family Life

Benjamin Schlesinger

SUMMARY. Important Canadian factors are discussed to obtain a profile of this country, its communities, and family trends. The challenges for Canadian families are presented and include the sandwich generation, seniors, effects of divorce and remarriage, and same-sex marriages. A review of existing studies related to the strengths of Canadian families is included. The need for families to be strengthened has led to a variety of social supports available to the families of Canada. doi:10.1300/ J002v41n03_03 *[Article copies available for a fee from The Haworth Document Delivery Service: 1-800-HAWORTH. E-mail address: <docdelivery@ haworthpress.com> Website: <http://www.HaworthPress.com> © 2007 by The Haworth Press, Inc. All rights reserved.]*

KEYWORDS. Canada, Canadian geography, Canadian population, family strengths

Benjamin Schlesinger is Professor Emeritus, University of Toronto, Faculty of Social Work.

Address correspondence to: (E-mail: rachels@yorku.ca).

The author thanks his wife, Rachel, for her help in developing this chapter.

[Haworth co-indexing entry note]: "Canada and Family Life." Schlesinger, Benjamin. Co-published simultaneously in *Marriage & Family Review* (The Haworth Press, Inc.) Vol. 41, No. 3/4, 2007, pp. 261-279; and: *Strong Families Around the World: Strengths-Based Research and Perspectives* (ed: John DeFrain, and Sylvia M. Asay) The Haworth Press, Inc., 2007, pp. 261-279. Single or multiple copies of this article are available for a fee from The Haworth Document Delivery Service [1-800-HAWORTH, 9:00 a.m. - 5:00 p.m. (EST). E-mail address: docdelivery@haworthpress.com].

Available online at http://mfr.haworthpress.com
© 2007 by The Haworth Press, Inc. All rights reserved.
doi:10.1300/J002v41n03_03

CANADA TODAY

Canada is a land of wilderness and rich farmland, of cosmopolitan cities, tiny fishing villages and industrial towns. It is a land of diverse communities and peoples, with six time zones and a variety of weather conditions. Given Canada's diversity, this cultural profile can provide only a glimpse of this large nation (University of Toronto, 2000).

Canada is the second-largest country in the world. It stretches more than 5,500 kilometers from Newfoundland on the Atlantic coast to Vancouver Island on the Pacific Ocean. The world's longest undefended border separates Canada from the United States to the south.

Canada is composed of ten provinces and three territories. The provinces are Alberta, British Columbia, Manitoba, New Brunswick, Newfoundland and Labrador. In Northern Canada are the territories: Yukon, Northwest Territories and the newest, Nunavut. Although the provinces have quite a bit of autonomy from the federal government, the territories do not. Most of the social programs of Canada are the responsibility of the provinces.

Over the centuries, Canada has witnessed different cultures coming together in conflict and compromise. Although the indigenous peoples showed the early explorers how to survive, many of them died of European diseases or in battles with the immigrants. The first immigrants were the French and the British, who arrived in the 17th century. After the American Revolution in the 18th century, they were joined by English-speaking Loyalists who moved north from the United States. During the 19th century, immigrants continued to come from Europe, Great Britain, Ireland and the United States. Chinese workers were brought to Canada to work on the railways. At the turn of the century, people from Northern and Eastern Europe helped settle the prairies, and immigrants from Asia settled on the West Coast.

The two World Wars brought refugees from Europe. Since the Second World War, Canada has welcomed immigrants from Africa, Asia, and Latin America, as well as Europe. Many come to find jobs, establish businesses or continue their education. Others have come to escape civil unrest or oppressive regimes in their home countries. Today, Canada's population includes people from more than 160 countries.

Landscape and Climate

Canada has six natural regions. The Atlantic Provinces have a mixture of fertile valleys, low mountains and rugged forests. The Canadian

Shield, which covers much of Ontario and Quebec, is the largest region, with rocky hills, evergreen forests and many lakes. To the south are lush forests and rich farmland along the Great Lakes and St. Lawrence River. This area is home to more than 60% of the population. The flat Prairie Provinces are known for their fields of wheat and canola. Further west are the high peaks, vast forests and rugged territory of the Rocky Mountains, which extend to the Pacific Ocean. In the Far North the ground is frozen year-round. No trees grow on the flat tundra. Each landscape has a characteristic climate. The Far North is like a cold desert. With low temperatures and little moisture, hardly any snow falls in this region, but the snow that does fall stays for many months. The West Coast has a milder climate and more rainfall than the rest of the country. Most Canadians experience four distinct seasons. Snow falls in the winter and the days are short and cold. In spring, the snow begins to melt and farmers plant their crops. Summers are hot and, in some regions, very humid. In fall, the nights are cold and the leaves turn red or yellow and drop from the trees.

Population Trends

Of Canada's total population, 79.7% live in urban areas, and 20.3% reside in rural areas. The total population consists of 33 million persons. Canada has an ethnically diverse population. Three Aboriginal groups make their homes in Canada. The largest group, the North American Indians, represent 62% of those who identified themselves as Aboriginal. The Metis represent 30% and the Inuit represent 5% of the Aboriginal population. Although the North American Indians and Metis live in several provinces and territories, one half of the Inuit population lives in the territory of Nunavut (Statistics Canada, 2001). Most assume that all three groups are part of the First Nations of Canada, however, the Inuit arrived later that the other two groups.

The Inuit comprise of 87% of the population in the capital of Nunavut, Igaluit. Almost half of the population of Igaluit are under the age of 19, with 51.2% aged 20-64, and 2.2% aged 65 +. The medium age is 22.1 years (Langlois, 2004). Inuit families are larger (33% have 3 or more children) than other Aboriginals (13%) or non-Aboriginals (11%) (Hull, 2006). Census data shows that the proportion of Canada's population who are foreign-born has reached its highest level in seventy years (Statistics Canada, 2003). Canada has a large immigrant population, numbering of 5.4 million persons (18.4% of the total population). Those from Asia and the Middle East comprise 60% of the immigrants.

In 2002, Canada admitted 25,111 refugees. Just over 11% of the population is known as "visible minorities." The Employment Equity Act has defined visible minorities as persons, other than Aboriginal peoples, who are non-Caucasian in race or non-white in color (Statistics Canada, 2003).

Communities

Language and Diversity. English and French are Canada's official languages. All Canadian government documents are written in both languages. Federal courts operate in French and English. Translators and interpreters work in Ottawa to ensure Canada's parliament functions in both languages. All goods sold in stores must be labeled in French and English. To be bilingual in Canada means to be able to speak both English and French. An Anglophone is someone whose mother tongue is English. A Francophone is a French speaker. The word *Allophone* is used in Quebec to describe someone whose mother language is neither English nor French. Not everyone speaks both languages. Most Canadians speak English. New Brunswick is the only officially bilingual province. Quebec is officially a French-speaking province. Four-fifths of Québécois speak French as their first language. Quebec has special language laws that promote the use of French. There are regional variations in the language. English speakers in some areas punctuate their sentences with the word *eh*. Quebec slang, which uses many English words, is called *joual*. Newfoundlanders use many words that are unique to their province. Immigrants to Canada bring their languages with them. After English and French, Cantonese and Mandarin are the most common languages spoken in Canada.

Canada's original peoples spoke more than 53 languages. Some of these are disappearing. The most common indigenous languages spoken today are Cree, Anishnaabe and Inuktitut. Language plays a significant role in the communities of Canada. The diversity of language and culture is known to effect ethnic identity. The Language of the Inuit is very sophisticated and important to the culture. The "Ningiqtuq" or sharing is imbedded with deep meaning and is used to pass on information and heritage among the Inuit people. Isajiw (1990) suggests that language is important to the development of the Canadian cultural identity. A major point of Canada's multiculturalism policy has been to support those of all ethnic groups in preserving and sharing their language, culture, and heritage while at the same time adapting to Canadian society. Although there is recognition that maintaining culture and language is important, research has found that Canadian immigrants who are able to speak English or French are more likely to identify themselves as Canadian (Pigott & Kalbach, 2005). Bauder and Sharpe (2002) found that the major cities of Canada have neither "ghettos" of minorities where they live together in one area nor are these ethnic minorities dispersed all over the city and isolated from their cultural groups. It does appear that at least in the major cities the visible minorities are realizing the success of Canada's multicultural policy.

Language also plays a role in the levels of education in Canada. Corbeil (2003) found that although the language groups of Anglophones, Francophones, and allophones, all have increased their levels of education over the past thirty years, that there are differences between the three groups.

Religion. There is no state religion in Canada. However, the Canadian Charter of Rights and Freedoms recognizes the supremacy of God and grants freedom to all Canadians to practice the religion of their choice. Roman Catholics constitute 43.6% of the population, Protestants 29.2%, others 10.7%, and 16.5% stated "no religion" in the last census. New immigrant populations have caused an increase in those who identify with the Muslim religion.

The last few decades have seen an increase in the number of Canadians who report having no religion and a decrease in those who attend religious services. Reports indicate, however, that while Canadians do not attend religious services, they do engage in religious practices on their own. Using the religiosity index, which includes the four dimensions of affiliation, attendance, personal practices and importance of religion, 40% of Canadians have a low degree of religiosity, 31% are moderately religious, and 29% are highly religious (Clark & Schellenberg, 2006).

In gathering data about religion, the reporting of some Aboriginal religions may not be accurate. Many followers of Native American Spirituality do not report their spiritual beliefs and practices as a religion but rather a part of their everyday lives. "Rather than going to church, I attend a sweat lodge; rather than accepting bread and toast [sic] from the Holy Priest, I smoke a ceremonial pipe to come into Communion with the Great Spirit; and rather than kneeling with my hands placed together in prayer, I let sweetgrass be feathered over my entire being for spiritual cleansing and allow the smoke to carry my prayers into the heavens. I am a Mi'kmaq, and this is how we pray" (Augustine, 2000).

Education. Canada spends more per capita on education than most other Western nations. Education is a provincial responsibility. The country has ten provincial school systems and three territorial systems.

Each system has its own approach to funding and administration. Elementary school includes Grade 1 to Grade 6, 7, or 8. Secondary school or high school continues to Grade 12. Public education is free until the end of secondary school. Some provinces require children to buy their own textbooks. Most provinces have a kindergarten program to prepare children for Grade 1.

Prior to WWII, comparatively few Canadians attended or completed high school but with the increasing need for skilled workers, the value of education has also increased. Although each province has different rates, overall dropout rates have decreased from approximately 17% in 1990-1991 to around 10% in the last three years. Males have higher dropout rates than girls and rates are higher in some parts of rural and small towns than in urban areas. Dropout rates are significantly higher among Aboriginal populations. One reason for the disparity in small towns and rural areas may include the idea that they see little by way of return on their investment in education, as job growth tends to be limited to urban areas. Among Aboriginal populations, more success has been shown in student retention when educational programs are community-based and relevant to employment as well as those that supports the cultural values and heritage of the student (Canadian Council on Learning, 2005).

Postsecondary education is available in most Canadian cities. Universities and community colleges are partially funded by the government, but students also pay tuition fees. Community colleges offer training in arts and trades as well as continuing education courses for working adults. There are 75 universities in Canada. There are 580,000 full-time and 246,000 part-time students in these institutions. Not unlike other countries with an open system of education, young people in Canada have high aspirations for higher education. Looker and Thiessen (2004) suggest that these aspirations result from Canada's high value of post-secondary education, parental encouragement, and the influence of peers.

Health Care. The introduction of a national hospitalization and national Medicare system through the Canadian Health Act is comparable to universal systems of Western Europe. Medical services are available to all citizens. Regular visits to the doctor and hospital stays are largely paid for by the government. Many employers sponsor additional health-insurance plans for their workers. Although Canadians are generally very proud of their comprehensive health-care and are committed to the fundamental principles of the system, a growing public dissatisfaction with some parts of the system beginning in the 1990s led to the need for changes that impact the families of Canada. Concerns include efficiency, quality, and delivery of services (Statistics Canada, 2005b).

Canadian Families

Family Trends. The report on Canadian families, *Profiling Canada's Families III* (Vanier Institute of the Family, 2004) revealed the top ten trends for families in Canada. Each trend that was identified including specifics about that trend lends understanding about the state of the family in Canada today.

1. *Fewer couples are getting legally married.* The 2001 census shows that an increasing amount of couples are choosing common-law relationships (cohabitation) without marriage (14%, up from 5.6% in 1981). As a result, the proportion of married couple families was down from 83% in 1981 to 70% in 2001 (Statistics Canada, 2002).
2. *More couples are breaking up.* Although the number of divorces has remained stable over the past few years (223.7 for every 100,000 people), there is an increase in the number of repeat divorces or those who have been divorces at least once before (Statistics Canada, 2005c)
3. *Families are getting smaller.* According to the 2001 census data, the average family size is 3.1 persons down from 4 in 1966 (Statistics Canada, 2001). The decline is due mostly to lower fertility rates as couples opt for fewer children and an increase in couples that choose not to have children (Statistics Canada, 2002).
4. *Children are experiencing more transitions.* The number of lone-parent families has increased from 9.4% in 1971 to 16% in 2001. Children are five times more likely to experience the separation of their parents than children in the 1960s which increases the likelihood that they will have multiple living situations throughout childhood (Human Resources Development Canada, 2002).
5. *Canadians are generally satisfied with life.* Despite the changes for families that appear to be negative, overall, 92% of Canadians report themselves to be either very satisfied or somewhat satisfied with their life (Mata, 2002).
6. *Family violence is under-reported.* Since 1999 there has been no change in the overall level of spousal violence reported by those who were married or living in a common-law relationship (7% of Canadians over 15 years of age), however, given the hidden

nature of domestic violence, measuring the prevalence of abuse is difficult as it is often not reported to the authorities. In addition, youth and the elderly are also unlikely to report abuse. Authorities estimate that the number of crimes that go unreported to police is considerable (Statistics Canada, 2004a).

7. *Multiple-earner families are now the norm.* The majority of young children have two parents working outside the home. Although women participate in the workplace less than men, 7.5 million women had jobs in 2004, twice as high as in the mid-1970s (Statistics Canada, 2006a). Among the countries in the European Union, Canada has one of the highest percentages of working mothers with young children (Human Resources Development Canada, 2002).

8. *Women do most of the juggling in balancing work and home.* Women still do most of the household work and tend to feel more stressed over it than men. Even though women's participation in the workforce has increased, their daily participation in housework (meal preparation, cleaning, and laundry) is at 85% (Statistic Canada, 2006b).

9. *Inequality is worsening.* Families are affected by inequality at many different levels in Canada. In the cities and urban areas, where most Canadians live, inequality is noted by the deterioration of economic welfare for immigrant (falling 35%), Aboriginal (falling 41.6%), and low-income families (falling 17.7%, 46.6% for lone-parents) while income rose for high-income families. A similar disparity in social well-being is also noted in affordable housing and healthcare (Heisz, 2005). In the northern rural areas, the Inuit face economic hardship because of the high cost of living, limiting their purchasing power (Hull, 2006).

10. *The future will have more aging families.* Although Canada's population is younger than most developed countries, its population is aging fast and senior citizens could outnumber children with in the decade. Projections show that as the baby boom cohort reaches 65 between 2011and 2031, their population will double from 13% to 25% (Statistics Canada, 2005a).

National Survey on Canadian Families

The majority of Canadians believe the traditional nuclear family is ideal, even though many do not live in such arrangements themselves (Bibby, 2004). In a national survey on family values and aspirations,

University of Lethbridge sociologist Reginald Bibby found the reality is often far from the dream. "The vast majority start off really wanting fairly traditional things, but it just doesn't often work out that way," he said in an interview. In the study, Professor Bibby also found that while most Canadians think the mom-dad-and-the-kids family model is best, many accept others' different arrangements. In the survey of more than 2,000 adults, he found just over half of Canadians wanted governments to give high priority to ensuring same-sex families receive the same benefits as others. Just under half believed gays and lesbians should be allowed to marry. About six in ten think homosexual couples can be good parents, and five in ten think they should be allowed to adopt children. But when asked for the *ideal* family arrangement, 58% answered a married man and woman with at least one child. Overall, the traditional family is seen as ideal by about 20% of gays and lesbians compared to approximately 60% of heterosexuals.

FAMILY CHALLENGES IN THE 21ST CENTURY

Canada faces some interesting family issues as we begin the 21st century. In addition to some of the challenges that were found among the trends mentioned previously, there are others that families in Canada will need to manage during this century.

The Sandwich Generation

The sandwich generation refers to those who are caught between the demands of raising their own children and caring for aging parents or other relatives. In Canada, almost three out of ten of those who are 45-64 with unmarried children still at home and who under age 25 were caring for an elderly person (Statistics Canada, 2004c). Although the sandwich generation is relatively small now, it is likely to grow as baby boomers age. One cause for the sandwich generation is the increase in the decision to delay marriage and childbearing. Births to mother 35 and older happen more frequently than the previous generation who now need their children's care. More adult children remain or return to their parent's home (up from 27% in 1981–see Table 1). In addition, over the past two decades, the care that seniors receive through institutions has been declining and of those who are not institutionalized, 45% are getting help from family and friends (Cranswick & Thomas, 2005).

TABLE 1. Percent of adult children living with parents.

Age	Percent of Adult Children
20-29	41%
20-24–men	64%
20-24–women	52%
25-29–men	29%
25-29–women	19%

Source: Boyd, M. & Norris, B. (1999). The crowded nest: Young adults at home. *Canadian Social Trends* (Spring), *52*, 2-6.

Women are more likely to be the ones who are sandwiched and often are the ones to change their work schedule or hours to accommodate the care. Statistics show that women spend an average of 29 hours a month in providing care to seniors as compared to 13 hours a month for males. Much of the tasks involved in caregiving remain the woman's responsibility. Caregiving includes personal care such as bathing, toileting, and dressing; care inside the home such as meal preparation, cleaning and laundry; care outside the home such as home maintenance and yard work; and transportation care such as shopping and running errands (Williams, 2005) Emotional care such as support and counseling, although not usually included in the discussion of tasks is certainly important and demands time from the caregiver.

Seniors

One of the fastest growing age groups in Canada are seniors who are 65 and over. Although most of the information provided about seniors is based on the 65 and over category, the Canadian government defines a "senior family" as a couple where at least one of the partners is 55 years of age or over. Of the total population, 13% are seniors, of whom 7% live in a health-care institution. Many seniors live with a spouse or partner, up from two decades earlier and over two-thirds own their own home. Living alone has also increased for both men and women and is common for those over 85 years old (Statistics Canada, 2002). Although more seniors are living longer and enjoying better overall health, the prevalence of chronic diseases such as diabetes, heart disease, hypertension and arthritis is increasing. Issues of special concern are inactivity and obesity. Overall health tends to decrease with income. In addition, Aboriginal seniors are more likely to report a lower health status than all Canadian seniors (30% vs. 44%) (National Advisory Council on Aging, 2006).

Income status for seniors has improved over the last few years, yet there are pockets of regional and cultural differences where senior incomes have not improved. Single senior women are also at-risk economically. Seniors who are recent immigrants are more likely to have the lowest incomes and must manage without government assistance because of residency requirements. Low-income seniors struggle with affordable housing, transportation, and safety (National Advisory Council on Aging, 2006).

Although being able to care for seniors seems to have important implications for Canadian families in the future, the challenge for all of Canada may be the implications for the work force when the first of the baby-boom cohort (those born in 1946) reaches 65 and when combined with other factors such as low fertility rates and increasing longevity (Statistics Canada, 2005a). The percentage of working seniors (the majority age 65-69) has increased from 6% in 2001 to 8% in 2005 (National Advisory Council on Aging, 2006).

The Effects of Divorce and Remarriage

On average there are about 72,000 divorces per annum. About 35,000 children are involved annually in divorces. Along with the number of divorces, children are experiencing divorce as increasingly earlier ages. Divorce has now replaced death as the number one reason for lone-parenting. The consequences for the family have been well documented in Canada as well as the U.S. and can include poverty for lone-parents with children (especially women) and environmental changes. Custody of the couple's children is granted in 27% of divorces. In 2001, over one million children (19%) did not live with both parents; most lived with their mother. (Statistics Canada, 2002).

Every year since the year 2000, about one third of marriages contained at least one person who was previously married. These figures represent and increase over a three-decade period (Statistics Canada, 2005c). Remarriage also involve children and represents about 12% of all Canadian couples with children (up from 10% in 1995) (Statistics Canada, 2002). Children have to adjust to this newly formed family pattern. Children in remarried families report less support from parents and more conflict with parents and siblings (Nilan, 2000).

Same-Sex Marriages

One of the most controversial family challenges is related to same-sex marriages. Statistics Canada has reported that 1% of Canadians say they are homosexual and 0.7% say they are bisexual (Statistics Canada, 2004b). The figures are interesting because they are lower than some figures that have been widely circulated. In 2004, the Supreme Court of Canada gave its blessing to the federal government's proposal to legalize same-sex marriage. The court said that the power to change the definition of marriage lies exclusively with the federal government, not the provinces, and that a proposed bill to legalize same-sex marriage is constitutional and fits smoothly within the evolution of the law. It also said churches cannot be forced to perform same-sex marriages.

But the court refused to state categorically whether it agrees with lower courts that the traditional man-woman definition of marriage is unconstitutional. That would have amounted to an unequivocal declaration that same-sex marriage must inevitably be the law of the land. Instead, the court deftly handed the politically explosive issue back to Parliament and put the onus to proceed with legislation on the prime minister.

The Civil Marriage Act enacted in July 2005 legalized same-sex marriage in Canada although court decisions had already legalized it in eight provinces and one territory. Passing same-sex marriage legislation made Canada one of the first, following the Netherlands, Belgium, and Spain, to make marriage for gays and lesbians the law of the land. However, in most Nordic countries, cohabitation or civil unions are on equal footing with marriage with the same rights and benefits. Religious spokesmen have said they will apply renewed pressure to politicians for a countrywide referendum on gay marriage and to vote against the proposed government legislation. However, a recent poll shows that 66% of Canadians do not want to bring the issue back to Parliament (CBC News, 2006). Supporters tend to be young and live in urban areas, while those who oppose the law tend to be older and live in rural areas.

CANADIAN FAMILY STRENGTHS

Definition and Assumptions

Family strengths may be defined as those relationship patterns, intrapersonal and interpersonal skills and competencies, and social and psychological characteristics that create: (1) a sense of positive family identity, (2) promote satisfying and fulfilling interaction among family members, (3) encourage the development of the potential of the family group and individual family members, (4) contribute to the family's ability to deal effectively with stress and crisis, and (5) function as a support/network to other families (King, 1983, p. 49).

Canadian Views on Family Strengths

Historically, Canadian researchers have been interested in the strengths of families. A pioneering Canadian study by Westley and Epstein (1969) examined the emotional health of families in Montreal. Their most important finding was that children's emotional health is closely related to the emotional relationship between their parents. When these relationships are warm and constructive, such that the husband and wife feel loved, admired, and encouraged to act in ways that they themselves admire, the children are happy and healthy. Couples who are emotionally close, meet each other's needs, and encourage positive self-images in each other, become good parents. Since they meet each other's needs, they do not use their children to live out their needs; since they are happy and satisfied, they can support and meet their children's needs; and since their own identities are clarified, they see their children as distinct from themselves. All this helps the children become emotionally healthy people.

The family with a balanced division of labor proved to be the only one in which the majority of couples had a vigorous sex life and experienced increasing satisfaction with the sexual relationship, had a good marital relationship, and had emotionally healthy children. Though it is true that this was also the only type of family in which the majority of husbands and wives were emotionally healthy, the researchers still found that there was a direct relationship between the division of labor and the emotional health of the children.

Cocivera (1982) at the University of Guelph conducted another Canadian study to determine the characteristics of a well-functioning family:

1. Role distinctions in a well-functioning family are clear and there is a distinct boundary between the integral family members and those in the extended family. The husband and wife in a two-parent family play dual roles. In the marriage relationship, as husband and wife, they provide each other with companionship, affection, sharing and sex. As parents, they play an executive or

managerial role in the nurturance, control and, later, the guidance of their children.

2. Individuality and a high degree of differentiation are encouraged in a successful family. The children and adults are able to develop their own interests. This leads to a continual tug and pull between separateness and mutuality. Conflict arises only if the family views individual expression as a threat.

3. Rules are clear and reasonable and change as the children mature. The punishment for breaking rules is humane and on a scale commensurate with the "crime." In families with rigid and unchallengeable rules, children either rebel or become passive and dependent.

4. Good communication is essential. All family members speak for themselves; children are listened to and their input respected.

5. Authority or power is clearly vested in individuals, with the tacit agreement of all family members. As the family moves through different stages in its life cycle and the children mature, there are shifts in the family's power base.

6. A full range of emotions is acceptable, appropriate and encouraged. Imposing taboos on expressing certain emotions leads to incongruity between emotions and behavior.

7. Conflicts are resolved through bargaining and negotiation, with all family members able to participate. This can be a highly constructive and satisfying approach to solving problems.

8. Tasks or chores are shared by family members, with a clear understanding of who performs which tasks; individuals can follow through in their own style and time. Flexibility is important. When a wife starts to work outside the home, some restructuring of chores is usually required. However, research consistently shows that neither the husband nor the children take on an equitable extra load under these circumstances.

9. Individual differences in energy levels, perception of time, and space requirements are respected. Families often have to adapt to the temporary challenge of long-term illness of a family member, and they also play an important role in nudging a disabled member to achieve as much as possible.

10. High esteem, both for the individual and the family, develops naturally in a well-functioning family. The well-functioning family isn't necessarily quiet, well-ordered and rational all the time. Amid the affection and companionship, children squabble, compete and get in each others' hair as they learn how to get

along with people. Negotiation, setting rules and challenging those rules also leads to some lively exchanges between parents and children.

The first Canadian study on lasting marriages was conducted by Schlesinger (1983) and examined 129 couples who had been married an average of 24 years. There were 19 items, which were chosen by more than 83% of the respondents as "extremely important" in helping marriages to last. The first ten, in order of importance were: respect for each other, trusting each other, loyalty, loving each other, counting on each other, considering each other's needs, providing each other with emotional support, commitment to make marriage last, fidelity, and give-and-take in marriage. An open-ended question dealt with the advice to be given to couples intending to marry. The most important items for the women (in order of importance) were: communication, respect, commitment, work at your marriage, and financial security. The men in our study gave the following items: communication, work at your marriage, commitment, financial security, and sharing.

Bibby (2004) recently completed a national study related to the strengths of families. In the forward to this publication, it states, "Canada will be shaped not only by the trends that are captured by statistical reporting but equally by the reactions, attitudes and opinions of citizens as they strive to understand and adapt to these trends" (p. v). This report reveals that Canadians view families as essential and value the family for its personal and social benefits. Results of the study show that Canadians regard the family as "a key source of love, support, stability, happiness and companionship, and as fundamental to optimum community and national life" (p. 9). Because most of the respondents believe that the traditional family is the ideal family form, one of the key questions that is raised by the findings of this study is how relationships can be strengthened regardless of what form they take. Table 2 contains the responses of 2,093 subjects to one of the questions about lasting relationships. These characteristics of lasting relationships are important in helping strengthen all lasting relationships. That is the challenge for Canadian family support in the future.

Societal Supports

In 1993, The Alberta Premier's Council in Support of Families (1993, pp. 19-20) made the following suggestions to strengthen Canadian families:

TABLE 2. Keys to a lasting relationship: Canadian study (N = 2,903) (in alphabetical order).

Acceptance	Give and take
Allowing your partner freedom	Honesty*
Being good friends	Ideas shared
Caring	Kindness
Common sense	Listening to each other
Commitment	Love*
Communication*	Mutual respect
Compatibility	Patience*
Compromise	Passion
Common interests	Respect for each other*
Consideration of partner	Soul mates
Confidence in each other	Stability
Dependability	Take care of your partner
Doing things together	Telling the truth
Equality	Trust
Faithfulness	Understanding
Flexible	Willingness to work through
Forgiveness	Working together on problems
Frankness	View work positively

*Top five responses
Source: Bibby, R. W. (2004). A survey of Canadian hopes and dreams. Ottawa: Vanier Institute of the Family, p. 33.

- Structure programs and services that respond to family needs, by ensuring collaborative, comprehensive services that focus on the whole family, in the areas of prevention, treatment and support. Current programs too often divide the problems of families and children into categories that fit the program mandate and requirements.
- Focus on community revitalization efforts, combining the efforts of governments, non-profit organizations, businesses, and communities in creating environments that support families.
- Focus on community-based program delivery to increase the probability of ease of access in order to be as responsive as possible to the families they serve.
- Encourage efforts of corporations to sponsor programs that enhance families and strengthen communities.
- Encourage workplaces to recognize the importance of policies that support families. Not only are families strengthened, but employee morale, motivation, loyalty and productivity are improved.
- Increase focus on self-help and other non-professionally-oriented mutual support networks that enhance and empower families.
- De-emphasize formal, categorical programs and increase involvement by communities, extended families, neighbors and churches.

These groups must reclaim their natural functions as agents of family support.

- Decrease attention on testing and assessment of problems in families and focus more on determining sources of family support and the context in which families live.
- Decrease adversarial approaches to addressing family issues and consider more efforts at mediation.

In 1994 The Canadian Association of Family Resource Programs (FRP Canada) was formed. FRP Canada is a national association that provides leadership to carry out social policy, conducts research, and offers resource development and training for those who help families to raise their children. FRP Canada is voluntary, not-for-profit, community-based organizations that support families by providing services that include information, referrals, networking, and material assistance. They reflect the needs of the families and communities where they serve and are known by a variety of different names depending on where they are located. FRP Canada works with other organizations that work with families such as child-care programs, early intervention programs, child protection agencies, Aboriginal family organizations, and national organizations with an interest in children and families.

There are many other family support agencies and groups across Canada such as not-for-profit groups, Family Service Canada and Child and Family Canada. The Canadian government agencies also include family services and have recently implemented initiatives to support families and children in the specific areas of early childhood development programs, extended parental benefits in the workplace, family tax benefits, funded research, Aboriginal programs and services, and healthy family initiatives.

CONCLUSION

Leo Tolstoy wrote "Happy Families are all alike, every unhappy family is unhappy in its own way." I do not believe that we can accept this quotation. All lasting families are unique in their own family life cycle. Each one manages to continue to grow in their unique style of living. It's time that we accentuate the positive aspects of family life and give credit to those Canadian families who manage to survive the day-by-day stresses and live in the 21st century as strong families.

REFERENCES

Alberta Premier's Council in Support of Families (1993, March). *Perspectives on family well-being.* Edmonton, Alberta.

Augustine, N. (August, 9, 2000). Grandfather was a knowing Christian, *Toronto Star,* Toronto ON Canada

Bauder, H., & Sharpe, B. (2002). Residential segregation of visible minorities in Canada's gateway cities. *The Canadian Geographer, 46,* 204-223.

Bibby, R. W. (2004). *A survey of Canadian hopes and dreams.* Ottawa: Vanier Institute of the Family.

Boyd, M., & Norris, B. (1999, Spring). The crowded nest: Young adults at home. *Canadian Social Trends, 52,* 2-6

Canadian Council on Learning. (2005). *Lessons in learning.* Ottawa, Ontario: Canadian Council on Learning.

CBC News. (January 24, 2006). Hungry for Change Fed Tory Vote: Poll.

Clark, W., & Schellenberg, G. (2006). *Canadian Societal Trends: Who's religious,* Ottawa, Ontario: Statistics Canada. Cat. # 11-008

Cocivera, M. (1982). *Normal families deserve support and encouragement.* Guelph, Ontario: University of Guelph, Fact Sheet.

Corbeil, J. (2003). 30 years of education: Canada's language groups. *Canadian Social Trends,* Ottawa, Ontario: Statistics Canada.

Cranswick, K., & Thomas, D. (Summer, 2005). Elder care and the complexities of social networks. *Canadian Social Trends,* Cat. no. 11-008, pp. 10-15. Ottawa, Ontario: Statistics Canada.

Heisz, A. (2005). *Ten Things to Know about Canadian Metropolitan Areas: A Synthesis of Statistics Canada's Trends and Conditions in Census Metropolitan Areas Series.* Ottawa, Ontario: Statistics Canada, Business and Labour Market Analysis Division.

Human Resources Development Canada (1996). *Growing up in Canada: National longitudinal survey of children and youth.* Ottawa, Ontario: Statistics Canada.

Human Resources Development Canada (2002). The well-being of Canada's young children. Ottawa, Ontario: Statistics Canada.

Hull, J. (2006). *Aboriginal Women: A Profile from the 2001 Census.* Ottawa, Ontario: Minister of Public Works and Government Services.

Isajiw, W. (1990). Ethnic identity retention. In R. Brenton, W. Isajiw, W. Kalbach, & J. Reitz (Eds.) *Ethnic identity and equality: Varieties of experience in a Canadian city* (pp. 34-82). Toronto: University of Toronto Press.

King, K. F. (1983). Recognizing family strengths. *Proceedings of the National Symposium on Family Strengths.* Oakville, Ontario: Sheridan College, 48-60.

Langlois, N. (Ed.) (2004). *Canadian global almanac.* Toronto, Ontario: John Wiley and Sons.

Looker, D., & Thiessen, V. (2004). Aspirations of Canadian youth for higher education. Gatineau, Quebec: Human Resources and Skills Development Canada.

Mata, F. (2002). A look at life satisfaction and ethnicity in Canada. *Canadian Ethnic Studies Journal, 34,* 51-65.

National Advisory Council on Aging. (2006). *Seniors in Canada: 2006 Report Card.* Ottawa, Ontario: Minister of Public Works and Government Services Canada.

Nilan, A. (2000). One hundred years of families. *Canadian Social Trends*. Ottawa, Ontario: Statistics Canada.

Pigott, B. S., & Kalbach, M. A. (2005). Language effects on ethnic identity in Canada. *Canadian Ethnic Studies Journal, 37*, 3-19.

Schlesinger, B. (1983, September). Lasting and functioning families in the 1980s. *Canadian Journal of Community Mental Health, 2*, 45-56.

Schlesinger, B. (1998). *Strengths in families: Accentuating the positive*. Ottawa, Ontario: Vanier Institute of the Family.

Statistics Canada (2001a). Canada yearbook 2001. Ottawa, Ontario: Statistics Canada, Cat #11-402-XP3.

Statistics Canada (2001b). Aboriginal peoples of Canada: A demographic profile. Ottawa, Ontario: Statistics Canada, Cat #96F003XIE2001007.

Statistics Canada (2002). Profile of Canadian families and households: Diversification continues. Ottawa, Ontario: Statistics Canada Cat. # 96F0030XIE2001003.

Statistics Canada (2003). Canada's ethnocultural portrait: The Changing mosaic. Ottawa, Ontario: Statistics Canada, Cat #96F0030XIE2001008.

Statistics Canada (2004a). Family violence in Canada: A statistical profile. Ottawa, Ontario: Statistics Canada, Canadian Centre for Justice Statistics. Cat # 85-224-XIE.

Statistics Canada (2004b). Canadian community health survey. Retrieved on August 26, 2006 from http://www.statcan.ca?Daily/English/040615/d040615b.htm, p. 7.

Statistics Canada (2004c). Study: The sandwich generation. The Daily, September, 28, 2004.

Statistics Canada (2005a). Population projections. The Daily. December 15, 2005.

Statistics Canada (2005b). Access to health care services in Canada. Ottawa, Ontario: Statistics Canada, Health Statistics Division, Cat # 82-575-XIE.

Statistics Canada (2005c). Divorces. The Daily, March 9, 2005.

Statistics Canada (2006a). Women in Canada: A gender-based statistical report. Ottawa, Ontario: Statistics Canada, Social and Aboriginal Statistics Division, Cat # 89-503-XPE.

Statistics Canada (2006b). General Social Survey: Paid and unpaid work. The Daily, July, 19, 2006.

University of Toronto, Faculty of Social Work (2000). *Canada: A cultural profile*. Toronto.

Vanier Institute of the Family (2004). *Profiling Canada's Families III*. Ottawa, Ontario: Vanier Institute of the Family.

Westley, W.A., & Epstein, N. B. (1969). *The silent majority*. San Francisco: Jossey-Bass.

Williams, C. (2005). The sandwich generation. *Canadian Social Trends*. Ottawa, Ontario: Statistics Canada.

doi:10.1300/J002v41n03_03

Family Strengths and Challenges in the USA

John DeFrain
Sylvia M. Asay

SUMMARY. Families in the United States are faced with many challenges both within the family and in the social environment. To balance this discussion of challenges, an exploration of how the strengths of families and couples–their positive abilities and attitudes toward life and each other–help to create an intimate family environment in which love, satisfaction, happiness, and comfort predominate. The discussion will focus on the work of two research teams whose work led to the development of the International Family Strengths Model by Stinnett, DeFrain, and their colleagues, and the development of the Couple and Family Systems Model (also known as the Circumplex Model) developed by Olson and his colleagues. Outcomes point out that though it is clearly important to learn and acknowledge dysfunction, it is also of utmost importance that we learn about family and couple strengths to develop

John DeFrain is Extension Professor of Family and Community Development, Department of Child, Youth, and Family Studies, 135 Mabel Lee Hall, City Campus, University of Nebraska, Lincoln, NE 68588-0236, USA (E-mail: jdefrain1@unl.edu). Sylvia M. Asay is Associate Professor of Family Studies, Otto Olsen 205A, University of Nebraska, Kearney, NE 68849, USA (E-mail: asays@unk.edu).

Address correspondence to: John DeFrain.

The authors offer special thanks to David H. Olson, Professor Emeritus of Family Social Science at the University of Minnesota at St. Paul, for his pioneering research on families.

[Haworth co-indexing entry note]: "Family Strengths and Challenges in the USA." DeFrain, John, and Sylvia M. Asay. Co-published simultaneously in *Marriage & Family Review* (The Haworth Press, Inc.) Vol. 41, No. 3/4, 2007, pp. 281-307; and: *Strong Families Around the World: Strengths-Based Research and Perspectives* (ed: John DeFrain, and Sylvia M. Asay) The Haworth Press, Inc., 2007, pp. 281-307. Single or multiple copies of this article are available for a fee from The Haworth Document Delivery Service [1-800-HAWORTH, 9:00 a.m. - 5:00 p.m. (EST). E-mail address: docdelivery@haworthpress.com].

Available online at http://mfr.haworthpress.com
© 2007 by The Haworth Press, Inc. All rights reserved.
doi:10.1300/J002v41n03_04

models of family dynamics that lead people to more satisfying relationships. doi:10.1300/J002v41n03_04 *[Article copies available for a fee from The
Haworth Document Delivery Service: 1-800-HAWORTH. E-mail address:
<docdelivery@haworthpress.com> Website: <http://www.HaworthPress.com>
© 2007 by The Haworth Press, Inc. All rights reserved.]*

KEYWORDS. Affection, appreciation, Circumplex Model, Couple and
Family Systems Model, couple flexibility, couple closeness, couple communication, commitment, family, International Family Strengths Model,
spiritual well-being, stress, crisis

INTRODUCTION

The United States is the third largest country in the world with a diverse
geography that includes mountains, plains, deserts, and arctic tundra.
The U.S. also has great diversity of people that has presented it challenges as well as a rich cultural tableau. About 300 million people live
in the United States, with a population growth rate of about 0.59% (U.S.
Bureau of the Census, 2006a). Before European colonization began at
the end of the 15th century, the U.S. was inhabited by Native Americans,
who arrived between 50,000 and 11,000 years ago (Smithsonian Institution, 1999), although they only represent a very small percentage of the
population today due to war, diseases transmitted from the European
colonists and the consequences of poverty. The United States is largely a
country of immigrants. Waves of immigrants from Europe, Asia, South
America and Africa have come (willingly and sometimes unwillingly,
as in the case of slavery) to build the diverse population of the U.S.
Although the majority of Americans are descendants of European
ancestry, this white majority, which has been declining since 1965, is
expected to be in the minority by 2050 if current immigration trends
continue. Although there is no official language in the U.S., English is
the most widely used. By 1900 the United States became the largest
industrial nation in the world and has been a leader in scientific and
technological research. This success has resulted in personal income
levels in the United States that are among the highest in the world; however, wealth is fairly concentrated, leaving poverty a national crisis.

In this chapter on families and couples in the U.S., we will offer a
balanced view, delineating the many challenges the outside world–the
social environment–presents with which families must contend. We will

balance this discussion of challenges with an exploration of how the strengths of families and couples–their positive abilities and attitudes toward life and each other–help to create an intimate family environment in which love, satisfaction, happiness, and comfort are ever-present.

Historically, *home* has been seen for us as a *haven in a heartless world*. The past three decades of research focused almost exclusively on family problems, and this has somewhat tarnished the image we have of the home. However, most people in the U.S. today still seek to make their family home a haven and they probably have done a reasonably good job of creating a caring environment for each other.

It is often said that people in the U.S. emphasize individuality over family and community, while in many other cultures around the world the emphasis is on family and community first. This is an easy box to fit American culture into, but it is a simplification of our country. It is probably true that political/social/media-level dialogue emphasizes individuality and the rights and responsibilities of the individual. The dominant discourse seems to be rugged individualism, which often demonstrates a genuinely mean streak: "I've got mine! Get your own!"

In spite of the talking heads on television and the blaring and aggressive verbiage in the headlines in the newspapers, there is always a kinder, gentler and more community-spirited dialogue going on in the United States. Though the aggression of our national politics can trickle down into our communities and our families, we believe the dominant discourse in our most intimate environments in the U.S. leans more toward the "*we*" side than the "*me*" side of the equation.

The fact is, our families, our neighborhoods, our schools, our communities simply could not function if aggressive and grasping individuality truly was the norm. The best way to learn about the United States is not to watch our movies, our television or read our newspapers, but to stay in the home of an American family. If visitors would eat dinner with our families, listen to our children talk about their lives, talk with our neighbors, go to school with family members, meet our colleagues and friends at work, and see how we spend our leisure time, a more positive image would emerge of couples and families in the U.S.

DEFINING FAMILY

We take an inclusive view when defining *family*, leaning toward the American Association of Family and Consumer Sciences (1975) definition:

A family is defined as two or more persons who share resources, share responsibility for decisions, share values and goals, and have a commitment to one another over time. The family is that climate that one comes home to and it is this network of sharing and commitments that most accurately describes the family unit, regardless of blood, legal ties, adoption, or marriage.

Newsweek reported a complementary but more streamlined definition of family from a random sample of 1,200 adults in the U.S. in a Massachusetts Mutual Life Insurance Company survey. The participants in the survey could choose from a wide variety of definitions of family. Some of the definition choices were very traditional, emphasizing blood and marriage. An alternative choice, however, emphasized the quality of the relationships among family members rather than biology and law. The vast majority of Americans opted for the most inclusive definition of family: 75% of the participants in the survey indicated that "a family is people who love and care for each other" ("Domesticated bliss," 1992). The essence of both of these definitions is on the strength of the relationships within the group–the social and psychological realities–rather than the structure of the group, blood, or legal ties.

CHALLENGES FAMILIES AND COUPLES FACE TODAY IN THE U.S.

The list of challenges American families and couples face is endless, and there is no genuinely objective way we know for generating such a list, ordering it or delimiting it. Every social observer's list will be different and the lists will change dramatically over time. The following are some of the challenges many Americans face today that we see regularly discussed in the media and around the breakfast table.

High Levels of Stress, Materialism and Competition

"Whatever you're doing," one anonymous observer in our country once wryly noted, "it's not enough." The velocity of life in the U.S. appears to many people to be increasing exponentially, urging us to produce and consume and this creates high stress. Stress is directly related to change and the greater the change, the higher the level of stress. The continuous cascade of new developments in society today is often defined broadly as progress, but many of these developments add stress to our lives. As a society, we also have a great appetite for material possessions. In fact, everything has to be new, if we were to believe media sales pitches: we need new cars, new houses, new clothes, perhaps a new nose. The business world is brimming with stories of corporate takeovers and downsizing. Companies come and go every day and workers are cast off like old furniture. In this kind of consumer culture, it is not such a stretch to imagine that finding a new partner is the easiest option when there are problems with the old relationship. In fact, we believe that our high divorce rate in America can be seen as a reflection of a consumer and cast-off society.

In many elements of the U.S. culture we do not seem to be content with who we are as an individual, but are continuously comparing ourselves to others. This competitiveness adds to the pace of life and generates anxiety and stress. A sports-type mentality pervades many of our institutions as we strive to reduce our lives to numbers and ratings that can be compared, making much of our lives a race to be run rather than an experience to be savored and loved. With all of these elements combined, technology, materialism and competition increase our level of stress in all areas of life. We feel pressured to do more and to have more–and to run faster while grasping for all of it. The first casualty in such an environment is our individual sense of well-being. The second casualty is our bonds of affection and closeness with each other.

Lack of Time for Oneself and One's Family

According to family researchers in America, one of the most difficult qualities to develop in many American families is the ability to spend enjoyable time together. Not only do we find ourselves challenged by a busy and competitive social environment outside the home, but once we return home, we need time to unwind from a hectic day before reconnecting with others. In today's society, the boundaries between the home and work are being blurred. As sociologist Arlie Hochschild (1997) observed, work becomes more like home and home becomes more like work. Caught in the time bind, the more time we work, the more stressful home life becomes. The more stressful home life becomes, the more we want to escape back to work. Hochschild argues that we must challenge the economic and social system that invites or demands long hours at work, and focus our efforts on investing less time in the job and more time in one's couple and family relationships.

Increasing Use of Child Care Outside the Family

One of the most challenging questions American parents face today is what to do with the children when both parents work. In 1940, only 10% of American children lived with a mother who was in the labor force. By 1990, nearly 60% of American children lived with an employed mother. This sixfold increase of mothers in the workplace over a fifty-year period fueled the steady increase of child care outside the family and the extended family, even for infants (Hernandez, 1997). Mothers and fathers, surrounded by the swirling controversy over child care, ask their own very personal questions such as: Do I really need to work outside the home? Is employment essential for our family's well-being? Will I be able to develop a bond with my child if she spends so much time away from me? How will the stresses of the job affect me or my family? Will my child receive good care? These are difficult questions many American parents have to answer.

A High Divorce and Remarriage Rate

Calculating divorce rates in the U.S. is a notoriously difficult and controversial task for statisticians in the government, but it has been estimated that about half of all first marriages and an even higher percentage of remarriages end in divorce (U.S. Bureau of the Census, 2000). Many observers have argued that our fast-moving and competitive social environment is directly related to the high rate of marital dissolution and the increase in single-parent families and stepfamilies. Although personality conflicts and troubles within a marriage clearly contribute to marital breakdown, societal factors and values also influence our intimate behavior. Many of our personal impressions come from the media. Married life on television and in the tabloid newspapers is far different from the average couple's life. It can be argued that the steady diet of extramarital affairs and marital conflict we receive from the media helps to create a *culture of divorce* in this country.

Violence, Criminal Victimization, and Fear

Violent and abusive behavior continues to be a major cause of death, injury, and stress and fear in our country. Crime victimizes millions annually. Statistics from the National Crime Victimization Survey indicate that 25.9 million violent and property victimizations occurred in 2001. There were 691,710 nonfatal violent victimizations committed by current or former spouses, boyfriends, or girlfriends of the victims that year. These crimes–intimate partner violence–usually involve female victims; 85% of the victimizations by intimate partners were against women. By contrast, intimate partners in the same year committed 3% of all nonfatal violence against men (U.S. Department of Justice, 2001).

Nation-wide, the most recent statistics available indicate an estimated 872,000 children were victims of abuse and neglect in 2004. Statistically, the 2004 victimization rate of 11.9 per 100,000 in population is lower than the 2001 rate of 12.5. During 2004, more than 60% of the victims suffered neglect; 18% were physically abused; 10% were sexually abused; 7% were emotionally maltreated; and 15% were associated with "other" types of maltreatment based on specific state laws and policies. A child could be a victim of more than one type of maltreatment. Girls were slightly more likely to be victims than boys. 1,490 children died due to child abuse or neglect. More than 80% of those children killed were younger than 4 years of age; about 12% were 4-7 years old; 4% were 8-11 years old, and 3% were 12-17 years old (Administration on Children, Youth and Families, 2006).

In *This Noble Land*, one of James Michener's last books before his death in 1997, Michener argued that America is becoming more and more violent. "The most instructive proof of our nation's increasingly vigorous move toward a macho society can be seen in our unique fascination with guns, our insistence on having them and our willingness to accept murder as a result of the huge number [of guns] we allow and even encourage private citizens to own" (1996, p. 176). In 2001 there were 29,573 firearm-related deaths in the U.S.: 16,869 (57%) from suicide; 11,671 (39%) from homicide (including 323 deaths due to legal intervention/war); and 1,033 (3%) undetermined/unintentional firearm deaths (Centers for Disease Control, 2003, p. 71). In the same year, 56% of all homicides and 55% of all suicides resulted from firearm use (U.S. Centers for Disease Control, 2003, p. 41). The rate of gun homicides in the U.S. per 100,000 people is almost 7 times higher than Canada; 28 times higher than England and Wales; and 198 times higher than Japan. (Educational Fund to Stop Gun Violence, 2002).

Sex as a National Obsession

Sex pervades the American social environment. It is a frequent topic on the radio, on television, on billboards, in movies, at the shopping mall, in the classroom, at the office, in churches, in our daily conversations, in government, in the White House. Sex has been big business in American culture for some time, but today it has reached the status of a national obsession and with the growth of the internet sex reaches deep into our homes causing concern about child exploitation on line (Congressional Internet Caucus Advisory Committee, 2004).

Some statistics in the area of sexuality in American culture:

- 49% of women in this country will have at least one unplanned pregnancy between the ages of 15 and 44. At current rates, 43% of American women will have had an abortion by age 45 (Alan Guttmacher Institute, 2000).
- More than half of all couples cohabit before marriage, and cohabitation is becoming more acceptable. Although cohabitation was once rare, a majority of young men and women of marriageable age will live together without being married for some time and about 40% of all children before reaching age 16 will spend some time in a cohabiting family (Bumpass & Yu, 1998, 2000). Recent research raises concerns for cohabitation in the areas of marital stability (Kamp Dush, Cohan & Amato, 2004), child well-being (Brown, 2004) and lower levels of personal commitment (Stanley, Whitton & Markman, 2004).
- Adolescent pregnancy, a long-standing social concern in the United States, has been one of the most frequently cited examples of perceived societal decay in this country. Fortunately, the rate of births to teenagers is lower today than it was throughout much of the 20th century (Coley & Chase-Lansdale, 1998). Between 1986 and 2000 the rate dropped 22%, and fell by 28% since peaking in 1990. The teen abortion rate in 2000 was 24.0 per 1,000 women aged 15-19. From 1986 to 2000 the total abortion rate in the U.S. dropped 43%; during the same period, the percentage of teenage pregnancies ending in abortion dropped from 46% to 33% (Alan Guttmacher Institute, 2004, p. 2).
- Extramarital sexual relationships are estimated to range from 30% to 50% for men and 10% to 40% for women (Atkins, Baucom, & Jacobson, 2001; Christopher, 2000; Laumann, Gagnon et al., 1995; Treas & Giesen, 2000).

To counter these challenges, couples need to create a loving and committed relationship in a social environment fascinated by sex and full of temptation and hypocrisy. For parents it will mean developing open and honest communication with their children on sexuality. This is a subject that few parents are really very good at talking about. There needs to be a more concerted effort to improve the quality of sex education in our schools, places of worship, and homes.

The High-Level Use of Alcohol, Tobacco and Other Drugs

The American social environment is dominated by advertising and a consumption-oriented approach to living. The advertising world has succeeded over the years in making alcohol and tobacco use look fun, sophisticated and sexy to countless young people who are lured to these dangerous drugs every day. But the dark side of these socially accepted and legal drugs is rarely portrayed. In fact, illegal drugs receive much more media attention, even though alcohol and tobacco kill approximately 30 times as many Americans as illegal drugs each year. More deaths and disabilities in the U.S. each year are attributed to substance abuse than any other cause. Approximately 18 million Americans have alcohol problems and 5 to 6 million more have other drug problems (Brandeis University, 1993, 2001). More than half of all adult Americans have a family history of alcoholism or problem drinking and more than 9 million children live with a parent who is dependent on alcohol and/or illicit drugs (Brown University, 2000). Alcohol contributes to the death of about 85,000 people each year in the U.S. (Centers for Disease Control and Prevention, 2004).

But alcohol-related deaths are dwarfed by deaths caused by tobacco in this country. In 2000, 435,000 people died from smoking tobacco, chewing tobacco and breathing other people's smoke. Illicit drugs, which receive so much media attention, claimed the lives of 17,000 Americans (Centers for Disease Control and Prevention, 2004). Thus, legal drugs (alcohol and tobacco) killed 520,000 people, more than 30 times as many as those killed by illegal drugs.

Changing Gender Roles and Power Issues in Marriages and Families

As we noted earlier, there has been a dramatic increase in the number of mothers working outside the home in America in the past four decades. This development has helped fuel an ongoing discussion of the roles of women and men in America and how power should be allocated in society as a whole and between household partners in particular. Although women have served as leaders of more than 20 countries around the world, a woman has yet to serve as president of the United States (Porter, 1999). Nevertheless, women are serving as associate justices in the Supreme Court, as senators and representatives of Congress and in countless other positions of power and influence in both government and the business world.

With the emergence of women in traditionally male roles, particularly in positions of power, gender roles are being redefined. Some observers argue that there has been a *masculine culture* in this country, which thrives on competition and the achievement of dominance, and a feminine *culture*, which aims at positive emotional connection and the creation of community. In their relatively new roles of authority, women are being encouraged to be more assertive and to let others know exactly where they stand. In contrast, males are being urged to be less aggressive and more honest and open about their feelings. American society in many corners is openly questioning the traditional role of the dominant male and the submissive female.

Just as *supermoms* struggle to find a meaningful balance between work and family, so, too, men are challenged by their own changing world. Years ago, a man's home was *his* castle; today it is an *egalitarian haven*. Just how fairly power and work should be shared in American households is a topic of considerable discussion today. Some observers suggest there is still a long way to go before true equality is reached in the home. Many maintain that women have been the true pioneers of the gender revolution, arguing that wives have more quickly changed their roles *outside* the home than men have changed their roles *inside* the home. Still others question how equal we really want males and females to be in our society. They assert that females and males are biologically different and that wives should stay at home to better socialize our children. Regardless of one's position, it is impossible to deny that gender roles and relationship power balances are evolving.

Urban Migration and Overcrowding

When farmers depended upon animals for work and transportation, small towns dotted the rural landscape in the heartland about six miles apart. Eventually, trucks and tractors replaced horses and mules, farms got bigger, and the number of farmers and farm families declined steadily over the years. Small towns also shrank in size. What do we lose when a small town vanishes? What do we lose when the kids grow up and leave the farm or ranch for the city? A realist, focusing solely on harsh economic forces, might say that the young person is leaving the farm to find work and a more stable life in an urban environment. An idealist might argue that we lose a little bit of the fabric of America, a small piece of the American dream. American rural societies tend to be caring environments in which many honest and hard-working individuals live and join together to help each other and their communities to succeed (Struthers & Bokemeier, 2000).

Another trend is that more people are moving away from the large cities to suburbs and small rural areas within commuting range to recapture that small town atmosphere. Others are beginning to realize that a village-like atmosphere can also be created in an urban neighborhood, in an apartment building, or among relatives and friends scattered about a city. Impersonal forces of urban living can be countered by the creation of village-like social structures in the neighborhood, in the workplace, in religious institutions, and in community settings. While it is possible to make these connections, there are many who continue to live a lonely and isolated existence surrounded by a sea of people.

Financial Problems, Overspending, Poverty and the Global Economy

Financial issues are the most common stressors couples and families face, regardless of how much money they make. Researchers have consistently found that economic distress and unemployment are detrimental to family relationships (Gomel, Tinsley & Clark, 1998). Estimates of homelessness in the U.S. indicate that over a five-year period, about 2-3% of the population (5-8 million people) will experience at least one night of homelessness (Substance Abuse and Mental Health Services, 2006). The nation's official poverty rate stood at 12.7% in 2004 (U.S. Bureau of the Census, 2006b), though many family economists argue that this number is unreasonably low. Over one in six children in this country live in poverty and more than one out of three of all poor people are children (U.S. Bureau of the Census, 2006c).

The number of children living in poverty is highly related to living in a single-parent versus a two-parent household in the United States but less so in other countries. In the United States, it has been estimated that nearly 60% of the children from single-parent households live in poverty, as compared to only 11% of children from two-parent households. In Western Europe in countries with stronger social welfare systems, the situation for single parents and their children is better. In Germany 43% of single mothers and their children lived in poverty compared to 4% of two-parent households; in Italy, 14% of single-parent families lived in poverty compared to 10% of two-parent households; and in Sweden, 6% of single-parent families lived in poverty compared to 2%

of two-parent families. The unfortunate fact of single parenthood in the United States is the lack of government support for these families that other Western countries are more likely to provide (Houseknecht & Sastry, 1996).

Though the rate of hunger in America dropped during the economic boom times of the late 1990s, 27 million people, including nearly 11 million children, were hungry or at least food-insecure in 1999, according to the U.S. Department of Agriculture ("Nation's hunger rate dropped 24 percent in the late 1990s," 2000). Later USDA figures from 2004 indicated 11.9% of American households were food-insecure and the prevalence of food insecurity with hunger was 3.9%. Data from 2004 indicated 15.7% of the nation's population is without health insurance coverage. This figure includes 8.3 million children without health insurance, an estimated 11.2% of all children under age 18 (U.S. Department of Agriculture, 2006).

Many Americans today are doing well financially, and yet many other Americans live close to the edge, lacking savings and chronically spending more than they earn. Easy credit lines have contributed to mounting debt, especially credit-card debt, which carries extraordinarily high interest rates. Debt threatens not only individuals but also the well-being of the lenders and, eventually, the economy as a whole. Many acknowledge the shrinking middle class and note the growing differences between the wealthy and lower classes. One reason for this may be middle-class workers who are being replaced by temporary workers who are willing to work for less money and demand fewer benefits.

Although economic survival is challenging for many people in the United States, residents of many countries around the world are in far worse straits. Nonetheless, their economic problems do not exist in isolation; as business commentators and politicians frequently point out, we are living in a global economy. The strength of the American economy is inextricably linked in complex ways to the economies of many other nations. The evolving global economy is a demon or a friend, depending upon who is talking. Economists seem to lean toward the brighter view of globalization, arguing that competition and market forces insure efficiency, cheaper goods, and a gradually unfolding better world for all. The economists, however, usually are looking at large-group data sets rather than listening closely to individuals and their families ("Special Report: Ten Years of NAFTA; Free Trade on Trial," 2004).

On the other hand, many people feel victimized by global market forces–the workers in a factory in the U.S. that is closing down and moving operations to Mexico, and the workers in a factory in Mexico that is closing down and moving operations to China. These are victims of global forces and the power of multinational companies that are not likely to be interested in theoretical long-term gain for the world in general or profits for large businesses in particular, but rather are most likely to focus on the pain of disruption in their personal lives and the lives of their families.

Ethnic/Cultural Tensions

American society continues to struggle over differences, often ignoring remarkable similarities and focusing instead on how we differ in terms of our political and economic systems, religious and social values, language, physical appearance, and a host of other points of contention. In our families, our most intimate environment and our most basic human social institution, we are much more alike than different, and a reasonable strategy for easing ethnic tensions would be to tap into our wonderful similarities as members of the human family. Some cultural anthropologists have argued that our attentiveness to differences has survival value in evolutionary terms. If your particular tribe looks the same as the tribe on the other side of the river except for the fact that *your* tribe wears yellow feathers and *their* tribe wears red feathers, and if their tribe will kill or enslave you if you are captured, it is in your best interest to be very attentive to the color of feathers. Americans remain extremely attentive to *tribal* differences today, whether we are talking about Democratic and Republican tribes, rich or poor tribes, black or white tribes, male or female tribes, countless religious tribes, and the innumerable and exhaustingly creative ways we as human beings have found to *tribalize* our country and separate ourselves from each other. Often times the tribal nature of our country leads us into trouble within our society and trouble with other cultures.

War and Terrorism

The events of September 11, 2001 have had a profound impact on Americans. As the world knows, about 3,000 people died that day in the attacks on the World Trade Center in New York City, at the Pentagon in Washington, D.C., and the plane crash in western Pennsylvania. The average American was shocked and stunned by the events of September 11th. Many Americans reacted with anger, wanting revenge against the attackers. And many Americans have reacted with sorrow, wondering what we could have possibly done to cause such hatred toward our country. Countless questions continue to be posed, swirling around issues of national identity: Is America a peace-loving nation, attacked for no legitimate reason by fanatics? Or, is it an imperial power with designs on global domination?

We believe that most Americans want peace in the world, and to live in a world where people from all nations get along with each other, share the earth's resources fairly, and where people of all cultures genuinely respect and appreciate the wonderful diversity we have in the world today. And many Americans are reaching out to people in other cultures and countries. But at the same time, many American families are feeling anxious and threatened. They worry about their own safety, especially when they travel and for the safety of their loved ones.

THE QUALITIES OF STRONG FAMILY AND COUPLE RELATIONSHIPS

As David H. Olson has said, "All the problems in the world seem to either begin in the family or end up in the family." Couples and families inadvertently create problems for themselves that they then have a diffi-cult time solving; or they are the recipient of problems from the outside world that demand immediate and careful attention. Life, however, is more than solving problems, even though human beings seem to have a proclivity for relentlessly focusing on difficulties while ignoring or neg-lecting or forgetting the good things that bring them joy and comfort–their strengths.

The first formal social science research on family strengths can be traced back to Woodhouse's study of 250 successful families during the depression in 1930; after that pioneering study, very little interest was shown. Fascination with a focus on family problems, however, has always dominated researchers' thinking. When Herbert Otto began his work on strong families and family strengths in the early 1960s, it became readily apparent that problems had proven far more interesting than strengths to a wide variety of professions (Gabler & Otto, 1964; Otto, 1962, 1963). Family strengths did not capture much interest again until Nick Stinnett began his work at Oklahoma State University in 1974 and moved to the University of Nebraska-Lincoln in 1977. Stinnett, DeFrain and their colleagues designed a series of studies focusing on various aspects of family strengths and among different ethnic/cultural groups, and they began publishing a continuous series of articles and books focusing on how families can succeed (Casas, Stinnett, DeFrain & Lee, 1984; DeFrain,

DeFrain, & Lepard, 1994; DeFrain & Stinnett, 2002; Stinnett & DeFrain, 1985; Stinnett, et al., 1999; Stinnett & O'Donnell, 1996; Stinnett & Sauer, 1977; Xie, DeFrain, Meredith & Combs, 1996).

A series of family strengths conferences beginning in 1978 proved to be a catalyst for research on strong families. Nine books of readings were published as a result of the National Symposium on Building Family Strengths series. An International Family Strengths Network (IFSN) began working on a series of family strengths gatherings in the late 1990s, and to date there have been more than 33 conferences held in North America, Asia and Australia. Upcoming conferences to be co-sponsored by the IFSN include a Middle Eastern International Family Strengths Conference, an American International Family Strengths Conference, a Korean International Family Strengths Conference, a Pan-African International Family Strengths Conference, and gatherings in Australia and Spain. (For the latest information on conference schedules, contact John DeFrain at <jdefrain1@unl.edu>.) In sum, a relatively small but dedicated number of researchers in the U.S. and around the world have been looking closely at what makes families work well, rather than focus all their attention on how families fail.

The simple genius of this focus on family strengths is to bring into a more reasonable balance our understanding of how families function in the face of life's inherent difficulties. By looking only at a family's problems and a family's failings, we ignore the fact that it takes a positive approach to be successful. In the case of a family in crisis, professionals sometimes seem to spend so much time focusing their fascination on the intricate details of the problem that they forget that problems are solved by a family using its own strengths effectively. In sum, to solve family problems, understand and use family strengths. What then are family strengths? What qualities make couple relationships strong? A number of models have been proposed over the years, and the fascinating aspect of all these models is how similar they are to each other. When studying Table 1 the reader will see how researchers use many different words to say very similar things.

We will focus our discussion here on the work of two research teams whose work led to the development of the International Family Strengths Model by Stinnett, DeFrain, and their colleagues, and the development of the Couple and Family Systems Model (also known as the Circumplex Model) developed by Olson and his colleagues. The models complement each other well, and that is why findings from the studies supporting them are presented together here in this chapter. To understand the work more fully, there are a number of useful sources (DeFrain, 1999;

TABLE 1. Dimensions of family strength as delineated by prominent researchers.

Theorists and Countries	Dimensions
Beavers and Hampson (1990). U.S.A.	Centripetal/centrifugal interaction, closeness, parent coalitions, autonomy, adaptability, egalitarian power, goal-directed negotiation, ability to resolve conflict, clarity of expression, range of feelings, openness to others, empathic understanding
Billingsley (1986). U.S.A.	Strong family ties, strong religious orientation, educational aspirations/achievements
Curran (1983). U.S.A.	Togetherness, respect and trust, shared leisure, privacy valued, shared mealtime, shared responsibility, family rituals, communication, affirmation of each other, religious love, humor/play
Epstein, Bishop, Ryan, Miller, and Keitner (1993). Canada.	Affective involvement, behavior control, communication
Geggie, DeFrain, Hitchcock and Silberberg (2000). Australia.	Communication (open, positive, honest, including humor), togetherness, sharing activities, affection, support, acceptance, commitment, resilience
Kantor and Lehr (1974). U.S.A.	Affect, power
Kryson, Moore and Zill (1990). U.S.A.	Commitment to family, time together, encouragement of individuals, ability to adapt, clear roles, communication, religious orientation, social connectedness
Mberengwa and Johnson (2003). Botswana.	Consensus as a means of settling differences, anger management, concern for the welfare of one's kin, valuing their culture, respect toward others, *kgotla* (community development associations) for strengthening neighborhoods
Olson, McCubbin, Barnes, Larsen, Muxen, and Wilson (1989); Olson and Olson (2000). U.S.A.	Strong marriage, high family cohesion, good family flexibility, effective coping with stress and crisis, positive couple and family communication
Otto (1962, 1963). U.S.A.	Shared religious and moral values; love, consideration and understanding; common interests, goals and purposes; love and happiness of children; working and playing together; sharing specific recreational activities
D. Reiss (1981). U.S.A.	Coordination, closure
Sani and Buhannad (2003). United Arab Emirates.	Patriarchal family structure; family-arranged marriages; gender-based rights, responsibilities and privileges; strong emotional family bonds (*muwada*); extended family (*dhurriyah*); living with or next extended family members; frequent consultation; elders as role models and advisors; crises are tests from Allah; Islamic beliefs (*taqwa*) and practices provide optimal guidelines; collectivism over individualism; the government is supportive of individual, couple and family well-being
Stinnett, DeFrain and their colleagues (1977, 1985, 2002). U.S.A.	Appreciation and affection, commitment, positive communication, enjoyable time together, spiritual well-being, effective management of stress and crisis

Theorists and Countries	Dimensions
Xia, Xie, and Zhou, Z. (2004); Xie, DeFrain, Meredith, and Combs (1996); Xu and Ye (2002). China.	Togetherness and time together across three generations; love, care, and commitment; communication; family support; spirituality (at peace with nature, at peace with oneself, at peace with others, at peace with the world); family oriented and harmonious
Yoo (2004); Yoo, DeFrain, Lee, Kim, Hong, Choi and Ahn (2004). Korea.	Respect, commitment, appreciation and affection, positive communication, sharing values and goals, role performing, physical health, connectedness with social systems, economic stability, ability to solve problems

DeFrain et al., 2006; DeFrain & Olson, 1999; DeFrain & Stinnett, 2002; Geggie, et al, 2000; Olson, 1996; Olson & DeFrain, 2006; Olson, Fye & Olson, 1999; Olson et al., 1989; Olson & Olson, 2000). First we'll look at the International Family Strengths Model, and then turn to recent research on couple strengths related to the Family Circumplex Model.

The International Family Strengths Model

An International Family Strengths Model has been developed over the past 30 years by Stinnett, DeFrain, and their colleagues. It is based on research with more than 24,000 family members in all 50 states of the U.S. and 28 other countries around the world. Each family's constellation of strengths is unique and different from every other family. Likewise, each culture's family strengths are unique and different from every other culture. But, family strengths from family to family and culture to culture are actually remarkably similar. In fact, we believe that family strengths when studying cultures comparatively are much more similar than different. In our most intimate of environments, what makes a family strong can be reduced to a handful of relatively simple concepts. These concepts are relatively easy to understand, but often-times difficult to put into practice.

There are six major qualities of strong couple and family relationships, then, in this particular model, and each of the six can be broken down further into sub-qualities: appreciation and affection; commitment to the family; positive communication; enjoyable time together; spiritual well-being; and effective management of stress and crisis. The elements of this model were delineated by collecting data from both *insider* and *outsider* perspectives. The research methodology in this work recognizes the validity of family members' perspectives from inside the family, and recognizes the validity of professionals' perspectives from outside the family. All of the family strengths are interconnected with each other, and actually are impossible to separate out. What unites all the strengths together is that each is founded upon a sense of *positive emotional connection*. People in strong families feel good about each other and work to insure each other's well-being. The following is a closer examination of the six family strengths:

Appreciation and affection. People in strong families deeply care for one another, and they let each other know this on a regular basis. They are not afraid to express their love. Some cultures appear to be better at this than others. We've seen many Americans who are not particularly adept in this regard, especially those that lean toward the strong-and-silent approach to life. By contrast, Latino families often seem more willing to outwardly express their inner emotions.

Commitment. Members of strong families are dedicated to one another's well-being, investing time and energy in family activities and not letting their work or other elements of their lives take too much time or emotional energy away from couple and family interaction. Commitment to the marital relationship is part of this.

Positive communication. Successful couple and family relationships are not simply about solving problems and resolving conflicts, though members of strong families are good at task-oriented communication, can identify difficulties, stay focused on them, and find solutions that work reasonably well for all family members. Strong families also spend time talking with and listening to one another just to stay connected.

Enjoyable time together. One fascinating element of our research and educational activities related to the international family strengths model has been to ask literally thousands of people to take *A Journey of Happy Memories*. We request people to go back in their memories of childhood and focus on *your happiest times*. The best times in life as a child, almost always, are family times. Some people have not grown up in a happy family, of course, and they are likely to describe good times with friends, favorite pets, or in solitude and communion with nature. Very few people in our investigations reply that money made an important contribution to their happy memories from childhood. Rarely, someone will talk about going to Disneyland or a fancy hotel for dinner. Most likely, they will talk about family gatherings at holiday times; games the family played together at the dining room table or outside; working on various projects that were fun; camping trips and adventures together in nature, or pleasant mealtimes. For most people, the happiest childhood memories they have are of the family being together and enjoying each other's presence.

Spiritual well-being. Perhaps the most controversial finding of the family strengths researchers is the importance of religion or spirituality in strong families. We use the term spiritual well-being to describe this concept, indicating that it can include organized religion, but not necessarily so. People in strong families describe this concept in many ways: some talk about faith in God, hope, or a sense of optimism in life; some say they feel a oneness with the world. Others talk about their families in almost religious terms, describing the love they feel for one another with a great deal of reverence. Others express these kinds of feelings in terms of ethical values and commitment to important causes. Spiritual well-being can be seen as the caring center within each individual that promotes sharing, love, and compassion. It is a feeling or force that helps people transcend themselves and their petty day-to-day hassles, and focus on that which is sacred to them in life.

Effective management of stress and crisis. Strong families are not immune to stress and crisis, but they are also not as crisis-prone as troubled families tend to be. Rather, they possess the ability to manage both daily stressors and difficult life crises creatively and effectively. They know how to prevent trouble before it happens, and how to work together to meet challenges when they inevitably occur in life. One tactic strong families use in difficult times is to search for new ways to define the situation. Therapists call this *reframing*. Basically, the family looks at the challenge from a different angle.

The Couple and Family Systems Model

Olson and his colleagues over the past 30 years have developed a Couple and Family Systems Model (also known as the Circumplex Model) that includes three major dimensions of cohesion, flexibility, and communication. *Cohesion* is a feeling of emotional closeness with another person. Four levels of cohesion can be described in couple and family relationships: disengaged, connected, cohesive, and enmeshed. The extreme low level of cohesion is called *disengaged*, and the extreme high level, *enmeshed*. The two middle levels of cohesion–*connected* and *cohesive*–seem to be the most functional across the life cycle, in part because they balance separateness and togetherness. Both connected and cohesive relationships are classified as balanced family systems.

Flexibility is the amount of change that occurs in leadership, role relationships, and relationships rules. Like cohesion, flexibility has four levels, ranging from low to high. Those levels are rigid, structured, flexible, and chaotic. The extreme types of family systems–the *rigid* and the *chaotic*–can work well in the short run, but they have difficulty adapting over time. Conversely, the balanced types–the *structured* and the *flexible*–are more able to adapt to change over the family life cycle.

Communication is the grease that smoothes frictions between partners and family members. Family communication is linear: The better the communication skills, the stronger the couple and family relationships. The following six dimensions are considered in the assessment of family communication: listening skills, speaking skills, self-disclosure, clarity, staying on topic, and respect and regard. Positive *listening skills* involve empathy and giving feedback. *Speaking skills* include speaking for oneself and using *I* statements rather than speaking for others. *Clarity* involves the exchange of clear messages. *Staying on topic* is another important aspect of interpersonal exchanges. Last, *respect and regard* reflect the good intentions of family members and keep communication positive.

Table 2 combines concepts from the Couple and Family Systems Model and the International Family Strengths Model, for the two models clearly complement each other.

The Couple and Family Systems Model also serves as the foundation for Olson's PREPARE/ENRICH educational programs for premarital and married couples. More than 50,000 counselors and clergy of all denominations have used this program with more than a million couples in the United States. A recent study involving 21,501 married couples from all 50 states in the U.S. sheds a good deal of light on couple strengths (Olson & Olson, 2000). The researchers used data collected using the

TABLE 2. Integrating the international family strengths model and the circumplex model.

Family Cohesion
Commitment
Enjoyable Time Together
Family Flexibility
Successful management of stress and crisis
Spiritual well-being
Family Communication
Positive communication
Appreciation and affection

195-item inventories called PREPARE/ENRICH that focus on 20 of the most important areas of a couple's relationship. The researchers looked in depth at 5,153 couples where both partners were happily married, and 5,127 couples where both partners were not happily married.

Table 3 lists the *Top Ten Stumbling Blocks for Couples.* These are the issues and problems that cause them difficulty in their relationship. These are typical issues that most couples in the U.S. report they have difficulty handling in their marriage.

Table 4 lists the *Top Ten Strengths of Happy Couples.* Table 4 includes the percentage of couples who believe they are happy together who agree on each of the strengths. Table 4 also includes the percentage of couples who believe they are unhappy but do agree that they have a particular strength. These strengths demonstrate the importance of communication, conflict resolution, closeness and flexibility in maintaining a strong marriage.

Why is it that some couples seem so happy, regardless of life situations, transitions, or circumstances they may encounter? Are they simply well-matched individuals? Are they doing something different from less happy couples? What is their secret? Olson and Olson (2000) believe the

TABLE 3. Top ten stumbling blocks for couples.

Issue/Problem	Percentage of Couples Having the Problem
1. We have problems sharing leadership equally.	93%
2. My partner is sometimes too stubborn.	87%
3. Having children reduces our marital satisfaction.	84%
4. My partner is too negative or critical.	83%
5. I wish my partner had more time and energy for recreation with me.	82%
6. I wish my partner were more willing to share feelings.	82%
7. I always end up feeling responsible for the problem.	81%
8. I go out of my way to avoid conflict with my partner.	79%
9. We have difficulty completing tasks or projects.	79%
10. Our differences never seem to get resolved.	78%

Note: Couples could check as many issues/problems that they believed they experienced.
Source: Olson & Olson (2000), p. 7.

TABLE 4. Top ten strengths of happy couples.

	Happy Couples PCA*	Unhappy Couples PCA*
1. I am very satisfied with how we talk to each other.	90%	15%
2. We are creative in how we handle our differences.	78%	15%
3. We feel very close to each other.	98%	27%
4. My partner is seldom too controlling.	78%	20%
5. When discussing problems, my partner understands my opinions and ideas.	87%	19%
6. I am completely satisfied with the amount of affection from my partner.	72%	28%
7. We have a good balance of leisure time spent together and separately.	71%	17%
8. My partner's friends or family rarely interfere with our relationship.	81%	38%
9. We agree on how to spend money.	89%	41%
10. I am satisfied with how we express spiritual values and beliefs.	89%	36%

* PCA = positive couple agreement
† This table lists the one item that best discriminates between happy and unhappy couples from the ten ENRICH categories.

Note: Couples could check as many strengths as they believed they had in their relationship.
Source: Olson & Olson (2000), p. 9.

three most important contributors to marital happiness, in order of importance, are *couple communication, couple flexibility,* and *couple closeness.* Happy couples in the study were clearly more satisfied with the various aspects of positive communication in their relationship than unhappy couples (90% to 15%). Happy couples were much more likely to agree that flexibility was a strength in their relationship when compared to unhappy couples (78% to 55%). And happy couples felt much closer to each other than unhappy couples (91% 35%) (Olson & Olson, 2000, pp. 10-11).

CONCLUSION

We believe that the focus of family research needs to shift from family and couple problems, and place more attention on family and couple strengths. Most of the research in the 20th Century in America focused on *why families fail*. We would like to see 21st Century research focus on *how families succeed.* A family strengths perspective does not deny the existence of family problems, but it comes from the optimistic world-view that seeks to learn *how families creatively and effectively meet challenges.* Though it is clearly important for our society to learn as much as we can about dysfunction, it is also of utmost importance that we learn about family and couple strengths so that we have models of family dynamics that can inspire and lead people to more satisfying relationships (DeFrain, 1999; DeFrain et al., 2006; Olson & DeFrain, 2006).

Because families, in all their diversity, are the basic unit of all cultures in the world, and because strong families around the world are remarkably similar, we would like to propose a joint effort uniting a global community of researchers, theoreticians, practitioners, and families to look closely at strong family and couple relationships. The advantages of linking our unique research, cultural traditions, and perspectives together would be considerable. Social scientists focusing on strong couple and family relationships can uncover powerful insights that can help families create a better world for themselves.

REFERENCES

Administration on Children, Youth and Families. (2006).*Child maltreatment 2004.* U.S. Department of Health and Human Services. Washington, DC: U.S. Government Printing Office.

Alan Guttmacher Institute. (2000). Induced abortion. Retrieved July 19, 2006, from http://www.guttmacher.org/

Alan Guttmacher Institute. (2004). U.S. teenage pregnancy statistics: Overall trends, trends by race and ethnicity and state-by-state information. Retrieved July 19, 2006, from http://www.guttmacher.org/

American Association of Family and Consumer Sciences (AAFCS). (1975). Definition of families. Cited in AAFCS Call for 2004 Program Proposals, 2. Washington, DC: http://www.aafcs.org/

Atkins, D. C., Baucom, D. H., & Jacobson, N. S. (2001). Understanding infidelity: Correlates in a national random sample. *Journal of Family Psychology, 15*(4), 735-749.

Beavers, W. R., & Hampson, R. B. (1990). *Successful families.* New York: Norton.

Billingsley, A. (1986). *Black families in White America.* Englewood Cliffs, NJ: Prentice Hall.

Brandeis University Institute for Health Policy. (1993). Substance abuse: The nation's number one health problem. Cited by National Council on Alcoholism and Drug Dependence: http://222.ncadd.org.

Brandeis University Institute for Health Policy. (2001). Substance abuse: The nation's number one health problem. Cited by National Council on Alcoholism and Drug Dependence: http://www.ncadd.org.

Brown, S. L. (2004). Family structure and child well-being: The significance of parental cohabitation. *Journal of Marriage and the Family, 66*(2), 351-368.

Brown University Center for Alcohol and Addiction Studies. (2000). Position paper on drug policy. Physician Leadership on National Drug Policy (PLNDP). Retrieved July 19, 2006, from http://www.ncadd.org.

Bumpass, L., & Lu, H. (2000). Cohabitation: How the families of U.S. children are changing. *Focus, 21*(1), 5-8.

Casas, C., Stinnett, N., DeFrain, J., & Lee, P. (1984). Family strengths in Latin America. *Family Perspective* (Winter).

Centers for Disease Control and Prevention. (2003, September 18). *National Vital Statistics Report, 52*(3). Retrieved July 19, 2006, from http://www.cdc.gov/nchs/data/nvsr/nvsr52/nvsr52_13.pdf

Centers for Disease Control and Prevention. (2004). Actual causes of death in the United States, 2000. National Center for Chronic Disease Prevention and Health Promotion. Retrieved July 19, 2006 from http://www.cdc.gov/

Christopher, F. S. (2000). Sexuality in marriage, dating, and other relationships: A decade review. *Journal of Marriage and the Family, 62*(4), 999-1017.

Coley, R. L., & Chase-Lansdale, P. L. (1998). Adolescent pregnancy and parenthood: Recent evidence and future directions. *American Psychologist, 53*(2), 152-166.

Congressional Internet Caucus Advisory Committee (2004). U.S. House of Representatives. Retrieved July 19, 2006, from http://www.netcaucus.org/statistics

Curran, D. (1983). *Traits of a healthy family.* Minneapolis: Winston Press.

DeFrain, J. (1999). Strong families around the world. *Family Matters: Journal of the Australian Institute of Family Studies, 53*(Winter), 6-13.

DeFrain, J., and the UNL for Families Writing Team. (2006). *Family treasures: Creating strong families.* Lincoln, NE: University of Nebraska Extension.

DeFrain, J., DeFrain, N., & Lepard, J. (1994). Family strengths and challenges in the South Pacific: An exploratory study. *International Journal of the Sociology of the Family, 24*(2), 25-47.

DeFrain, J., & Olson, D. H. (1999). Contemporary family patterns and relationships. In M. Sussman, S. Steinmetz, & G. W. Peterson (Eds.), *Handbook of Marriage and the Family.* New York: Plenum.

DeFrain, J., & Stinnett, N. (2002). Family strengths. In J. J. Ponzetti et al. (Eds.), *International encyclopedia of marriage and family* (2nd ed.). New York: Macmillan Reference Group, pp. 637-642.

Domesticated bliss: New laws are making it official for gay or live-in straight couples. (1992, March 23). *Newsweek.*

Educational Fund to Stop Gun Violence (2002, July). Update: Closing Illegal Markets. Retrieved July 19, 2006, from http://www.csgv.org

Epstein, N. B., Bishop, D. S., Ryan, C., Miller, L., & Keitner, G. (1993). The McMaster model of family functioning. In F. Walsh (Ed.), *Normal family processes* (pp. 138-160). New York: Guilford Press.

Gabler, J., & Otto, H. (1964). Conceptualization of family strengths in the family life and other professional literature. *Journal of Marriage and the Family, 26*, 221-223.

Geggie, J., DeFrain, J., Hitchcock, S., & Silberberg, S. (2000, June). Family strengths research project: Final report to the Australian Commonwealth Government Ministry of Family and Community Services, Canberra, A.C.T. Callaghan, N.S.W., Australia: Family Action Centre, University of Newcastle.

Gomel, J. N., Tinsley, B. J., Parke, R. D., & Clark, K. M. (1998). The effects of economic hardship on family relationships among African American, Latino, and Euro-American families. *Journal of Family Issues, 19*(4), 436-476.

Hernandez, D. J. (1997). Child development and the social demography of childhood. *Child Development, 68*(1), 149-169.

Hochshild, A. (1997). *The time bind: When work becomes home and home becomes work.* New York: Metropolitan Books.

Houseknecht, S. K., & Sastry, J. (1996). Family decline and child well-being: A comparative analysis. *Journal of Marriage and Family, 58,* 726-739.

Kamp Dush, C. M., Cohan, C. L., & Amato, P. R. (2004). The relationship between cohabitation and marital quality and stability: Change across cohorts? *Journal of Marriage and the Family, 65*(3), 539-550.

Kantor, D., & Lehr, W. (1974). *Inside the family.* San Francisco: Jossey-Bass.

Krysan, M., Moore, K. A., & Zill, N. (1990). *Identifying successful families: An overview of constructs and selected measures.* Washington, DC: Child Trends, Inc. [2100 M St., NW, Suite 610] and the U.S. Department of Health & Human Services, Office of the Assistant Secretary for Planning and Evaluation.

Laumann, E. O., Gagnon, J. H., Michael, R. T., Michaels, S., & Kolata, G. (1995). *Sex in America: A definitive survey.* Boston: Little, Brown.

Mberengwa, L. R., & Johnson, J. M. (2003). Strengths of Southern African families and their cultural context. *Journal of Family and Consumer Sciences, 95*(1), 20-25.

Michener, J. A. (1996). *This noble land: My vision for America.* New York: Random House. Nation's hunger rate dropped 24 percent in late 1990s. (2000, September 9). *Lincoln* [NE] *Journal Star,* p. 1.

Olson, D. H. (1996). Clinical assessment and treatment using the Circumplex Model. In F. W. Kaslow (Ed.), *Handbook in relational diagnosis* (pp. 59-80). New York: Wiley.

Olson, D. H., & DeFrain, J. (2006). *Marriages and families: Intimacy, strengths, and diversity* (5th Ed.). New York: McGraw-Hill.

Olson, D. H., Fye, S., & Olson, A. K. (1999). *National survey of happy and unhappy married couples.* Roseville, MN: Life Innovations.

Olson, D. H., McCubbin, H. I., Barnes, H., Larsen, A., Muxen, M., & Wilson, M. (1989). *Families: What makes them work* (2nd Ed.). Los Angeles, CA: Sage.

Olson, D. H., & Olson, A. K. (2000). *Empowering couples: Building on your strengths* (2nd Ed.). Roseville, MN: Life Innovations.

Otto, H. A. (1962). What is a strong family? *Marriage and Family Living, 24,* 77-81.

Otto, H. A. (1963). Criteria for assessing family strength. *Family Process, 2,* 329-339.

Porter, J. (1999, January 10). It's time to start thinking about electing a female president. *Lincoln* [NE] *Journal Star,* p. 6D.

Reiss, D. (1981). *The family's construction of reality.* Cambridge, MA: Harvard University Press.

Sani, A. & Buhannad, N. (2003). Family strengths in Islam: Perceptions of Women in the United Arab Emirates. National Council on Family Relations *Report, 48*(4), F12-F15.

Smithsonian Institution (1999). Paleoamerican origins. Retrieved May 2, 2006, from http://www.si.edu/resource/faq/nmnh/origin.htm

Special report: Ten years of NAFTA, Free trade on trial. (2004, January 3). *The Economist*, pp. 13-16.

Stanley, S. M., Whitton, S. W., & Markman, H. J. (2004). Maybe I do: Interpersonal commitment and premarital or nonmarital cohabitation. *Journal of Family Issues*, *25*(4), 496-519.

Stinnett, N., & DeFrain, J. (1985). *Secrets of strong families*. Boston: Little, Brown.

Stinnett, N., & O'Donnell, M. (1996). *Good kids*. New York: Doubleday.

Stinnett, N., & Sauer, K. (1977). Relationship characteristics of strong families. *Family Perspective*, *11*(3), 3-11.

Stinnett, N., Stinnett, N., Beam, J., & Beam, A. (1999). *Fantastic families*. Lafayette, LA: Howard.

Struthers, C. B., & Bokemeier, J. L. (2000). Myths and realities of raising children and creating family life in a rural county. *Journal of Family Issues*, *21*(1), 17-46.

Substance Abuse and Mental Health Services Administration. (2006). Homelessness statistics and data. U.S. Department of Health and Human Services. Retrieved July 18, 2006, from http://www.samhas.gov?Matrix/statistics_homeless.aspx

Treas, J., & Giesen, D. (2000). Sexual infidelity among married and cohabiting Americans. *Journal of Marriage and the Family*, *62*(1), 48-60.

U.S. Bureau of the Census. (2000). *Statistical abstract of the United States* (120th ed.). Washington, DC: U.S. Government Printing Office.

U.S. Bureau of the Census. (2006a). U.S. and world population clocks–POPclocks. Retrieved July 19th, 2006, from http://www.census.gov/main/www/popclock.html

U.S. Bureau of the Census. (2006b). U.S. Census Bureau News. Retrieved July 18, 2006, from http://www.census.gov/Press-Release/www.releases/archives/income_wealth/005647.html

U.S. Bureau of the Census. (2006c). American Fact Finder. Retrieved July 19, 2006, from http://factfinder.census.gov/jsp/saff/SAFFInfo.jsp?_content=su2_new_features_0406.html

U.S. Department of Agriculture. (2006). Food security in the United States. USDA Economic Research Service. Retrieved July 18, 2006, from http://www.ers.usda.gov/briefing/FoodSecurity/

U.S. Department of Justice. (2001, June). Criminal victimization 2000: Changes 1999-2000 with trends 1993-2000. Retrieved July 19th, from http://ojp.usdoj.gov/bjs/

Woodhouse, C. G. (1930). A study of 250 successful families. *Social Forces*, *8*, 511-532.

Xia, Y., Xie, X., & Zhou, Z. (2004). Case study: Resiliency in immigrant families. In V. L. Bengtson, A. Acock, K. Allen, P. Dilworth-Anderson, & D. Klein (Eds.), *Sourcebook of family theory and research* (pp. 108-111). Thousand Oaks, CA: Sage.

Xie, X., DeFrain, J., Meredith, W., & Combs, R. (1996). Family strengths in the People's Republic of China. *International Journal of the Sociology of the Family*, *26*(2), 17-27.

Xu, A., & Ye, W. (2002). Quality of marriage: Major predictors of stability. Shanghai *Research Quarterly*, *4*, 103-112.

Yoo, J. J. (2004). A study of the development of the Korean Family Strengths Scale for strengthening the family. *Journal of the Korean Association of Family Relations*, 9(2), 119-151.

Yoo, Y. J., DeFrain, J., Lee, I., Kim, S., Hong, S., Choi, H., & Ahn, J. (2004, June). Korean family strengths research project: A national project funded by the Korea Research Foundation. Seoul, Korea: Institute of Korean Family Strengths and Kyunghee University.

doi:10.1300/J002v41n03_04

LATIN AMERICA

Strengths and Challenges of Mexican Families in the 21st Century

Rosario Esteinou

SUMMARY. This article will analyze some of the strengths and challenges for Mexican families in the beginning of this century. It will start with a description of some of the characteristics of the country, and then will deal with some of the most important challenges families face. Challenges are divided in two categories: external and internal, including in the first one the economic context, poverty, migration and cultural change; in the second one, we consider symbolic and cultural differentiation, the impact of the secularization of values, changes in role structures and changes among generations. The presentation will proceed with a description of some of the strengths Mexican families have, including those based on institutional grounds and based on expressive and individual elements. Throughout the article we will try to consider other family forms, including their challenges and strengths. doi:10.1300/J002v41n03_05

Rosario Esteinou is Family Sociologist Researcher, Centro de Investigaciones y Estudios Superiores en Antropología Social, Juárez 87, Tlalpan, 14000 México D.F. (E-mail: esteinou@ciesas.edu.mx).
Author note: My daughter Ana, a light of joy, helps me understand the importance of strong families.

[Haworth co-indexing entry note]: "Strengths and Challenges of Mexican Families in the 21st Century." Esteinou, Rosario. Co-published simultaneously in *Marriage & Family Review* (The Haworth Press, Inc.) Vol. 41, No. 3/4, 2007, pp. 309-334; and: *Strong Families Around the World: Strengths-Based Research and Perspectives* (ed: John DeFrain, and Sylvia M. Asay) The Haworth Press, Inc., 2007, pp. 309-334. Single or multiple copies of this article are available for a fee from The Haworth Document Delivery Service [1-800-HAWORTH, 9:00 a.m. - 5:00 p.m. (EST). E-mail address: docdelivery@haworthpress.com].

Available online at http://mfr.haworthpress.com
© 2007 by The Haworth Press, Inc. All rights reserved.
doi:10.1300/J002v41n03_05

[Article copies available for a fee from The Haworth Document Delivery Service: 1-800-HAWORTH. E-mail address: <docdelivery@haworthpress.com> Website: <http://www.HaworthPress.com> © 2007 by The Haworth Press, Inc. All rights reserved.]

KEYWORDS. Family challenges, family cohesion, family communication, family flexibility, family strengths, Mexican families, secularization

GENERAL BACKGROUND OF MEXICO

Mexico is located in North America. Our neighbors are the United States on the north and Guatemala and Belize on the south. On the east we have the Atlantic Ocean and on the west the Pacific Ocean.

According to the 2000 population census (Inegi, 2003), there are 97.5 million people in Mexico. We have grown very rapidly. In 1900 there were 13.6 million, in 1950 we reached 25.8 million, but the highest population growth rate was reached in 1970 when there were 48.2 million. At this point we were growing at a rate of 3.4 percent per year. By the year 2000 we had a diminished rate of growth of 1.9 percent due to a strong family planning policy. Of these 97.5 million, 5% (6.8 million) are older people, 65 years of age or more; 60% (58 million) are adults between 15 and 64 years old; and 34% are children between 0 and 14 years old. Thus, with this population structure we face a strong demand for services for the adult population.

Mexico is a country with considerable cultural diversity. There are more than eight million indigenous people, so approximately one out of ten persons is indigenous. Sixty-four Indian languages have been identified, but the main groups in which these are concentrated are seven languages, of which nahua, maya and mixteco are the most important. These groups are concentrated in the southwest and southeast part of the country. In regard to religion, 89% of the population is Catholic. Catholic people tend to concentrate in the center of the country and non-Catholics tend to be in the south and north of the country. Today, Mexico has a democratic political system, constituted by a party system in which three main parties contend to rule the government. In 2000, after 70 years of being ruled by the Institutional Revolutionary Party, another party, the National Action Party, won the elections.

Concerning education, we have reached important goals. About 90% of the population 15 years of age and above can read and write and is therefore literate. About 92% of the population between 6 and 14 years of age go to school. The national average number of years of study is 7.6.

So, today, we are facing an important demand for high school and higher education for the population.

A number of measures give us an understanding of the extent of access to services and how well equipped households are, by looking at some articles. Table 1 shows us that around 86% of the households have television, 10% have computers, about one out of three households has a car and a telephone, 40% have a VCR, one out of two has a washing machine, two out of three have a refrigerator and 85% have a radio.

Access to public social security services is an important aspect of social policy. What appears amazing, as shown in Table 2, is that 57% of the population does not have access to these services; only 32% have access to the main social security service (Instituto Mexicano de Seguridad Social), and 6% are state workers who have access to the state social security service (Instituto de Seguridad Social al Servicio de los Trabajadores del Estado). What these percentages tell us is that we have a very weak public social security system and consequently a very weak family policy.

TABLE 1. Percentage of households owning the listed domestic appliances.

Type of domestic appliance	Percentage of household ownership
Television	86
Computer	10
Car	32
Telephone	36
VCR	40
Washing machine	52
Refrigerator	69
Radio	85

Source: INEGI, Population Census, 2003.

TABLE 2. Percentage of population according to entitlement to social security services, 2000.

Type of service	Percentage of population in receipt of service
No access to any service	57
IMSS	32.3
ISSTE	5.9
Others	2.2
Unspecified	2.9

Source: INEGI, Population Census, 2003.

The nuclear family structure developed as the main important family form since the colonial period in the sixteenth century. But, modern internal family relations associated with the modern nuclear family only began to appear at the end of the nineteenth century (Esteinou, 2005). The extended family has had an important presence in Mexican society and it represents an important pattern among rural and indigenous families. It is really in the twentieth century when modern family relations developed.

The economically active population is composed of 70% men who work and around 30% women who carry out economic activity. The increase of women in the labor force has been very important and had important consequences on family life, as dual-earner or dual-career families are increasing very rapidly. There have been some changes in the last 30 years in the types of households represented. Table 3 shows that approximately 67% of households are nuclear families but this type of household has been decreasing; extended households have increased, reaching 31%. One-person households have also increased, composing today 1.5% of the households. Another important characteristic of households is that one out of five is led by a woman. There has been an important increase in single-parent families headed by women.

CHALLENGES FAMILIES FACE
IN THE TWENTY-FIRST CENTURY

In the 21st century families face a series of important challenges. Some of these can be classified as external and others come from their internal features of the family. Poverty, migration and cultural change can be considered challenges families face at the external level. Secularization, symbolic differentiation, changes in role structure, and changes

TABLE 3. Percentage of population according to type of household, 2003.

	Year	
	1990	2000
Household type		
Nuclear	73.9	66.9
Extended	24.4	31.4
One-person	1.0	1.5

Source: INEGI, Population Census, 2003.

among generations are some of the main challenges families face coming from their internal features and dynamics.

Despite the high value attributed to the family by Mexicans, family life today faces many challenges and strains. Especially in the last three decades, Mexican society has experienced many rapid changes, and for the members of families it is difficult to cope. In an increasingly modernized society, tradition is losing ground, and certainty in many aspects of life becomes fragile. At the same time, family matters require more effort and attention in order to sustain them and there are no other institutions which give families substantial support. The diminishing role of the state in social life, represented by the weak social security system, has also resulted in families having to face all the problems and strains basically on their own. Families, therefore, live with high levels of stress.

Economics and Family Life

Mexico has experienced in the last three decades various economic crises which have deteriorated the standard of living and quality of life. Since 1976 there has been a decrease in real income, unemployment has increased at different times, and formal employment has faced important reductions. Since the 1980s the state has implemented an economic policy of stabilization and structural adjustment; however, these tendencies continue to develop. The increase of inequalities was the main risk of the continued growth in these tendencies and this has been reduced by the rapid development of the informal economy. As a consequence of stabilization and structural adjustment measures, income distribution became more unequal, and increasing informality and flexibility in the labor market led to a situation in which many workers have lost job stability. Very low wages are paid to non-qualified workers and precarious working conditions proliferate (Cortés, 2000; Gordon, 2002; Esteinou, 2008). Therefore, families have faced income deterioration and to overcome it they have developed different strategies to manage and increase their resources. One of the answers to these problems that families have designed is the maximization of the family labor force, through the intensification of work as well as the development of an additional economic activity or longer working hours for the head of the household. In other words, families have increased the number of family members in the labor market or they have intensified their work by taking on additional jobs (Cortés, 2000; Molina & Sánchez, 1999; García & de Oliveira, 1994). But the incorporation of more members of the family into the labor markets, especially women, constitutes one of the most important results. The presence of women in the labor markets is significant: while in 1940 the figure was 8%, in 1993 female participation rates in the economically-active population ranged between 24% and 41% in different states of the country and according to projections for the year 2010 this figure will increase to between 28% and 45% (Conapo, 1998). This tendency presents a relevant characteristic: it is constituted not only by single, widowed, separated and divorced women, but also by mothers/housewives. Within this group, those in the central age groups with small children, who before constituted a very small proportion of the economically-active population, have increased considerably in the last decades (García & de Oliveira, 1994). The growth of married women in the workforce has increased so fast that by 2003 it reached almost 32% (Inegi, Instituto Nacional de las Mujeres, 2004) and in 1995 for divorced and separated women was 68.9% and 73.9% respectively (López, 1998). The most relevant consequence of this fact is that role structuring within the family is changing, as we shall see further and new family forms, such as dual-career and dual-earner families are emerging in greater proportions. These new forms, although they may have a nuclear structure, in their relationships tend to imply different forms of organization and value orientations.

Besides changes in organization and role structuring, these economic tendencies have had as an outcome an important problem of poverty, both in urban and rural areas, though it is deeper in the latter areas. Some characteristics that poor families have are: they tend to be extended families; their size is greater than the national average; the number of members who depend economically on one member is greater; they tend to live in a crowded dwelling; they have a greater number of children under 12 years old; children attend schools less; a greater proportion of adolescents work; the heads of the households have a low level of formal education and they tend to be young (Cortés, Hernández, Hernández, Székely & Vera, 2002; Esteinou, 2008).

Migration

The difficult socioeconomic conditions many Mexicans face have contributed to an increase in migration, mainly to the United States of America, up to the point that it has become an important national issue. It is estimated that throughout the 1970s around 30,000 persons migrated annually to the United States while this increased up to 360,000 during the last five years of the 1990s. The population of Mexicans born in Mexico and those of Mexican origin born in the United States of America and living in the United States rose in the year 2000 to a little over 23 million, composing the biggest group within the Hispanic population (Tuirán, 2002; Esteinou, 2008).

Migration is having a great impact on family life. Some of the changes it is influencing in small towns are:

1. Courtships are more open, even though they are maintained over long distances. Given the contact young men have with North American culture and given the greater opportunities women have of meeting men, courtships have become more open, decreasing practices such as "stealing the bride," which was very common in the past decades in rural areas. This practice consists of the groom taking ("stealing") the bride (in the past could be without her consent, in more recent times it is usually with her consent) to live with him at his parents´ house without the consent of her parents in order to avoid the usual ritual of asking for their permission to marry and the expensive costs of the wedding.
2. Marriage rituals tend to take place during specific seasons. Weddings usually take place in December since young men come home for vacation at this time.
3. Exogamy is increasing. Even though the expectation of marrying someone from their own ranch or town is still high, migration has brought more opportunities to meet girls or boys from other places.
4. Increase in the age of marriage. Women and men prefer to wait longer before marrying. They want to study or work in order to help their families and get ahead in life.
5. There is a decrease in patrilocal post-marital residence and an increase in the neolocal. Many migrants buy their own house before they marry with the remittances they send, thus neolocal residence after marriage is becoming more common (Mummert, 1996; Esteinou, 2008). This is an important change since the patrilocal post-marital residence use to be a very common family pattern in rural areas. These changes reveal the development of modernization tendencies regarding family formation and family life. However, these tendencies coexist with traditional patterns, so individuals and families experience serious challenges concerning how to manage patterns coming from tradition with those coming from new modern conditions.

Migration has become an important strategy which families implement and it has been positive in gathering more economic resources, but it puts a lot of stress on families. Since one or more members spend long periods of time away from home, the risk of family disintegration is high. The pressures to maintain family functions usually fall on the women, bringing additional problems in parenting, in taking care of the elderly, and in managing daily survival. Members of the family have to adjust emotionally to the new conditions.

Cultural Changes in Family Life

Secularization. Cultural changes have acted not only to promote positive outcomes, but as challenging factors in family life as well. Four decades ago, families used to have more stability as a result of a strong communitarian culture and traditions reproduced through the generations. Although this communitarian culture was not completely homogeneous, since we have a long history of cultural diversity due to the indigenous population, Mexicans could say that they lived in a relatively unique world where very few principles of social organization structured social and cultural life. In the last three decades we have experienced a deeper modernization process, especially in the private sphere. In a different context, Berger, Berger, and Kellner (1973) pointed out three decades ago in *The Homeless Mind* the process by which modernization impacted social and cultural life.

Following their ideas, it can be said that Mexican society has experienced the diffusion of a process of rationalization by which individuals and families are inluenced more than in the past by individualism, globalization, rational thinking and the world of work. For example, it is more common today to make a list of the groceries to buy for the whole week, instead of going almost every day to the market to buy what is needed for the day, as it used to be in the past. To plan the day, the week's activities, or even the course of our future life is much more common today than it was in the past, and this is clearly an influence of rational thinking. Also, Mexicans, especially middle class, today believe more in the values associated with the free market, democracy and the importance of scientific thinking, rather than a religious perspective when solving problems. For example, mothers use contraceptive methods to control birth rather than controlling it following in the religious beliefs. In fact, in the last three decades a strong secularization process in private life has developed.

Besides secularization and rationalization, Berger, Berger, and Kellner (1973) pointed out that in modern societies there has been a process pluralization of meaning worlds, not only in the public sphere but also in the private one, therefore impacting family life. This means that there is a multiplicity of social and cultural meanings in family life, making it more difficult for individuals and families to follow social and cultural standards to orient their behavior today, in contrast to the relatively few social and cultural standards which oriented their behavior in the past. For example, in the past Mexican individuals had a clearer picture of what was considered to be a *good* family and they tried to orient their behavior in order to adhere to this model. Today the possibilities of being a *good* family are differentiated: nuclear families, extended families, single-parent families, step families, lesbian or gay families, and so forth. All these familiy types are plausible and coexist. None of them is *healthier* or *better* than the others. This plurality of types weakens the certainty about only one being valid. In the past most families were alike and we felt that this way of making a family was a natural fact and normal. Today individuals feel that they can choose different paths to form a family and they are not certain which one is the best. Besides this, pluralization often implies that these different meaning worlds are not compatible with each other, and frequently are not integrated or coherent. Thus, we can observe, for example, that values associated with the free market are not compatible with the particularistic values of family life. Each meaning world has a cognitive style and other elements which make *sense* in this particular world but not in another (Esteinou, 1999).

Pluralization. Pluralization in the private sphere or as Sciolla (1983) has labeled this process, symbolic differentiation, has deepened in such a way that it has affected primary socialization, basic formation of self and subjective world processes. For a long time it has been assumed that private life and the family are central sense sources which face the hostility and discrepancy of public meaning worlds. The individual tries to build and maintain a *domestic world* which can be a meaningful center, a place of certainty, for his life in society. Berger, Berger and Kellner (1973) observe that in modern societies the individual is unlikely to find in the private world such *certainties*, because individuals are exposed from the very beginning of their social experience to a multiplicity of worlds. From their perspective, individuals have never possessed an integrated and uncontested *domestic world*. The exposure to such multiplicity has at the same time two consequences: on the one hand, it *broadens the individuals' thinking*, but on the other hand, it weakens at the same time the integrity and plausibility of their domestic world. For these reasons, it is a risky and precarious task to try to build and maintain an integrated and uncontested domestic world. In the past, for example, Mexican families believed that it was enough to send children to school to get the proper education in skills, training, and in value orientations. The school would give the children adequate tools to face the external world, but the family remained the main institution in charge of giving core values and moral education. This was accomplished basically by the uncontested authority parents had over their children.

Today this idea is fading away, especially among urban middle-class groups, and in its place there has been a multiplication of moral and instrumental standards and agencies regarding education. Parents have different options to choose in order to raise their children. Stimulation centers for children at an early age have proliferated, which is a new outcome in the education of children. After that experience, parents can choose from a wide variety of schools to send their children: a school which follows the Montessori pedagogical method or an active education program; a center for the integral development of the child; a private, rigid catholic school; a non-Catholic public school; a bilingual (Spanish-English) secular school; a non-secular private school, and so on. The differentiation of options runs along with a strong tendency to try to complement the education given in schools. Middle- and upper-class parents spend a lot of time, money, and energy trying to look for a good complementary education. In the afternoons they send their children to music, sports, art lessons, and to different types of therapy. These tendencies have resulted in children who are exposed more than in the past to a diversification of cultural models, which are present in their interaction spheres of life and these models compete with each other for supremacy (Esteinou, 1999). The generation of the 1950s, for example, was raised in a relatively homogeneous world. All children had similar worlds and families (Catholic, many brothers and sisters with a short distance between their ages, non-divorced parents). Today, children are raised in a context of diversity: a child can have as a classmate a child from divorced parents, a child who belongs to a single-parent family, a child with different religious beliefs or whose family values are more secular.

But symbolic differentiation manifested through the multiplication of socialization agencies implies another important aspect concerning the relationship between the parent's authority and the school's authority. In the past, this relationship supposed a delicate balance between the different functions each institution should develop and a precise, implicit limit about their competencies. The definition between education in the family and in school implied a delicate equilibrium between parents' and school's authority. Parents' authority used to be respected by the school. Today, the incorporation of psychology and pedagogy within the administration and management of schools has had an important impact on parents' authority. The assimilation of psychology in educational agencies has implied a widening of the field of scientific competencies. Schools today are concerned not only for the development of technical and professional skills, but they also have become active and vigilant in regard to children's psychological and emotional development and how these impact on their performance in school. This surveillance is not new. For example, in the past it was present in schools with a Catholic orientation. But it existed under different parameters and maintained a relatively clear separation between scientific competency fields and of other areas. In the education of the child, science had an important role concerning professional education. With the development of skills and abilities, ethical, moral, and psychological development had a very minor role.

However, as noted by Berger and Berger (1984), with the development of science and the enlargement of its spheres of application, the individual, the family and the private spheres have been incorporated as *quantification and scientific experimental* objects. A *good family*, *healthy sexuality*, a *normal childhood*, and *good parental function* are objects defined according to quantifiable criteria and have become objects of experimentation by purported experts, who claim jurisdiction over these areas. Consequently, individuals and families are judged under the lens of these supposedly scientific criteria.

In the case of Mexican schools, the broadening of scientific areas of competence as part of the development of students has expressed itself not only in a more rational performance of the school's authority, but also in an increase of competency among the socialization agencies to perform its function. This has led to a relative weakening of parents' authority, in the sense of a decrease in the performance that a parent used to hold in a privileged way. Parents compete with the different socialization agencies, which define their own socialization criteria and models, especially in regard to the modern school. This situation has become more problematic and the *equilibrium* of the relationship between both institutions is more delicate.

The greater influence that the school's authority has, the more the family experiences it as an *invasion* of the parent's intimate domain. It can also be seen by parents as an attitude which emphasizes guilt and stigmatization. In fact, the school assumes a scientific or specialized character when observing the development of children. It stands as an authority in the sense that it knows the family dynamics which can generate student behaviors labeled as *pathological*. This, along with the different assimilation of scientific knowledge about child development, produces tension between both institutions, and questions parental authority. The certainties parents had before over how to raise their children are now questioned under the lens of this scientific authority the school represents. Although there is evidence that this is a challenge faced mainly by middle-class families (Esteinou, 1996), it is probably a challenge faced by other social groups, since there is a general trend in schools to include the scientific perspective of psychology and pedagogy.

Concerning role structure, we can say that the majority of families follow a traditional pattern in which adult women perform their main roles of being housewives and mothers, and adult males are the fathers and breadwinners. There is also an alternative pattern, although in a minor proportion of the population, in extended families where role structure is more complex and the division of labor is distributed among the different members. But there is an important change that we pointed out earlier related to the increasing proportion of married women who are involved in labor force activity. One out of three married women has a job. This fact has had important implications, from a sociocultural point of view, in role structuring and in the configuration of new family forms, specifically dual-earner and dual-career families. Although these changes still need to be analyzed in depth, we can describe some important tendencies which reveal challenges families are facing.

Important shifts have been observed in the configuration and meanings regarding the mother and housewife roles and in the husband, father and breadwinner roles that are influenced by expectations and practices of the female labor role. We have had a long tradition in which the role of the mother has been so highly valued and worshiped that it constituted the main space of performance and personal development socially recognized. Even when mothers were employed, it was symptomatic that in the censuses, for example, when they were asked about their occupation, many would answer: "the home and the children." It was said that they were the "queens of the house," and in that expression there was an acknowledgment of their position in the family and in society. This configuration of the mother and housewife role was reinforced through different social-control mechanisms, such as the negative sanctions by close relatives and friends when the mother/housewife worked. Phrases such as, "This man is supported by his housewife," and "Look! He put his wife to work because he cannot support his family," noted men's "failure" as a breadwinner, but also the incursion of mothers into the world of work. There were others which sanctioned (and still do) the mother's labor role negatively: "She is neglecting her children," and

"She is selfish, her duty is first with her kids." Only in the exceptional cases of economic need in situations of abandonment, separation, and widowhood was it accepted that the mother worked. From this perspective of disapproval, it meant an inversion of roles among genders which distorted the normative and cultural standards. In this sense, the value of being a mother was not compatible with that of work outside the home; or in other words, the latter was not a value orientation. Besides appreciation for the motherhood role, it was normatively chained with another role, the housewife, in such a way that these roles socially demarcated a women's life horizon and social status.

The strict bond established normatively and culturally between these two roles has been eroded and is part of a process which is weakening the traditional conjugal nuclear family as a symbolic and normative referent. In contrast to what happened 30 years ago, female work in general and particularly mother's work is becoming an expectation and a value orientation for multiple social groups (Beltrán, Castaños, Flores, Meyenberg, & del Pozo, 1996). Women's expectation horizons, including those of mothers with dependent children, are diversifying in such a way that a woman's economic contribution to family welfare through economic activity is more accepted today than in the past. Women's work is not only justified by an economic need but also for personal or professional fulfillment. Women's roles are configured in a more open way toward the external world, due to economic activity, and present challenges for men and women concerning how they face and conciliate different values as a couple and as a family. At least three situations have been observed:

1. Men and women maintain the traditional value orientations and incorporate women's work as a practical matter. In this case women usually experience role overload, because they have to cover the traditional family roles and the new role that is an additional one. They usually incorporate this new value within their value framework denying it or neutralizing it. Women's real economic contributions are taken as secondary aspects, which do not change the traditional role structure. It remains as a latent aspect which can produce tension and conflict.

2. Men and women as a couple maintain different conceptions about role structuring. Men usually have a traditional conception and women have a different one due to their work role, which modifies their conception of family roles. When women strive for a more equal division of labor tension and conflict occur.

3. Both members of the couple accept women's labor role and modify their family value orientations regarding role structure. The traditional values are considered in a relative way and they are not considered as the main sources of identity and social status. In the last two situations there is flexibility in role structuring (Esteinou, 2004a).

As part of cultural change that Mexican society is undergoing, there is an important challenge families face regarding the generations and parenting. Relationships among generations within the family are becoming more conflictive. Parents face problems regarding how to maintain their authority in a society where children's opinions and decisions count more and they have difficulties coping with the values in which they were raised with and a culture that gives more freedom to children. In the past, parent's authority had a hierarchical base which gave them particular tools to face and guide children's behavior. With symbolic differentiation, this hierarchical pattern is being eroded but parents find themselves often without the proper skills and tools to face and solve their children' demands and problems (Esteinou, 2004a).

THE STRENGTHS OF MEXICAN FAMILIES

Despite the fundamental importance family has for Mexicans, scientists have not developed research based on family strengths perspectives. In this section, thus, we will try to point out some of the strengths we can gather through the knowledge we have about Mexican families. To be able to describe some of these strengths, we will need to discuss what the term *strength* means. Olson and DeFrain (2006) note that researches have suggested three broad clusters which identify the main family strengths in different countries or in social groups with different ethnic backgrounds. These clusters are family cohesion, family flexibility, and family communication.

This is a useful framework to be explored in other contexts. Nevertheless, we have to be careful when we use it in the Mexican case, because it has some characteristics which come from a specific social and cultural context. Consequently, we do not necessarily find them in Mexican families. For example, the sources of family cohesion, family flexibility, and family communication may have some similarities, but also important differences between cultures. In cultures in the United States, it seems that individualism plays an important role while in Mexican culture it is not so wide-spread and communitarism still plays an important role.

Family Cohesion

In general terms we can say that Mexican families are strong. We can take the first cluster of qualities Olson and DeFrain (2006) identify, cohesion, and analyze the Mexican case in contrast. The authors include in this cluster commitment to the family (considering trust, honesty, dependability, and faithfulness), spending enjoyable time together manifested in committing a considerable amount of quality time to sharing activities, feelings and ideas, and enjoying each other's company (Olson & DeFrain, 2006, pp. 39-40). Mexican families have a high level of cohesion in the sense that family members are strongly oriented to the family. We can say that individuals trust and depend on each other, but we do not know for sure the level of honesty and faithfulness they have with each other. We know also that members of the family usually spend a lot of time together but we do not know the quality of it. Therefore, when we talk about cohesion as a strength, we have to look for the sources of it.

One thing that we can gather from different studies is that there is a high level of commitment among family members, but that this commitment comes more from the strengths of normative standards and a communitarian culture and not, as it seems it is in the United States and other industrialized countries, from a commitment agreed upon by individuals. In Mexican culture the main source of family cohesion comes from a communitarian institutional base and in industrialized societies it seems to come from an individualism institutional base. Communitarism puts emphasis on the group and not individual interests and usually has an important level of cohesion. This is an important aspect we have to consider when we talk about strengths.

There are strengths which reinforce the group but restrain the development and demonstration of the individual's interests and feelings. In a communitarian culture, family cohesion demarcates the parameters in which an individual can be happy or satisfied. The level and quality of satisfaction and happiness Mexicans have within a communitarian family cohesion remains a point to be analyzed.

Along with this communitarian family cohesion pattern, there is another one based on individualism with an institutional base, which has similar characteristics to the industrialized societies. This type of cohesion is less common, but it is developing mainly among urban middle-class families, especially in dual-earner and dual-career families, where there are high levels of education. In these families, individualism is becoming an important rule which orients behavior. Cohesion is not a result of the external force of the group which limits individuality, but from a process of negotiation among individuals. Cohesion does not result from the force of the group and tradition, but it can be questioned, analyzed and agreed upon by individuals.

In Mexican society, cohesion is related to another important strength, that is, familism. In fact, a survey by Beltrán and colleagues (1996) has revealed that the family among Mexicans is highly valued and the majority of them perceive it as an institution on which they can rely and in which they can trust its members. From the family, they get their main economic support, emotional support and personal satisfaction. Mexicans associate the word family with highly-positive connotations, such as love, bonds, children, home, welfare, parents, and understanding.

Taking the different components of familism pointed out by Hennon, Peterson, Polzin and Radina (2008), we observe that Mexican families promote different types of familism as sources of cohesion. The most important of them and more pervasive is normative familism. For many Mexicans, the family is a solidarity unit, implying a series of commitments toward its members and the relations which are beyond the individual interests have supremacy.

We can observe also an instrumental familism as a source of cohesion. From an economic perspective, there have been numerous studies which point out that the family is a fundamental organizational economic unit (Lehalleur & Rendón, 1988; Salles, 1988; De la Peña, Escobar, & Duran, 1999; Molina & Sánchez, 1999). During economic crises and difficult times the family is revealed as a strong institution capable of overcoming economic adversity through cohesion. Family members can contribute by using the labor force to acquire more resources, family units can exchange economic resources between them, or they can even change their structure in order to gather more resources. The latter is observed in the 2000 census information. In the 1990s, extended families have increased and nuclear families have decreased (Inegi, 2003) as a result of the difficult economic conditions. Families responded to difficult economic problems by incorporating other relatives to maximize their resources and changing their structure from nuclear to extended.

As we have said before, family cohesion may come from different sources, according to different social contexts and social groups. These may vary not only between countries but also within a specific one, so that in Mexico the sources of family cohesion vary in different social groups. One important source of cohesion related to another type of familism comes from the kinship network. This has been labeled behavioral familism (Hennon, Peterson, Polzin & Radina, 2008) and concerns the interaction between the family and the kinship networks. The individuals feel compelled toward relatives and develop feelings and attitudes. Kinship networks constitute an extension of nuclear family cohesion. It implies a broader system. Kinship networks play an important role in many social groups with different ethnic and class backgrounds.

Research on an elite family with Spanish backgrounds (Adler & Perez-Lizaur, 1987) found that although they followed a neolocal residence pattern after the marriage, the different nuclei of the Gómez family tended to live close to one another, on the same land, block or neighborhood. As part of their ideology and myths, they encouraged assistance between rich uncles and poor nephews or between close kin in general. Material resources were not the only thing they exchanged. There was a flow of information between the Gómez relatives which contributed toward the construction of a cognitive kinship map that was shared by the members of the kinship group. They developed a series of family rituals which reinforced the family and kin as a big group, such as meeting on weekends to eat together, on birthdays and other celebrations. Kin bonds were very important and established a series of mutual obligations. For example, if an aunt was in the hospital, she would receive the visits of close-kin relatives, who brought her presents and company. Cohesion was so strong among the kinship group that it manifested itself in the fact that they sent their children to the same school or club.

Today some of these traits are diminishing, particularly in the big cities in Mexico, due to the changes in urban structure and development, as well as the long distances which cause difficulties. This pattern still continues to prevail to some extent not only among rich families, but also among middle class social groups. Adler and Pérez-Lizaur (1987) proposed that in Mexico the three-generation family system, with its strong kin network, provides economic, social and emotional security to the group and individuals and also places heavy restrictions upon individuals who thus tend to lack personal freedom. It seems that cohesion, in Mexican society, is strongly associated with low freedom of choice for individuals, as we have seen before.

In another study, Lomnitz (1977) found that families in a context of marginality also develop important kinship networks in order to survive. In these groups, as well as in other social classes with low socioeconomic position, kinship networks perform an active role for economic and service support. Among these families, economic support is given very frequently, not as much in the form of money but in-kind services.

One important form it takes is through the caring for children. Women who work lean on their mothers for the care of their offspring. Considering that the Mexican state provides very few social services to meet this need, the use of the kin network constitutes an important strength that families demonstrate (Inegi, Instituto Nacional de las Mujeres, 2004). As in upper- and middle-class families, low-socioeconomic families still tend to regroup in the neighborhood, living nearby each other. This allows them to support each other and reproduce rituals and values that generate strong cohesion.

In other social classes such as the peasants in rural areas, another pattern of cohesion adds to the previous ones and is related to the structural type of familism. This type refers to the tendency to form extended and multigenerational households which delimit the social setting where behaviors occur. This pattern comes from a traditional source associated to the indigenous world. Families tend not only to live nearby, usually on the same land or close to each other, but also the sons go to live in the same house of their father when they unite or marry. They take their wife with them and she becomes subordinate to her mother-in-law's authority. This patrilocal pattern implies strong family cohesion among different family units, but also implies strong inequalities among its members, especially between genders and generations.

The son is also under his father's authority, so the new couple has little freedom to behave as they want. These families form a domestic group and perform important economic and social functions as a whole. They have specific ways of transmitting and inheriting property among members of the domestic group. They follow a collective way of production and have specific rituals and normative standards that reproduce these in the groups. There is a vast amount of literature which illustrates this pattern in different indigenous communities (Franco, 1992; Robichaux, 1996; Millán & Valle, 2003; Arizpe, 1973; Lehalleur, 1988; Salles, 1988). It is interesting to observe that this pattern has been impacted by migration. In the past when migration took place one of the members, usually a man, went to the United States to work but did not take his wife with him. As the patrilocal residence had strict rules to follow, when they united or married men used to leave their women *in the charge* of his family, especially under the surveillance of his mother. This would avoid the temptations to establish new relationships with other men. At the same time, family cohesion was maintained, in spite of the physical distance.

Although this pattern still persists, there is a tendency among couples today for both to migrate to the United States, establishing a new neolocal residence pattern. In the new generations the compulsive need to maintain family cohesion has motivated men to bring not only their wives with them, but also their children and even their parents, especially their mothers so they can care for the children while the young couple works (Mummert, 1999; D'Aubeterre, 2000).

Family Flexibility

According to Olson and DeFrain (2006), the second cluster of strengths families have, whatever their ethnic identification or country of origin, is constituted by flexibility. This is

> ... *the ability to change and adapt when necessary*. Flexibility also relates to dealing effectively with stress and having helpful spiritual beliefs. Coping abilities include using personal and family resources to help each other, accepting crises as challenges rather than denying them, and growing together by working through crises. Spiritual well-being includes happiness, optimism, hope, faith, and a set of shared ethical values that guide family members through life's challenges. (Olson & DeFrain, 2006, p. 39)

This definition implies an important ingredient of individualism in the sense that the strength lies within individuals. The resolution of family conflicts and crises depends a great deal on the skills and capabilities of individuals. In this context, individuals have developed personal resources in order to meet their needs, a great sense of individuality, and a sense of freedom of action within the context of the family. Negotiation in this context becomes the field where differences are resolved. In Mexican society, as we have said, personal freedom is developing among certain social groups, but also coexists with a strong communitarian pattern that structures social life, including the family. Although there is no detailed knowledge about coping skills to face crises and conflict, we can say that Mexican families rely basically upon the strength the family has as an institution. Social normative standards, such as *the family has to be kept united* and *the family group is more important than individual interests* guide to a great extent the way conflicts and crises are faced.

This means that individuals can act and move their personal resources within the limits set by the group. One way to see how individuality still has a discrete place within the family is through the level of the divorce rate. In the past, the divorce rate was very low: in 1950 it was 4.4% (Inegi, 1996). In recent decades it has increased considerably, especially in urban areas. Although we do not have precise information about the rate, it has been estimated that in 1999, the separation and divorce rate was around 14.5% (Conapo, 1999). What the low divorce rates could tell us is that the members of the family prefer to solve their conflicts and crises following the traditional way, which puts an emphasis on keeping the group together in spite of individual interests. Nevertheless, this pattern, plus symbolic differentiation and rationalization have favored the development of a tendency among certain social groups, such as the urban middle classes and among younger generations, in which individuality counts more than in the past and thus divorce rates are increasing. In these groups, individuals and families rely on personal resources.

The description of flexibility by Olson and DeFrain (2006) includes spiritual well-being of the family members. On this point there is important evidence about the source of spiritual well-being for Mexican families. But it is important to observe that this source emphasizes, again, the institutional dimension of the family and the group over the individual. In general, Mexican families have strong beliefs coming mainly from the Catholic religion, which reinforces the group and marriage as a long-term institution.

Happiness, optimism, hope, faith, and a set of values which guide family members through life's challenges can be met following the precepts established by this particular religion. In fact, according to the 2000 census, 89% of Mexicans practice Catholicism (Inegi, 2003). Other studies have also indicated the importance of Catholic religion in family life (Beltrán et al., 1996). In spite of the importance Catholic religion plays in family life, in recent decades an important process of secularization has developed in a way that each day more individuals tend to distance themselves from Catholic norms. This opens the way for individuals to identify with other beliefs which erode traditional values (Fortuny, 1999). This is a point which has not been explored and merits more intensive study in order to assess how Catholicism may or may not mold family normative standards of action.

The definition of family flexibility by Olson and DeFrain (2006) implies another important element, that is, role flexibility. Members of the family are able to change some tasks and roles in order to respond to certain situations. Therefore, a rigid pattern or role structuring is not compatible with flexibility. In México, there is vast evidence that the majority of families follow a rigid pattern of role structuring in which the adult males develop an instrumental role, being the breadwinners of the family and the adult women develop an expressive role, taking care of the children and emotional balance of the family (De Barbieri,, 1984; Benería & Roldán, 1992; García & de Oliveira, 1994; Esteinou, 1996;

Inegi & Instituto Nacional de las Mujeres, 2004). Most of these works have focused on inequalities in the division of labor between genders, but very little has been done concerning the role balance between the couple and other members of the family, which transcends the division of labor. In spite of this lack of information, there are a few studies, focused mainly on the middle class, which observe flexibility in family role structures, particularly in dual-earner and dual-career families. In these families, fathers and husbands develop other activities associated before as women's roles, such as becoming involved in the care of children (Esteinou, 1996). Although it remains an area to be studied in depth, there are some signs in everyday life which point to a growing flexibility of roles in other social groups, especially in urban areas. However, we can say that role structure flexibility in Mexican families is not a very common strength.

Family Communication

The third cluster of family strengths, following the characterization made by Olson and DeFrain (2000), focuses on family communication, emphasizing appreciation and affection among the members of the family.

> Positive communication includes having open, straightforward discussions, being cooperative rather than competitive, and sharing feelings with one another. Appreciation and affection includes kindness, mutual caring, respect for individuality, and a feeling of security. (Olson & DeFrain, 2006, pp. 39-40)

The majority of these qualities have not been studied in Mexican families. One thing that has been widely stated is the great level of solidarity that family units have and the strong sense of cooperation that prevails (Lomnitz, 1977; Salles, 1988; Franco, 1992). We can also say that since the family is highly valued and since individuals have stated in some surveys (Beltrán, et al., 1996) that they recieve a great level of satisfaction from the family, we can assume that there is some sort of communication that positively holds the family together. Members of the family show great levels of appreciation, affection and a sense of security. In fact, the Mexican family is an important institution of solidarity.

But this positive outcome is demonstrated within a special context. We have said before that social and cultural standards of action and role structuring in the past used to be strongly authoritarian. Couple relationships and parent-child relationships used to be non-egalitarian and hierarchical. Within this culture, social standards were clearly rigid with regard to communication. Individual interests and the expression of feelings were attached to role competencies and to hierarchies, so within this pattern women used to be the leaders in the process of family communication. Authoritarianism also limited communication as a resource and confined the expression and discussion of certain themes, such as sexuality. This culture, in general, was present in all social groups, so we can say that communication was not a strength among Mexican families. However, this pattern has been eroding and Mexicans are developing communication as a resource for the management of relationships, using more skills within a more open culture that gives more space and freedom to individuals. Esteinou (2004a) found that in middle-class families there is a shift from the use of orders to that of greater communication as a main resource for socializing the young. Giving advice, for example, is much more prevalent and there is more frequent use of open communication about such matters as sexuality and emotions. Open communication is becoming the main resource and is used instead of scolding and punishing. Also, emotional communication represents an important change, particularly for male youth. This is especially true compared to the previous generations, who in the past tended to be distant, expressed limited affection and restricted their emotionality. In contrast, in recent generations, fathers are much more expressive, not only verbally, but also through physical contact (Esteinou, 2004b). Parent-child communication is becoming more important than punishment for younger generations and there is evidence that youth feel that there is a process of democratization and growing flexibility in parent-child relationships (ENJ, 2000; Esteinou, 2004b).

CONCLUSION

As we have seen, Mexican families have valuable strengths, many of them coming from a communitarian culture. The most important are family and kinship cohesion, family networks and familism. Most of these strengths are found in the institutional base where the group is dominant over individuals and social standards make individuals strongly family oriented. But there are other strengths which are developing due to modernization, secularization, and the symbolic differentiation processes. These strengths are similar to others present in industrialized societies. The prevalence of individual interests, freedom of action, negotiation, flexibility and open communication are some of the strengths that are becoming more common each day, not only among middle-class families, but also in other social groups. It is interesting to observe that even though these strengths are based on a culture of individualism, as families develop these strengths they are confronted with other challenges, such as how to keep the group together when individuality is emphasized.

Besides the challenges faced by Mexican families related to developing a culture of individualism and a symbolically-differentiated society, there are other important challenges they face, such as poverty and migration. Therefore, in the future we will probably be experiencing the mixture of both tendencies: one toward keeping traditions and another promoting modernization. Families will have to deal with both and will have to build their strengths in order to overcome the resulting challenges.

REFERENCES

Adler, L. & M. Pérez-Lizaur. (1987). *A Mexican elite family. 1820-1980*. Princeton: Princeton University Press.

Arizpe, L. (1973). *Parentesco y economía en una sociedad Nahua*. México D. F.: Colección Secretaría de Educación Pública, Instituto Nacional Indigenista. [Kinship and economy in a Nahua society].

Bazán, L. (1999). Los recursos de los desempleados de Pemex en la ciudad de México. *Estudios Sociológicos*, XVII, *50*, 473-498. [The resources of Pemex unemployed workers in Mexico city].

Beltrán, U., Castaños, F., Flores, J., Meyenberg, Y. & del Pozo, B. (1996). *Los mexicanos de los noventa*. México D. F.: Instituto de Investigaciones Sociales de la Universidad Nacional Autónoma de México. [The Mexicans of the nineties].

Bebería, L. & M. Roldán. (1992). *Las encrucijadas del género: Trabajo a domicilio, subcontratación y dinámica de la unidad doméstica en la ciudad de México*. México D. F.: El Colegio de México, Fondo de Cultura Económica. [Gender crossroads. Home work in service and dynamics of domestic units in Mexico city].

Berger, P. & B. Berger. (1984). *In difesa della famiglia borghese*. Bologna, Italy: Il Mulino.

Berger, P., Berger, B. & Kellner, H. (1973). *The homeless mind*. New York: Vintage.

Conapo (Consejo Nacional de Población). (1999). *La situación demográfica en México 1999*.

México D. F. (1999). Consejo Nacional de Población. [The demographic situation 1999].

Conapo (Consejo Nacional de Población). (1998). *La situación demográfica en México 1998*. México D. F.: Consejo Nacional de Población. [The demographic situation in Mexico 1999].

Cortés, F. (2000). *La distribución del ingreso en México en épocas de estabilización y reforma económica*. México D. F.: Centro de Investigaciones y Estudios Superiores en Antropología Social/Miguel Angel Porrúa. [Income distribution in Mexico in stabilization and economic reform periods].

Cortés, F., Hernández, D., Hernández, E., Székely, M. & Vera, H. (2002). Evolución y características de la pobreza en México en la última década del siglo XX. In Consejo Nacional de Población, *La situación demográfica de México 2002* (pp. 121-137). México D. F.: Consejo Nacional de Población. [Evolution and characteristics of poverty in Mexico in the last decade of the XX century].

D'Aubetterre, M. E. (2000). *El pago de la novia. Matrimonio, vida conyugal y prácticas transnacionales en San Miguel Acuexcomac, Puebla*. Zamora, Michoacán, Mexico: El Colegio de Michoacán, Benemérita Universidad Autónoma de Puebla, Instituto de Ciencias Sociales y Humanidades. [The bride´s payment: Marriage, conjugal life and transnational practices in San Miguel Acuexcomac, Puebla].

De Barbieri, T. (1984). *Mujeres y vida cotidiana*. México D. F.: Fondo de Cultura Económica, Secretaría de Educación Pública. [Women and every day life].

De la Peña, G., Escobar, A. & Duran J. M. (Eds.). (1990). *Crisis, conflicto y sobrevivencia: Estudios sobre la sociedad urbana en México*. Guadalajara, Mexico: Universidad de Guadalajara, Centro de Investigaciones y Estudios Superiores en Antropología Social. [Crises, conflict and survival: Studies about urban society in Mexico].

ENJ (2000). *Encuesta Nacional de Juventud: Resultados generales*. México D. F.: Secretaría de Educación Pública, Instituto Mexicano de la Juventud. [Youth national survey. General results].

Esteinou, R. (2008). Mexican families: Sociocultural and demographic patterns. In C. Hennon and S. W. Wilson (Ed.). *Handbook of families in cultural and international perspective*. New York: Haworth Press.

Esteinou, R. (2005). The emergence of the nuclear family in Mexico. *International Journal of Sociology of the Family, 31*, 1-18.

Esteinou, R. (2004a). La parentalidad en la familia: Cambios y continuidades. In M. Ariza & O. de Oliveira (Coords.), *Imágenes de la familia en el cambio de siglo: Universo familiar y procesos demográficos contemporáneos* (pp. 251-282). México D. F.: Instituto de Investigaciones Sociales, Universidad Nacional Autónoma de México. [Parenting in Mexico: Changes and continuities].

Esteinou, R. (2004b). Parenting in Mexican society. *Marriage and Family Review, 36*, 7-30.

Esteinou, R. (1999). Familia y diferenciación simbólica. *Nueva Antropología, XVI, 55*, 9-26.

Esteinou, R. (1996). *Familias de Sectores Medios: Perfiles organizativos y socio-culturales*. México D. F.: Centro de Investigaciones y Estudios Superiores en Antropología Social. [Middle class families: Organizacional and sociocultural profiles].

Fortuny, P. (1999). *Creyentes y creencias en Guadalajara*. México D. F.: Centro de Investigaciones y Estudios Superiores en Antropología Social, CONACULTA, Instituto Nacional de Antropología e Historia. [Believers and beliefs in Guadalajara].

Franco, V. M. (1992). *Grupo doméstico y reproducción social: Parentesco, economía e ideología en una comunidad otomí del valle del Mezquital*. México, D. F.: Centro de Investigaciones y Estudios Superiores en Antropología Social. [Domestic group and social reproduction. Kinship, economy and ideology in a Valle del Mezquital otomi community].

García, B. & de Oliveira, O. (1994). *Trabajo y vida familiar en México*. México D. F.: El Colegio de México. [Work and family life in Mexico].

Gordon, S. (2002). Desarrollo social y derechos de ciudadanía. In C. Sojo, *Desarrollo Social en América Latina* (pp. 151-214). México D. F.: Facultad Latinoamericana de Ciencias Sociales /Banco Mundial. [Social development and citinzenship rights].

Hennon, C. B., Peterson, G. W., Polzin L. & Radina E. (2008, in press). Familias de ascendencia mexicana residentes en Estados Unidos: recursos para el manejo del estrés parental. In R. Esteinou (Ed.) *Fortalezas y desafíos de las familias en dos contextos: Estados Unidos de América y México*. México D. F., Manuscript. [Families of Mexican heritage living in the United States: Sources of managing parental stress].

Inegi (Instituto Nacional de Estadística, Geografía e Informática). (2003). *Censo Nacional de Población, 2000*. Mexico City: Instituto Nacional de Estadística, Geografía e Informática. [2000 Population Census].

Inegi (Instituto Nacional de Estadística, Geografía e Informática). (1996). *Estadísticas de matrimonios y divorcios, 1996-1997*. México D. F.: Instituto Nacional de Estadística, Geografía e Informática. [Marriage and divorce statistics, 1996-1997].

Inegi (Instituto Nacional de Estadística, Geografía e Informática), Instituto Nacional de las Mujeres. (2004). *Mujeres y hombres de México*. México D. F.: Instituto Nacional de Estadística, Geografía e Informática), Instituto Nacional de las Mujeres. [Women and men of Mexico].

Lehalleur, M. P. & Rendón, T. (1988). Reflexiones a partir de una investigación sobre grupos domésticos campesinos y sus estrategias de reproducción. In O. Oliveira, M. P. Lehalleur & V. Salles (Eds.). *Grupos domésticos y reproducción cotidiana* (pp. 107-126). Mexico City: Coordinación de Humanidades de la Universidad Nacional Autónoma de México, El Colegio de México, Miguel Angel Porrúa. [Reflections from a research on peasant domestic groups and their reproduction strategies].

Lomnitz, L. (1977). *Networks and marginality: Life in a Mexican shantytown*. New York: Academic Press.

López, M. P. (1998). Género y familia. In Sistema Nacional para el Desarrollo Integral de la Familia, *La familia Mexicana en el Tercer Milenio* (pp. 28-40). México D. F.: Sistema Nacional para el Desarrollo Integral de la Familia. [Gender and family].

Millán, S. & Valle, J. (Eds.). (2003). *La comunidad sin límites: Estructura social y organización comunitaria en las regiones indígenas de México*. Mexico D. F.: Instituto Nacional de Antropología e Historia. [The community without limits. Social structure and communitarian organization in the indigenous regions of Mexico].

Molina, V. & Sánchez, K. (1999). El fin de la ilusión: Movilidad social en la ciudad de México. *Nueva Antropología, XVI, 55*, 43-56. [The end of illusion: Social mobility in Mexico City].

Mummert, G. (1999). "Juntos o desapartados": Migración transnacional y la fundación del hogar. In G. Mummert (Ed.), *Fronteras fragmentadas*. Zamora, Michoacán, Mexico: El Colegio de Michoacán, Centro de Investigación y Desarrollo del Estado de Michoacán. ["Together or dis-together": Transnational migration and home foundation].

Mummert, G. (1996). Cambios en la estructura y organización familiares en un contexto de emigración masculina y trabajo asalariado femenino: Estudio de caso en un valle agrícola de Michoacán. In M. P. López (Coord.), *Hogares, familias: desigualdad, conflicto, redes solidarias y parentales* (pp.39-46). México D. F.: Sociedad Mexicana de Demografía. [Changes in structure and family organization in an emigration male context and female salaried work: A case study in an agricultural valley of Michoacán].

Olson, D. H. & J. DeFrain. (2006). *Marriages and families: Intimacy, diversity and strengths.* New York: McGraw-Hill Higher Education.

Robichaux, D. (1996). Un modelo de familia para el "México profundo." *Miscelanea Antropológica.* México D. F.: Centro de Investigaciones y Estudios en Antropología Social, 1-22. [A family model for the "México profundo"].

Salles, V. (1988). Una discusión sobre las condiciones de la reproducción campesina. In O. Oliveira, M. P. Lehalleur & V. Salles (Eds.). *Grupos domésticos y reproducción cotidiana* (pp. 127-160). Mexico City: Coordinación de Humanidades de la Universidad Nacional Autónoma de México, El Colegio de México, Miguel Angel Porrúa.

Sciolla, L. (1983). Differenziazione simbolica e identitá. In *Rassegna italiana di sociologia*, XXIV, *1*. [Symbolic differenciation and identity].

Tuirán, R. (2002). Migración, remesas y desarrollo. In Consejo Nacional de Población, *La situación demográfica de México 2002* (pp. 77-87). México D. F.: Consejo Nacional de Población. [Migration, remmitances and development].

doi:10.1300/J002v41n03_05

Culture-Related Strengths
Among Latin American Families:
A Case Study of Brazil

Gustavo Carlo
Silvia Koller
Marcela Raffaelli
Maria R. T. de Guzman

SUMMARY. We provide an analysis of culturally-specific strength characteristics associated with families in Brazil. The focus is on familism and familial interdependence, the role of the extended family, cooperative and prosocial tendencies, a collective orientation, and the closing

---

Gustavo Carlo is Professor of Psychology, 320 Burnett Hall, Department of Psychology, University of Nebraska-Lincoln, Lincoln, NE 68588 (E-mail: gcarlo1@unl.edu). Silvia Koller is Professor of Psychology, Caixa Postal 9001, 90040-970, Instituto de Psicologia, Universidade Federal do Rio Grande do Sul, Porto Alegre, RS, Brazil (E-mail: silvia.koller@pesquisador.cnpq.br). Marcela Raffaelli is Professor of Psychology and Ethnic Studies, 321 Burnett Hall, Department of Psychology, University of Nebraska-Lincoln, Lincoln, NE 68588 (E-mail: mraffaelli1@unl.edu). Maria R. T. de Guzman is Adolescent Development Extension Specialist and Assistant Professor of Family and Consumer Sciences, 256 Mabel Lee Hall, Department of Psychology, University of Nebraska-Lincoln, Lincoln, NE 68588 (E-mail: mguzman2@unl.edu).

Address correspondence to: Gustavo Carlo.

Funding support was provided by a grant from the National Science Foundation (BNS 0132302) to the first author and a Tobacco Settlement Fund grant from the Office of Sponsored Research at the University of Nebraska-Lincoln to the first and third authors.

[Haworth co-indexing entry note]: "Culture-Related Strengths Among Latin American Families: A Case Study of Brazil." Carlo, Gustavo et al. Co-published simultaneously in *Marriage & Family Review* (The Haworth Press, Inc.) Vol. 41, No. 3/4, 2007, pp. 335-360; and: *Strong Families Around the World: Strengths-Based Research and Perspectives* (ed: John DeFrain, and Sylvia M. Asay) The Haworth Press, Inc., 2007, pp. 335-360. Single or multiple copies of this article are available for a fee from The Haworth Document Delivery Service [1-800-HAWORTH, 9:00 a.m. - 5:00 p.m. (EST). E-mail address: docdelivery@haworthpress.com].

Available online at http://mfr.haworthpress.com
© 2007 by The Haworth Press, Inc. All rights reserved.
doi:10.1300/J002v41n03_06

gender gap. The article is divided into four sections. First, we provide some background information on the demographics and history of Brazil. Second, the family strength characteristics are discussed. Third, case studies are briefly presented to illustrate the protective role of the characteristics. And fourth, we discuss the implications of the strengths-based approach to studying families for theories, research, and program development. doi:10.1300/J002v41n03_06 *[Article copies available for a fee from The Haworth Document Delivery Service: 1-800-HAWORTH. E-mail address: <docdelivery@haworthpress.com> Website: <http://www.HaworthPress.com> © 2007 by The Haworth Press, Inc. All rights reserved.]*

KEYWORDS. Culture, gender, families, Latin America, prosocial behaviors

INTRODUCTION

The family unit serves multiple purposes in societies and families are defined in varied ways across cultures (LeVine, 1988). However, the central role of the family in the health and well-being of children has long been acknowledged by scholars. Today, as in the past, families help to shape and define the unique characteristics of cultures worldwide. Culturally-shared beliefs and practices continue to evolve to provide children and families optimal and adaptive chances for success.

The present chapter provides an analysis of culturally-specific characteristics associated with families in Brazil. Though the focus is on Brazil, many of the cultural features are also evident in families from other Latin American societies (and some non-Latin American societies as well). Although there are other unique characteristics of Brazilian families and society, we chose to focus our analysis on familism and familial interdependence, the role of the extended family, cooperative and prosocial tendencies, a collective orientation and the closing gender gap. We view these characteristics as strengths–characteristics that are adaptive and serve to enhance optimal success for individuals in those societies. These characteristics can also be conceived as resilience or buffer factors (i.e., factors that protect individuals from high-risk environments or adverse conditions).

The article is divided into four sections. First, we provide some background information on the demographics of Brazil. Second, the family strength characteristics are introduced and discussed. Third, case studies of real families are briefly presented to illustrate the protective role of the culture-specific characteristics. And fourth, we conclude by discussing the importance for theories, research, and program development of the strengths-based approach to studying families.

BACKGROUND AND SOCIODEMOGRAPHIC CONTEXT

The Context of Families in Brazil

Brazil is an immense country that covers 3,285,618 square miles and spans four time zones (CIA, 2005). It has the world's fifth largest population (over 172 million) and eighth largest economy (in terms of GNP). Brazil's present-day characteristics reflect events that occurred over 500 years, since the arrival of the Portuguese in 1500. Reflecting generations of intermarriage between European settlers, indigenous tribes, and enslaved Africans, as well as large-scale migration from Europe in the late 1800s and early 1900s, the population is racially diverse. In the 2000 Census, 54% of the population self-identified as White, 38.5% as mixed, 6% as Black, and 1.5% as other (Japanese, Arab, indigenous).

Brazil shares borders with every South American country except Chile and Ecuador, and is divided into five regions that are geographically, culturally, and economically distinct (PAHO, 2001). The seven states of the Northern region are the most sparsely populated (3.3 inhabitants per square kilometer), encompassing the Amazon basin, and occupy 45% of Brazil's national territory. The Northeast region consists of 9 states (18% of the nation's territory and 28% of the population), and is characterized by high levels of poverty. In the center of the country, three sparsely populated states and the federal district (established in 1960) make up the Central-East district. The four states of the industrialized Southeastern region, which includes Rio de Janeiro and Sno Paulo, are characterized by the nation's highest population density (77.9 inhabitants per square kilometer). Finally, the Southern region encompasses just three states and is characterized by a temperate climate (contrasting with the rest of the nation, which is tropical) and a relatively high standard of living. The five regions have experienced different histories, settlement patterns, and economic development that profoundly affect the experiences of families.

In part because of regional disparities, Brazil is a country of contradictions. Its major cities possess modern infrastructures, including state-of-the-art transportation systems, advanced medical and educational systems, and technology- and service-oriented industries. On many social indicators, Brazil's citizens are comparatively well off. For example, life.expectancy is 68 years, adult literacy for both men and women is 85%, fertility rates are 2.2 (lower than the regional average of 2.6) and 95% of children attend primary school (UNICEF, 2004). The country has a well-established public health system; as a result, vaccination rates are high (over 95%), 86% of pregnant women have prenatal care, and 88% of births are assisted by a skilled birth attendant (UNICEF, 2004). Women are not disadvantaged compared to men in terms of life expectancy or secondary school enrollment, and the maternal mortality ratio (annual number of maternal deaths per 100,000 live births) of 160 is lower than the regional rate (190), although still far higher than is seen in industrialized nations (12) (UNICEF, 2004).

Despite these relative advantages, many Brazilian families experience serious challenges. Some are in situations of pervasive poverty that result from high levels of income inequality and lack of government-sponsored welfare programs. In 2000, the poorest 40% of the Brazilian population received just 8% of the nation's total income, whereas the richest 20% received 64% of the nation's wealth (UNICEF, 2004). Another challenge stems from Brazil's extremely high external debt, which has resulted in a succession of economic measures to curtail spending. Brazil's debt service (expressed as a percent of exports of goods and services) was 78% in 2000, which was considerably higher than the regional average (34%), is the highest in the world. As a result of family poverty, many young people do not complete their education. Only two-thirds of primary school entrants reach grade five (UNICEF, 2004), just over a third (35%) graduate from secondary school, and fewer than 10% of the working age population has any postsecondary education (World Bank, 2003).

Other challenges to Brazilian families of all socioeconomic levels are high urbanization rates, linked to rapid and often uncontrolled growth of mega cities in the past few decades (Gilbert, 1996). Rural migrants are attracted to large cities by the possibility of jobs but often find themselves working in the informal economy as street vendors or day laborers while living in the areas surrounding the slums that are controlled by drug gangs and characterized by high levels of violence (Krug, Dahlberg, Mercy, Zwi, & Lozano, 2002). In 2001, 81% of Brazil's population lived in urban areas, compared to the regional average of 76% (UNICEF, 2004). Poverty and lack of economic opportunities have been linked to high levels of urban violence in Brazil (Balán, 1996). In reaction to heightened levels of violence in Brazilian cities, the rich are increasingly segregating themselves in gated communities, venturing forth only in armored cars. Rich families are increasingly using secure spaces for leisure, such as malls, recreation settings, or clubs that are protected by armed guards. In contrast, the children of the poor typically play in the streets. The division of the country into rich and poor, and increasing separation of families at different socioeconomic levels during work and leisure represent major threats to the health of the nation.

The current situation of Brazilian families must be understood in light of the country's recent past. In 1964, a military dictatorship was established that shaped the country's political, social, and economic systems for over two decades. Brazil's political system under military rule was characterized by repressive measures intended to preserve order and discourage expressions of discontent (Diversi, Moraes & Morelli, 1999). The rigid controls resulted in policies that undermined the quality of life for most Brazilian families during that historical period. Although many policies have been modified or eliminated, their legacy continues to impact the quality of life for families even today.

There are at least two reasons for the continued impact of past policies. One major factor is that the economic situation in Brazil continues to fluctuate since the restoration of civilian rule, and although the economy is improving, investments in social programs have not been substantial enough to bring about significant improvement in families. A second related factor is the lack of an organized welfare system to deliver services. For many years, the Brazilian government never developed a social welfare system to help families and individuals who could not take care of themselves. Instead, non-governmental organizations and religious agencies formed the basis for the social welfare system (Diversi, et al., 1999). Improvements in government policies are slow to change the situation. For example, in some locations families can apply for scholarships so children are able to attend school rather than work to help feed their families. However, despite the development of such programs, in many parts of the country families are little better off than they were under military rule.

One tragic consequence of the poverty conditions, inadequate government policies, and ineffective social welfare programs in Brazil (as well as in some other Latin American countries) is the large number of street children. Nearly half of the world's street youth are found in Latin American countries (Raffaelli, Koller, Reppold, Kuschick, & Bandeira, 2000). In many families, poverty creates strong pressures for children to live on their own or to work on the streets under high-risk conditions. Although economic and demographic factors are often cited as causes of street and homeless children, family circumstances are also relevant. For example, family disruptions such as parental death or absence, job loss, rural-to-urban migration, and family violence have been associated with street children and homelessness (see Raffaelli, 1997).

In summary, Brazil is a complex society. There is abundant wealth, industrialization, and modernization, as well as advanced educational and medical systems (especially in major cities). However, there is also much poverty throughout the country and there are large rural, less structurally developed regions in the country. The challenges of families in Brazil are many and multifaceted; however, there are a number of culturally-related resources that protect and buffer many children and adolescents from maladjustment and factors that threaten family well-being.

CULTURE-RELATED STRENGTH CHARACTERISTICS

Despite the multicultural heritage and the diverse demographic of families in Brazil, there are pervasive strength themes that are common to many Brazilian families. These themes are common throughout many other Latin American countries as well. Most importantly, these themes serve to protect and buffer many Brazilian children and adolescents from the possible adverse conditions of their communities. The present chapter will focus on five of the commonly identified themes: familism and familial interdependence, the role of the extended family, cooperation and prosocial behaviors, a collectivist group orientation, and the closing gender gap.

It is important to note that although there are unique characteristics associated with specific Latino and Latin American populations, most of the existing research that focuses on Latinos (in the United States) has been conducted with Mexicans and Mexican Americans (Raffaelli, Carlo, Carranza, & Gonzalez-Kruger, 2005). Furthermore, in many studies, Latinos from different countries of origin are grouped and not differentiated. Finally, for the present article, we use the term Latino in the broadest sense–individuals from Latin American countries. This is distinct from other terms such as Hispanics, which are often used to depict individuals from Spanish-speaking countries. As will be noted, there is sparse research that directly examines the central role of the family in the well-being and adjustment of Brazilians. In light of these limitations, the bulk of the research reviewed here should be interpreted with much caution.

Familism and Familial Interdependence

Family plays a central role in shaping Latinos' experiences (Azevedo, 1994; Carlo, Carranza, & Zamboanga, 2002; Fuligni, Tseng, & Lam, 1999; Knight, Bernal, & Carlo, 1995; Korin, 1996). One of the hallmark characteristics of many Latino families is the strong value of family unity and connection. This value is reflected in familism the strong identification with, and attachment and loyalty to, one's family, which has also been well-documented among Latinos in other studies (e.g., Sabogal, Marin, Otero-Sabogal, Marin, & Perez-Stable, 1987; Suárez-Orozco & Suárez-Orozco, 1995). A somewhat distinct but related notion is familial interdependence, or the notion of developing and maintaining close physical and psychological family ties (see Knight et al., 1995; McDade, 1995; Zayas & Solari, 1994).

Relative to other societies (such as the United States), Brazilian and Latino parents strongly guide and encourage their children to stay physically and psychologically close to family through frequent social interactions and close physical proximity. Research indicates that Brazilian youth do not show individuation from parents or increased conflict during adolescence, and report a continued high rate of social support from both parents and peers (Van Horn & Marques, 2000). In many Latino families, older and extended family members maintain active roles in family activities. There is an emphasis on the importance of contributing to the family by assigning responsibility for household chores and tending to young children (Delgado-Gaitan, 1994; Zayas & Solari, 1994). Young family members might be raised not only by parents but by siblings, aunts, uncles, and grandparents. Respect toward adult family members is strongly reinforced and there are usually clear rules and consequences (e.g., social disapproval, shame) when respect is violated. Moreover, even when children enter adulthood, parents (and grand-parents) are sought as sources for financial, instrumental and emotional support. These socializing actions and behaviors serve to strengthen an orientation towards familial interdependence, which serves as the basic foundation of a social support network.

There is a strong theoretical basis to expect that familial interdependence should bolster the well-being of family members (especially children). Attachment theorists suggest that the development of a close, nurturing parent-child relationship fosters a positive internal working model (see Thompson, 1998). Internal working models reflect the sense of security about one's self and their social world. Securely attached, as opposed to insecurely attached children, are likely to develop positive developmental outcomes as a result of their ability to explore and interact successfully with their social environment. Furthermore, maintaining close and supportive family relationships undoubtedly impacts parent-child relationships beyond childhood and adolescence. Moreover, researchers on parenting styles and practices suggest that close and supportive parenting styles are associated with social competence and well-being (Baumrind, 1991; see Eisenberg & Murphy, 1995, and Maccoby & Martin, 1983).

Somewhat surprisingly, despite the preponderance of scholarly discussion of the importance of familial interdependence and familism among Latino families, direct research is relatively sparse. There is some research that shows that Latinas (relative to Latinos) remain closely monitored by their parents and maintain close relationships with their parents (see Carlo Fabes, Laible, & Kupanoff, K. (1999). Suárez-Orozco and colleagues (Suárez-Orozco, Todorova, & Louie, 2002) also reported that Latinos strongly endorse the notions of familism and familial interdependence. Recently, de Guzman and Carlo (2004) showed that family adaptability was associated positively with prosocial behaviors in a sample of Latino adolescents. Laible, Carlo, and Roesch (2004) found that close, supportive relationships with parents were associated with self-esteem in a sample of mostly Latino college students. The finding suggests that, among Latinos, families who are flexible in their roles and in responding to the youth's specific circumstances may be more adept at fostering prosocial behaviors. Perhaps more importantly, there is research that suggests the important role of strong familial interdependence in fostering well-being in Latino families. Furthermore, studies suggest that parents may still be influential even in adolescence (Carlo et al., 1999; Laible et al., 2004) and this might be particularly true among some Latinos.

There is other research that shows that positive family relationships can help protect Latino adolescents from becoming involved in problem behaviors. A number of studies have shown that higher family support, strong family connectedness, and higher parental monitoring is associated with lower alcohol and substance use and less gang involvement among Latinos (Frauenglass, Routh, & Pantin, 1997; Kerr, Beck, Shattuck, Kattar, & Uriburu, 2003). A study with Latino adolescents revealed a significant relation between familism and lower levels of lifetime marijuana use (Ramirez, Crano, Quist, Burgoon, Alvaro, & Grandpre, 2004). Although we might expect similar findings in Brazilian samples, as is evident from the review, research directly relevant to Brazilian families is sorely lacking (see also Carlo & Koller, 1998).

The Role of the Extended Family

Closely tied to the notions of familism and familial interdependence, is the prominent role of extended family members. For Brazilians (and many other Latinos and Latin Americans), the notions of familism and familial interdependence extend to family members other than the nuclear family (Fonseca, 1991). Furthermore, extended family members have major roles and responsibilities in various aspects of domestic life. The encouragement of maintaining and valuing close family ties is often manifested in life decisions regarding careers, family planning, education, and childcare. Usually, strong familism tendencies result in more consideration to maintain close proximity in choosing schools and careers. It can also impact decisions to have children (and the timing of children) and there might be a strong pull to ask extended family members to assist in childcare.

Scholars have long acknowledged the central role of social support in buffering and protecting individuals from adverse, high risk conditions (Barrera & Li, 1996; Cohen & Wills, 1985; Sarason, Sarason, & Gurung, 1997). One important source of social support for Latinos is parents and family (Raffaelli et al., 2005). As noted earlier, attachment theorists note the powerful affective, cognitive, and behavioral systems responsible for the development of secure caregiver-child attachment relationship. Although the systems function mostly between caregivers and their children, there is reason to believe that similar mechanisms foster secure relationships among siblings and extended family members. Clearly, frequent contact with extended and nuclear family members provides ample opportunities for multiple attachment relationships to develop.

There is research that shows that Latinos report stronger obligations and more support from their family than European Americans (Freeberg & Stein, 1996; Fuligni et al., 1999). Evidence on the impact of attachment and supportive relationships on well-being and health among family members in Brazilian families is scant. However, research on North American samples of Latinos suggests links between secure attachment and children's empathy and social competence (Eisenberg & Fabes, 1998; Thompson, 1998).

Cooperative and Prosocial Tendencies

The development and maintenance of close positive family relationships is facilitated by frequent cooperative and prosocial behaviors among members. Prosocial behaviors are defined as actions designed to benefit others (Eisenberg & Fabes, 1998). Prosocial behaviors are varied but include behaviors such as altruism (i.e., behaviors whose primary intention is to benefit others while often incurring a cost to the self), compliant (i.e., asked for helping behaviors), dire (i.e., helping under emergency situations), and cooperative (i.e., behaviors that mutually benefit individuals). For example, sharing, nurturance, and comforting behaviors are two types of behaviors that foster close family relationships. Frequently, prosocial behaviors trigger reciprocal prosocial behaviors and promote trust and positive affect, basic characteristics of close, intimate relationships.

What is of particular interest, however, is that despite the almost universal propensity and strong biological basis for prosocial tendencies (Braten, 1996; de Guzman, Edwards, & Carlo, 2005; Zahn-Waxler, Friedman, & Cummings, 1983; Zahn-Waxler, Radke-Yarrow, & King, 1979; see Carlo, 2005; Eisenberg & Fabes, 1998), wide individual and group differences in prosocial behaviors are also evident. The evidence for variation in frequency and types of prosocial behaviors across cultures is also evident. For example, in one of the early cross-cultural studies of socialization practices, Barry, Child, and Bacon (1959) showed that agricultural-based economy societies valued nurturance and co-operation (compliance) more so than hunting-fishing based economy societies. Other early studies (Munroe & Munroe 1977; Shapira & Madsen, 1969, 1974; also see Whiting & Edwards, 1988) and more recent observational and self-report investigations corroborate those findings, both cross-nationally and cross-ethnically (Suzuki & Greenfield, 2002; Knight & Kagan, 1982; Rotheram-Borus & Phinney, 1990). What accounts for these cultural variations?

Although there are undoubtedly complex interactions between biology and environment that help to account for variations among families, cultural psychologists have noted socialization practice differences by people from different societies that shape children's development (Edwards, Knoche, Aukrust, Kumru, & Kim, 2006; Whiting & Whiting, 1975). For example, in some societies, young children are assigned household duties and responsibilities that foster social responsibility and prosocial behaviors. In other societies, prosocial behaviors are encouraged through formal curriculum requirements in early education programs. Even across early education programs, there are differences in the aspects of morality that are emphasized: some might focus on empathy and respect and others might focus on reasoning and problem solving (Whiting & Edwards, 1988). The impact of these and other wide-ranging socialization practices and experiences on prosocial development in different societies, however, is little understood.

In their classic study of six cultures, the Whitings and their colleagues found cultural variations in levels of exhibited prosocial behaviors (Whiting & Whiting, 1975; see also Whiting & Edwards, 1988). For example, cultures that exhibited higher levels of prosocial behaviors tended to have larger families, placed greater importance on the nurturing role of women, had less specialized careers, and less centralized governments. In addition, gender differences in prosocial behaviors were more pronounced in those cultures. The gender differences favoring women were attributed to greater responsibility for the welfare of the family (e.g., younger siblings) and to the assignment of responsible, household chores early in life. Although direct research on Brazilian families is sparse, Brazilian families are characterized by relative large families (although this has declined in recent years; Marteleto, 2005) and by the central role of women in the welfare and responsibility of the family.

Several studies of prosocial and care-based moral reasoning and motives also suggest an emphasis on cooperation and prosocial tendencies among Brazilian families and youth (see Carlo & Koller, 1998). For example, recent investigators of cooperative behaviors found greater emphasis on cooperative behaviors and less emphasis on competitive behaviors among children from Brazil than among children from the US (Carlo, Roesch, Knight, & Koller, 2001). Furthermore, researchers have found that Brazilian children and adolescents frequently report needs-oriented and empathic and internalized modes of prosocial moral reasoning (Carlo, Koller, & Eisenberg, 1996; Eisenberg, Guthrie et al., 2002). Perhaps more importantly, these same researchers showed that prosocial moral reasoning was positively associated with prosocial behaviors. In a study of late adolescents, Brazilians frequently rejected hedonistic forms of prosocial moral reasoning (i.e., self-oriented concerns) in resolving moral dilemmas (Carlo, Roesch, & Koller, 1999). Finally, among institutionalized Brazilians, low SES Brazilian adolescents reported higher level prosocial moral reasoning than delinquent or orphaned Brazilian adolescents (Carlo, Koller, &

Eisenberg, 1998). Taken together, these studies suggest that cooperative and prosocial behaviors are highly valued by many Brazilian children
and adolescents.

Collectivist Orientation

One aspect of many Latino societies including Brazil is the strong
collectivist orientation. Collectivism refers to an emphasis and focus on
consequences to the broader social group, including family and community (Triandis, 1994). Many scholars have noted that collectivist-oriented
societies value cooperative behaviors more than individualistic-oriented
societies (Hofstede, 2001; Knight , Bernal, & Carlo,1995; Triandis, 1994).
The emphasis on cooperation and maintenance of close family relationships in agricultural based societies is thought to be adaptive for the
enhancement of the community. Based on the work of several scholars
(Hofstede, 2001; Trianidis, 1994; Schwartz, 1992), many individuals from
Latin American countries, including Brazil (Gouveia, Albuquerque,
Clemente, & Espinosa, 2002) are considered oriented toward collective
goals and concerns. Collectivist tendencies would be expected to foster
and nurture close, strong relationships with others, which provide an
important source of social support.

Consistent with this notion, there is evidence that Brazilians are oriented, and concerned with, collective goals and issues (Bontempo, Lobel &
Triandis, 1990). Moreover, there is an abundance of empirical evidence
that shows relatively high levels of cooperative behaviors among individuals from Latin American countries as compared to individuals from
individualistic-oriented countries (Carlo et al., 2001; see Knight et al.,
1995, for a review). For example, Carlo and colleagues (2001) found that
children from Brazil exhibited higher levels of cooperative behaviors
than children from the United States. Furthermore, among college students, Brazilians frequently reported empathic and internalized modes
of prosocial moral reasoning (though relatively less than European
Americans; Carlo et al., 1999). Thus, the existing research suggests that
many Brazilians endorse a collectivist orientation and are cooperative with
others; however, research on the direct impact of cooperative tendencies
and a collectivist value orientation in Brazilian families is lacking.

The Closing Gender Gap

Similar to many countries around the world, there is a long tradition
in many Latino countries for gender-based inequities based on strong

gender-based stereotypes. The tradition stems in part from practical economic considerations and strong religious beliefs that advance somewhat narrow conceptions of masculinity and femininity. Masculinity and femininity are associated with notions of instrumentality, agency, expressiveness, and communion (Huston, 1983). At the extreme end of masculinity is the notion of *machismo*–commonly referred to as a strong societal expectation that men dominate social relationships (DeSouza, Baldwin, Koller, & Narvaez, 2004). Closely related to machismo is the notion of marianismo, that women should be submissive, a good mother and wife, and self-sacrificing to men. These notions are transmitted across generations and are powerfully maintained, at the macro-societal level, by social, economic, and educational forces. They are also promoted by more proximal socialization agents such as parents, siblings, peers, and the media (e.g., television, radio, magazines, books, the Internet). In a recent study of gender equality in 58 countries around the world, using five indicators (political empowerment, educational access, health and well-being, economic participation, economic opportunity), Brazil ranked 51st (Lopez-Carlos & Zahidi, 2005)–ranking lower than other Latin American countries such as Venezuela, Chile, and Argentina.

Like many other Latin American countries, gender-typed notions have been characterized as strong and rigid in Brazil (e.g., the notion of a machismo-oriented society). Although some scholars have pointed out that there might be some positive consequences of machismo (e.g., honor, responsibility, protection of the family), strong, stereotyped, gender-based conceptions can seriously limit and restrict the role of women and men (DeSouza, Baldwin, Koller, & Narvaz, 2004).) For example, the traditional feminine-typed expectation that women are nurturant, expressive and communal might restrict career aspirations and opportunities for women. Similarly, masculine-typed notions of lack of expressiveness might limit opportunities for care-related career opportunities and hamper the development of healthy intimate relationships for men. These restrictions might have consequences for long-term health and well being.

However, Brazilian families are quite varied and corresponding gender roles are equally complex. Traditional patriarchal families are still common but there are increasing numbers of single-parent families and there are scores of co-equal couple families (Azevedo, 1994). These different family systems are linked directly to economic and socio-demographic factors (e.g., urbanization, industrialization) (Bock, Iutaka, & Berardo, 1975; Fonseca, 1991). For example, co-equal couple families endorse less traditional gender-role stereotypes and are more likely to agree that there are equal rights between the sexes. Furthermore, women in single-parent households (e.g., when husbands leave the home to work in other regions) and women in middle- class households tend towards matriarchy (Azevedo, 1994). Thus, it is possible that the closing gender gap is most relevant in specific sociodemographic demographic parts of Brazil. Unfortunately, the scarcity of research on these varied family structures seriously limits our understanding of possible changing gender roles in families.

To date, there is mixed evidence on whether strong gender-typed notions are becoming diluted and that the gender gap is closing among Brazilians. At the societal level, ongoing sociopolitical movements (e.g., the feminist movement) and new government laws and policies have expanded sociopolitical, educational, and economic opportunities for women (DeSouza et al., 2004). Researchers have noted that Brazilians are no more likely to endorse gender stereotypes than individuals from other countries (see DeSouza et al., 2004, for a review). For example, Hutz, Koller, and Biaggio (1992) found evidence that Brazilians might be rejecting the rigid gender-typed notions and more accepting of flexible gender typologies. However, other researchers noted that strong gender-role stereotypes and gender differences are still prevalent among Brazilian children and adolescents (Carlo et al., 2001; de Guzman, Carlo, Ontai, Koller, & Knight, 2004). Raffaelli and Koller and their colleagues (2000) noted that although street girls and boys did not differ on many family circumstances, girls were more likely than boys to have left home because of family violence and more negative relationships with their parents. Fonseca (1991) reported that most Brazilian slum women cited their responsibility to their children as the primary reason for not seeking employment.

Although there is promise regarding a rapidly closing gender gap in Brazil, caution is needed in over-simplifying or over-generalizing the impact of those changes (see Sturm, 1991). It is likely that the somewhat mixed findings are due to differences in the study populations and the specific topic of study. Therefore, more research examining gender-role disparities across different behavioral domains and with different populations is needed. Furthermore, it is also important to note that there will likely be a time lag in observed changes as a result of expanded opportunities for women. Moreover, similar to the situation in many other countries around the world, gender-based prejudice and discrimination (e.g., pay inequities) and family violence mostly directed at women still exists. Nonetheless, a closing gender gap holds great promise for the future well being and health of Brazilian families.

BRAZILIAN FAMILY CASE STUDIES

The next section presents two case studies of families in different situations. As will be seen, each family brings their own unique talents, skills, and resources to deal with challenges and demands. However, there are pervasive cultural-related strength characteristics that serve to protect and enhance the individuals' well being and health.

A Situation of Challenge: Maria's Family

Maria was born 33 years ago, in a rural city and moved to the capital with her family when she was nine years old. Due to the family's financial difficulties, she went to live with an upper-middle-class couple. It was not an adoption; Maria performed domestic chores in exchange for a place to live. She remembers that the couple gave her affection and offered the possibility to have a career, but these opportunities were not valued by her at that time. When she was 16 years old, she abandoned the fourth grade and the home where she was living due to a pregnancy. She started to live with her son and relatives in the slums. At that time, she held sporadic jobs until her 24th birthday, when she became involved with a man who was 20 years older and her life changed dramatically.

Maria separated from her child and went to live with this man, a drug dealer who pretended to be a taxi driver to hide his real occupation. The atmosphere was characterized by violence and constant police inspections. In the beginning, there was a seductive involvement between the partners; however, in due course, and culminating with Maria's second pregnancy, the relationship became more and more violent. Beatings with pieces of wood and iron marked her body, and kicks revealed that her pregnancy was not wanted by the father. Although Maria did not use or traffic in drugs, she experienced increasing stress from drug-related death threats and the possibility of arrest and imprisonment. She started to have heart problems that resulted in a bypass operation when she was 28 years old. Maria continued to be abused by her partner. After several violent episodes, she shot and killed him in self-defense. Although acquitted of the killing, Maria was not free. In spite of his death, her husband continued to threaten her well-being: Maria had been infected with HIV, the virus that causes AIDS. This could have been the end of Maria's story; however it is just the beginning of the story of a new and resilient family.

Today, Maria lives with her eight-year-old daughter Ana and two orphan nieces, Tereza (age nine) and Joana (age seven), in a small cottage in a slum community in the state capital. The cottage has three rooms–a bedroom, a kitchen and a bathroom–and there are no internal doors. Although their home is rudimentary, the family keeps it clean and organized. Maria also teaches the girls to take care of themselves and to value personal hygiene. Despite the cold winter weather and lack of central heating, family members bathe every day. The children are responsible for domestic tasks such as cooking, washing, and organizing the house; for example, Ana was taught to prepare meals at the age of five. The three girls study at a public school, and Maria says that education is essential to have a career in the future. Ana now knows how to read and says that she will be a confectioner when she is older. Maria's 16-year-old son frequently visits the family and his presence is always a reason for happiness.

Tereza and Joana are the daughters of Maria's sister. The girls' father was murdered at age 19 in an assault. Two years ago they lost the mother, 26 years old, to meningitis–she was also infected with HIV. After their mother's death, the girls went to live with a couple of uncles in an environment characterized by conflict and physical aggression. During this time, Tereza went to school, and her school performance was low. The family decided that the girls should be moved to Maria's home. The nieces have lived with their aunt for less than one year. This change transformed their lives in a positive way. Today, they are good students, their grades are above average, and they amicably share tasks and the family atmosphere. In spite of the difficulties that Maria faces–her body weakened by the terminal disease, the responsibility for her daughter's and nieces' education, and the lack of financial stability–she is optimistic and happy. Maria knows that she is preparing her girls to have a better life than she had. She says that her family cannot be considered to be dysfunctional, because she is a vigilant caregiver and the needs of her daughter and nieces are the main focus of her everyday life.

In the path of life for Maria, Ana, Tereza and Joana, it is possible to identify many risk factors such as poverty, low level of education, the loss of significant people, Maria's physical disease, the restricted space of the home, and exposure to chronic violence and drugs in the slum community. In the past, Maria faced many challenges as she moved from a rural area to the state capital, as she yearned to create intimate relationships, and as she struggled through an adolescence marked by pregnancy and an unstable and violent relationship. Maria's daughter, Ana, bore witness to these conditions. Maria's nieces, Joana and Tereza, experienced the loss of their parents. Moments marked by vulnerability and high risk were constant in this family.

Despite the great hardships, there were many strength characteristics associated with her culture that benefited Maria's family. Maria has restructured her life armed with a set of personal and environmental characteristics that have resulted in a strong will and conviction to supercede her challenges. She has thrived under the rubric of her personal characteristics (e.g., autonomy, self-control, and self-efficacy) and her social support and family cohesion. Her social support network, including her family, friends, and her religion, supplies the material, emotional and spiritual comfort necessary so that the family may face daily difficulties. Within the family, with her daughter and nieces, the dialogue is constant. The most painful themes, such as the losses of family members, are openly approached. This attitude is only possible because there is strong cohesion in the family group.

Positive changes have resulted from Joana and Tereza's transfer to Maria and Ana's home. Maria has created a relatively safe environment that nurtures and protects her daughter and nieces. The strength and closeness of the group reinforces in each one of them positive values of themselves and of the world. Maria encourages the girls to share, learn, and study in preparation for a career. She promotes the healthy aspects of mutual cooperation and values that favor adaptation and trust among family members. The girls are being prepared to manage their lives without the presence of their terminally-ill caregiver.

Maria could have abdicated her nieces' care to improve her financial conditions; however, she opted to care for her family and to work to maintain a strong family connection. The positive and nurturing environment rewards reciprocal practices by her nieces and has become an affirmation of family acceptance. In this family, the structuring of their relationships favors resilient aspects that reduce the impact of the risks to which family members are exposed. This can be observed, for instance, in the girls' concern with Maria's medication schedule and her well-being. The mother receives the children's affection, is fortified emotionally by this affection and care, which in turn strengthens her will to battle her disease.

The many protective factors that increase the resilience of Maria's family are evident in the quality of their interactions and relationships. Maria's family has benefited from strong familism and familial interdependence, a collectivist orientation towards the good of the group (i.e., family), support of extended family members, a desire to overcome rigid gender-stereotyped submissive behaviors, and frequent prosocial and cooperative behaviors that serve to constantly reinforce and maintain their strong bonds. In this family, it is possible to observe these strength characteristics. Maria, Ana, Tereza and Joana have formed a family built on the available strength characteristics that are nurtured and promoted by their culture.

A Family of Privilege: Jorge's Family

The Silvas are descendants of a Portuguese family that arrived in Brazil in the beginning of the last century. Jorge, 50 years old, is an administrator employed by a large company. His wife, Carmen, is 45 years old and is a nurse who works at the hospital of a public university. They met during their college graduation year and were married soon after, with the full support of their families. Two years later the first son Rodrigo was born. Today, Rodrigo is 20 years old and is studying to be a physician at an expensive private university. Rodrigo is an exemplary student and receives financial support from his parents so he can devote his time to his studies. Ana was born one year after Rodrigo and is getting ready to study psychology at a public university. She will also likely receive full financial support from her parents so she can dedicate her time to study.

The family is in a good financial condition. For example, before Rodrigo entered university, the family had built a nice and comfortable house. In addition, each family member has a car and the family spends vacations at a small beachfront cottage. The family usually gathers together on weekends for family lunches with the couple's parents, siblings, nephews and nieces. Since their home is very spacious and, at the same time, cozy, Jorge and Carmen insist on hosting these extended family gatherings. During these frequent gatherings, family members cook traditional recipes, sing Portuguese songs, and tell stories about the family.

Recently, due to the need to reduce expenses in Jorge's company, there was a mass dismissal of employees, which affected primarily the most senior employees. Jorge is quite frightened about this situation, because he has large responsibilities with his family and wants to maintain the good standard of living that they have always had. Carmen's job is relatively secure and she receives a good salary, but her salary alone would not be sufficient to maintain the family's current standard of living.

Jorge wanted to avoid showing the family his concern about the difficulties in his company, but his wife and the children observed that he had been somewhat depressed. Recently, Jorge did not want to host their family at home for the family's traditional lunch gathering, alleging physical fatigue. However, this unusual event generated a series of phone calls from their relatives and friends inquiring about the well-being and needs of Jorge's family.

After some insistence by Carmen and the children, Jorge revealed his concerns during one of their family dinners. Immediately after he finished disclosing the situation, he heard his children's manifestation of solidarity and support. They said they could change their spending habits and get part-time jobs to help with expenses. Ana, his daughter, offered to sell her car. Carmen, his wife, suggested that they could get some money by renting the cottage at the beach instead of spending vacations at the cottage. Several options were discussed among the family members. This left Jorge feeling much more calm and at ease about their situation.

Coincidentally, during their conversation, Carmen's mother called to inquire about her daughter and her grandchildren. Hearing about the pressing family situation, she also offered her support and solidarity to the family and reassured them that they would also received support from other members of their family.

The situation for Jorge's family was clearly very different than that of Maria's family. However, as in Maria's family, one could observe pervasive strength characteristics that serve to buffer Jorge's family from potential challenges. The strong family bonds reflective of their familism and familial interdependence, the supportive role of extended family members, the collectivist orientation toward the good of the group, the flexible gender-type orientation that promotes achievement, and the cooperative and prosocial practices of support and comfort, are all reflected to some degree in maintaining the well-being and health of the individual family members. Even in a relatively privileged family environment, these strength characteristics are reinforced and encouraged.

The Future of Research on Families: A Strengths-Based Approach

In the present chapter, we briefly summarized some of the strength characteristics of many families in Brazil. Although there are other strength characteristics (e.g., religion) that could be reviewed in more depth, it is important to note that all families have strength potential. That is, all families have individual and environmental resources that can potentially enhance and strengthen the well-being and health of families and their members. We attempted to show that strength characteristics can be manifested across families living in different, and sometimes challenging, circumstances. Moreover, strength characteristics can be culture-specific or they can be evident across cultures. There is a need for future researchers to identify culture-specific strength characteristics–lest we assume that strength characteristics serve the same function across cultures.

Unfortunately, our understanding of strength characteristics among Brazilian (and Latin American) families is limited. There are many research gaps perhaps due to the traditional overemphasis on deficiencies and "deficit model" approaches in studying ethnic group families and individuals (McLoyd, 1998; Raffaelli et al., 2005). Similarly, there has been much research on negative and high-risk factors among families and individuals from ethnically-diverse groups in the U.S. (Raffaelli et al., 2005). This research has increased our understanding of these problem behaviors and conditions that stimulate problem behaviors and mental illness. However, we have little understanding of strength conditions and the strength conditions that stimulate positive social outcomes and well-being. As several scholars have noted (e.g., Raffaelli et al., 2005; The Consortium on Social Competence, 1994), our understanding of problem and high-risk environments do not necessarily further our understanding of positive and low-risk environments–studies are needed to focus on each set of behaviors and environments. We hope this chapter helps to invigorate research programs to examine the personal and environmental factors that contribute to health and well-being among families.

An approach that focuses and emphasizes the strength among families is not just an argument for scholars to view issues from a "glass half full" perspective. Rigorous and programmatic strengths-based research will be needed to provide critical information for more effective intervention programs. A strengths approach to studying families offers a qualitatively distinct approach and methodology. For example, furthering our understanding of strengths promotes the development of prevention programs aimed at enhancing and nurturing existing family strength characteristics rather than an emphasis on post-hoc intervention programs designed to fix manifested problems and pathology. Furthermore, we can develop diagnostic tools to identify existing strengths among individuals and families so that these strengths can be channeled more effectively.

In our increasingly global society, it is important to cross national boundaries in our research to further our understanding of families. Furthermore, at a time when much of the national and international media focus is on negative social behaviors, it is important for social science scholars to provide a balanced perspective on strengths as well as risks for families. Moreover, families, however they are defined, serve multiple functions and are complex systems shaped by the interplay of biology and environment. A strengths-based approach offers an opportunity for scholars to adequately account for the multidimensional complexity of family systems. Ultimately, our theories, research programs, and intervention programs will need to fully account for the real-world complexity of families in order to adequately address the challenges and promote the promise and hopes of future families.

REFERENCES

Azevedo, H. S. (1994). The family in Brazil. *Canadian Home Economics Journal, 44*, 111-114.

Balán, J. (2002). Introduction. In S. Rotker (Ed.), *Citizens of fear: Urban violence in Latin America* (pp. 1-6). New Brunswick, NJ: Rutgers University Press.

Barrera, M. & Li, S. A. (1996). The relation of family support to adolescents' psychological distress and behavior problems. In G. R. Pierce, B. R. Sarason, & I. G. Sarason (Eds.), *Handbook of social support and the family* (pp. 313-343). New York: Plenum.

Baumrind, D. (1991). The influence of parenting style on adolescent competence and substance abuse. *Journal of Early Adolescence, 11*, 56-95.

Barry III, H., Child, I. L., & Bacon, M. K. (1959). Relation of child training to substinence economy. *American Anthropologist, 61*, 51-63.

Bock, E., Iutaka, S., & Berardo, F. M. (1975). Maintenance of the extended family in urban areas of Argentina, Brazil, and Chile. *Journal of Comparative Family Studies, 6*, 31-45.

Bontempo, R., Lobel, S., & Triandis, H. (1990). Compliance and value internalization in Brazil and the U.S. *Journal of Cross-Cultural Psychology, 21*, 200-213.

Braten, S. (1996). When toddlers provide care: Infants' companion space. *Childhood, 3*, 449-465.

Carlo, G. (2005). Care-based and altruistically-based morality. In M. Killen & J. G. Smetana (Eds.), *Handbook of moral development* (pp. 551-579). Mahwah, NJ: Lawrence Erlbaum Associates.

Carlo, G., Carranza, M., & Zamboanga, B. L. (2002). Culture and ecology of Latinos on the Great Plains: An introduction. *Great Plains Research, 12*, 3-12.

Carlo, G., Fabes, R. A., Laible, D. J., & Kupanoff, K. (1999). Early adolescence and prosocial/moral behavior II: The role of social and contextual influences. *Journal of Early Adolescence, 19*, 133-147.

Carlo, G., & Koller, S. (1998). Desenvolvimento moral pro-social em criancas e adolescentes: Conceitos, metodologias, e Pesquisas no Brazil (Prosocial development in children and adolescents: Concepts, methodologies, and research in Brazil). *Psicologia: Teoria e Pesquisa (Psychology: Theory and Research), 14*, 161-172.

Carlo, G., Koller, S. H., & Eisenberg, N. (1996). A cross-national study on the relations among prosocial moral reasoning, gender role orientations, and prosocial behaviors. *Developmental Psychology, 32*, 231-240.

Carlo, G., Koller, S., & Eisenberg, N. (1998). Prosocial moral reasoning in institutionalized delinquent, orphaned, and noninstitutionalized Brazilian adolescents. *Journal of Adolescent Research, 13*, 363-376.

Carlo, G., Roesch, S. C., Knight, G. P., & Koller, S. H. (2001). Between- or within-culture variation? Culture group as a moderator of the relations between individual differences and resource allocation preferences. *Journal of Applied Developmental Psychology, 22,* 559-579.

Carlo, G., Roesch, S., & Koller, S. H. (1999). Cross-national and gender similarities and differences in prosocial moral reasoning between Brazilian and European-American college students. *Interamerican Journal of Psychology, 33,* 151-172.

CIA. (2005). *The world factbook–Brazil.* Retrieved on November 21, 2005, from http://www.cia.gov/cia/publications/factbook/print/br.html.

Cohen, S. & Wills, T. A. (1985). Stress, social support, and the buffering hypothesis. *Psychological Bulletin, 98,* 310-357.

The Consortium on the School-Based Promotion of Social Competence. (1994). The school-based promotion of social competence: Theory, research, practice, and policy. In R. J. Haggerty, L. R. Sherrod, N. Garmezy, & M. Rutter (Eds.), *Stress, risk, and resilience in children and adolescents: Processes, mechanisms, and interventions* (pp. 268-316). Cambridge: Cambridge University Press.

de Guzman, M. R. T. & Carlo, G. (2004). Family, peer, and acculturative correlates of prosocial development among Latino youth in Nebraska. *Great Plains Research, 14,* 185-202.

de Guzman, M. R. T., Carlo, G., Ontai, L. L., Koller, S. H., & Knight, G. P. (2004). Developmental and gender differences in friendship nominations and ratings among Brazilian children. *Sex Roles, 51,* 217-225.

de Guzman, M. R. T., Edwards, C. P., & Carlo, G. (2005). Prosocial behaviors in context: A study of the Gikuyu children of Ngecha, Kenya. *Journal of Applied Developmental Psychology, 26,* 542-558.

Delgado-Gaitan, C. (1994). Socializing young children in Mexican-American families: An intergenerational perspective. In P. M. Greenfield & R. R. Cocking (Eds.) *Cross-cultural roots of minority child development* (pp. 55-86). Hillsdale, NJ: Lawrence Erlbaum.

DeSouza, E. R., Baldwin, J., Koller, S. H., & Narvaz, M. (2004). A Latin American perspective on the study of gender. In M. A. Paludi (Ed.), *Praeger guide to the psychology of gender* (pp. 41-67). Westport, CT: Praeger Publishers.

Diversi, M., Moraes, N., & Morelli, M. (1999). Daily reality on the streets of Campinas, Brazil. In M. Raffaelli & R. W. Larson (Eds.), *Homeless and working youth around the world: Exploring developmental issues* (pp.19-34). San Francisco: Jossey-Bass.

Edwards, C. P., Knoche, L., Aukrust, V., Kumru, A., & Kim, M. (2006). Parental ethnotheories of child development: Looking beyond independence and individualism in American belief systems. In U. Kim, K. Yang, & K. Hwang (Eds.), *Indigenous and cultural psychology: Understanding people in context* (141-162). New York: Springer.

Eisenberg, N., Guthrie, I. K., Cumberland, A. Murphy, B. C., Shepard, S. A., Zhou, Q., & Carlo, G. (2002). Prosocial development in early adulthood: A longitudinal study. *Journal of Personality and Social Psychology, 82,* 993-1006.

Eisenberg, N. & Fabes, R. A. (1998) Prosocial development. In N. Eisenberg & W. Damon (Eds.), Handbook of Child Development, Vol. 4: Social, emotional and personality development (5th ed., pp. 701-778) New York: John Wiley & Sons, Inc.

Eisenberg, N. & Murphy, B. (1995). Parenting and children's moral development. In M. H. Bornstein (Ed.), *Handbook of parenting, Vol. 4: Applied and practical parenting* (pp. 227-257). Hillsdale, NJ: Lawrence Erlbaum Associates, Inc, 1995. pp. 227-257.

Frauenglass, S., Routh, D. K., Pantin, H. M. (1997). Family support decreases influence of deviant peers on Hispanic adolescents' substance use. *Journal of Clinical Child Psychology, 26*, 15-23.

Freeberg, A. L. & Stein, C. H. (1996). Felt obligations towards parents in Mexican-American and Anglo-American young adults. *Journal of Social and Personal Relationships, 13*, 457-471.

Fonseca, C. (1991). Spouses, siblings, and sex-linked bonding: A look at kinship organization in a Brazilian slum. In E. Jelin (Ed.), *Family, household and gender relations in Latin America* (pp. 133-160). London, UK: Kegan Paul International and UNESCO.

Fuligni, A. J., Tseng, V., & Lam, M. (1999). Attitudes toward family obligations among American adolescents with Asian, Latin American, and European backgrounds. *Child Development, 70*, 1030-1044.

Gilbert, A. (1996). The Latin American mega-city: An introduction. In A. Gilbert (Ed.), *The mega-city in Latin America* (pp. 1-24). United Nations University Press.

Gouveia, V. V., de Albuquerque, F. J. B., Clemente, M., & Espinosa, P. (2002). Human values and social identities: A study in two collectivist cultures. *International Journal of Psychology, 37*, 333-342.

Hofstede, G. (2001). National cultures revisited. *Behavior Science Research, 18*, 285-305.

Huston, A. C. (1983). Sex-typing. In P. H. Mussen (Ed.), *Handbook of Child Psychology: Vol. 4 Socialization, personality, and social development* (pp. 387-467). New York : Wiley.

Hutz, C. S., Koller, S. H., & Biaggio, A. M. (1992). *Attitudes toward adultery, violence, and neglect in Brazilian men and women.* Paper presented at the Meeting of the American Psychological Association, Washington, D. C.

Kerr, M. H., Beck, K., Shattuck, T. D., Kattar, C., & Uriburu, D. (2003). Family involvement, problem and prosocial behavior outcomes of Latino Youth. *American Journal of Health Behavior, 27 (Supplement 1)*, S55-S65.

Knight, G., Bernal, M., & Carlo, G. (1995). Socialization and the development of cooperative, competitive, and individualistic behaviors among Mexican American children. In E. E. Garcia & B. M. McLaughlin (Eds.), *Meeting the challenge of linguistic and cultural diversity in early childhood education, Vol. 6: Yearbook in Early Childhood Education* (pp. 85-102). New York: Teachers College Press.

Knight, G. P., & Kagan, S. (1982). Siblings, birth order, and cooperative-competitive social behavior: A comparison of Anglo-American and Mexican-American children. *Journal of Cross-Cultural Psychology, 13*, 239-249.

Korin, E. C. (1996). Brazilian families. In M. McGoldrick, J. Giordano, & J. K. Pearce (Eds.), *Ethnicity and family therapy, 2nd ed.* (pp. 200-213). New York: Guilford Press.

Krug, E. G., Dahlberg, L. L., Mercy, J. A., Zwi, A. B., & Lozano, R. (Eds.) (2002). *World report on violence and health.* Geneva, Switzerland: World Health Organization. Retrieved January 6, 2005, from http://www.who.org.

Laible, D. J., Carlo, G., & Roesch, S. C. (2004). Pathways to self-esteem in late adolescence: The role of parent and peer attachment, empathy, and social behaviours. *Journal of Adolescence, 27,* 703-716.

LeVine, R. A. (1988). Human parental care: Universal goals, cultural strategies, individual behavior. In R. A. LeVine, P. M. Miller, & M. M. West (Eds.), *Parental behavior in diverse societies: New direction for child development, Vol. 40* (pp. 3-12). San Francisco: Jossey-Bass.

Lopez-Carlos, A. & Zahidi, S. (2005). Women's empowerment: Measuring the global gender gap. Retrieved January 30, 2006, from the World Economic Forum, http://news.bbc.co.uk/2/shared/bsp/hi/pdfs/16_05_05_gender_gap.pdf.

Maccoby, E. E., & Martin, J. A. (1983). Socialization in the context of the family: Parent–child interaction. In P. H. Mussen (Ed.) & E. M. Hetherington (Vol. Ed.), *Handbook of child psychology: Vol. 4. Socialization, personality, and social development* (4th ed., pp. 1-101). New York: Wiley.

Marteleto, L. (2005). Family size, demographic change, and education attainment: The case of Brazil (Population Studies Center Research Report No. 05-0584). Retrieved January 30, 2006, from http://www.psc.isr.umich.edu/pubs/pdf/rr05-584.pdf.

McDade, K. (1995). How we parent: Race and ethnic differences. In C.K. Jacobson. (Ed.), *American families: Issues in race and ethnicity* (pp. 283-300). New York: Garland Publishing.

McCloyd, V. C. (1998). Changing demographics in the American population: Implications for research on minority children. In V. C. McCloyd & L. Steingberg (Eds.), Studying minority adolescents (pp.3-28). Mahwah, NJ: Erlbaum.

Munroe, R. L., & Munroe, R. H. (1977). Cooperation and competition among East African and American children. *Journal of Social Psychology, 101,* 145-146.

PAHO. (2001). *A saúde no Brazil–2002* [Health in Brazil–2002]. Brazilia, DF: Pan American Health Organization.

Raffaelli, M. (1997). Family situation of street youth in Latin America: A cross-national review. *International Social Work, 40,* 89-100.

Raffaelli, M., Carlo, G., Carranza, M. A., & Gonzales-Kruger, G. E. (2005). Understanding Latino children and adolescents in the mainstream: Placing culture at the center of developmental models. In R. Larson & L. Jensen (Eds.), *New horizons in developmental research: New directions for child and adolescent development* (pp. 23-32). San Francisco: Jossey-Bass.

Raffaelli, M., Koller, S. H., Reppold, C. T., Kuschick, F. M. B. K., & Bandeira, D. R. (2000). Gender differences in Brazilian street youth's family circumstances and experiences on the street. *Child Abuse and Neglect, 24,* 1431-1441.

Ramirez, J. R., Crano, W. D., Quist, R., Burgoon, M., Alvaro, E. M., & Grandpre, J. (2004). Acculturation, familism, parental monitoring, and knowledge as predictors of marijuana and inhalant use in adolescents. *Psychology of Addictive Behaviors, 18,* 3-11.

Rotheram-Borus, M. J., & Phinney, J. S. (1990). Patterns of social expectations among Black and Mexican-American children. *Child Development, 61,* 542-556.

Sabogal, F., Marin, G., Otero-Sabogal, R., Marin, B. V., & Perez-Stable, E. J., (1987). Hispanic familism and acculturation: What changes and what doesn't? *Hispanic Journal of Behavioral Sciences, 9,* 397-412.

Sarason, B.R., Sarason, I. G., & Gurung, R. A. R. (1997). Close personal relationships and health outcomes: A key to the role of social support. In S. Duck (Ed.), *Handbook of personal relationships: Theory, research and interventions* (2nd ed., pp. 547-573). Hoboken, NJ: John Wiley.

Schwartz, S. H. (1992). Universals in the content and structure of values: Theoretical advances and empirical tests in 20 countries. In M. P. Zanna (Ed.), *Advances in experimental social psychology, Vol. 25* (pp.1-65). Orlando, FL: Academic Press.

Shapira, A., & Madsen, M. C. (1969) Cooperative and competitive behavior of kibbutz and urban children in Israel. *Child Development, 40,* 609-617.

Shapira, A., & Madsen, M. C. (1974). Between- and within-group cooperation and competition among kibbutz and non-kibbutz children. *Developmental Psychology, 10,* 140-145.

Sturm, F. G. (1991). Epilogue. In M. L. Conniff & F. D. McCann (Eds.), *Modern Brazil: Elites and masses in historical perspective* (pp. 265-280). Lincoln: University of Nebraska Press.

Suárez-Orozco, C. & Suárez-Orozco, M. M. (1995). Transformations: Immigration, family life, and achievement motivation among Latino adolescents. Stanford: Stanford University Press.

Suárez-Orozco, C., Todorova, I. L. G., & Louie, J. (2002). Making up for lost time: The experience of separation and reunification among immigrant families. *Family Process, 41,* 625-643.

Suzuki, L. K., & Greenfield, P. M. (2002). The construction of everyday sacrifice in Asian Americans and European Americans: The roles of ethnicity and acculturation. *Cross-Cultural Research, 36,* 200-228.

Thompson, R.A. (1998). Early sociopersonality development. In W. Damon (Series Ed.) & N. Eisenberg (Vol. Ed.), *Handbook of child psychology (5th ed.). Vol. 3. Social, emotional, and personality development* (pp. 25-104). New York: Wiley.

Triandis, H.C. (1994). Theoretical and methodological approaches to study of collectivism and individualism. In U. Kim, H. C. Triandis, C. Kagitcibasi, S. Choi, & G. Yoon (Eds.), *Individualism and collectivism: Theory, method, and application* (pp. 19-41). London:

UNICEF (2004). *State of the World's Children 2003.* Available at http://www.unicef.org.

Van Horn, K. R. & Marquez, J. C. (2000). Interpersonal relationships in Brazilian adolescents. *International Journal of Behavioral Development, 24,* 199-203.

Whiting, B. B., & Edwards, C. P. (1988). *Children of different worlds: The formation of social behavior.* Cambridge, MA: Harvard University.

Whiting, B. B., & Whiting, J. W. M. (1975). *Children of six cultures: A psycho-cultural analysis.* Cambridge, MA: Harvard University Press.

World Bank. (2003). *Overview: Poverty in Latin America and the Caribbean.* Retrieved January 6, 2005, from http://www.worldbank.org/lacpoverty.

Zahn-Waxler, C., Radke-Yarrow, M., & King, R. A. (1979). Child rearing and children's prosocial initiations toward victims of distress. *Child Development, 50,* 319-330.

Zahn-Waxler, C., Friedman, S. L., & Cummings, E. M. (1983). Children's emotions and behaviors in response to infants' cries. *Child Development, 54,* 1522-1528.

Zayas, L. H., & Solari, F. (1994). Early childhood socialization in Hispanic families: Context, culture and practice implications. *Professional Psychology: Research and Practice, 25,* 200-206.

doi:10.1300/J002v41n03_06

EUROPE

Russian Families:
Historical and Contemporary Perspectives
on Problems and Strengths

Vladimir Zubkov

SUMMARY. The Russian Federation (Russia) is the largest country in land mass and its population is seventh in the world. The historical development of the Russian family is connected, first of all, with Russian Orthodoxy. After the October revolt of 1917 socialism began and the bases of the traditional family were abolished. However, since the 1930s the family was still formally recognized as *a primary cell* of Soviet society. In modern Russia the demographic data show the tendencies of a decrease in the number of concluded marriages and an increase in the number of divorces, one-child and childless families. Nevertheless,

Vladimir Zubkov is Professor in Sociology, Youth Policy and Social Technologies Institute of the Russian State Technological University named in honor of K.E. Tsiolkovsky, 121552 Moscow, Orshanskaya st., 3, Russia (E-mail: v.zubkov@rambler.ru).

[Haworth co-indexing entry note]: "Russian Families: Historical and Contemporary Perspectives on Problems and Strengths." Zubkov, Vladimir. Co-published simultaneously in *Marriage & Family Review* (The Haworth Press, Inc.) Vol. 41, No. 3/4, 2007, pp. 361-392; and: *Strong Families Around the World: Strengths-Based Research and Perspectives* (ed: John DeFrain, and Sylvia M. Asay) The Haworth Press, Inc., 2007, pp. 361-392. Single or multiple copies of this article are available for a fee from The Haworth Document Delivery Service [1-800-HAWORTH, 9:00 a.m. - 5:00 p.m. (EST). E-mail address: docdelivery@haworthpress.com].

Available online at http://mfr.haworthpress.com
© 2007 by The Haworth Press, Inc. All rights reserved.
doi:10.1300/J002v41n03_07

according to representative opinion polls, the family is highly valued in Russian society. What modern challenges worry members of Russian strong families the most and how do they manage these challenges? To answer these questions, we have undertaken qualitative sociological research. doi:10.1300/J002v41n03_07 *[Article copies available for a fee from The Haworth Document Delivery Service: 1-800-HAWORTH. E-mail address: <docdelivery@haworthpress.com> Website: <http://www.HaworthPress. com> © 2007 by The Haworth Press, Inc. All rights reserved.]*

KEYWORDS. Challenges of modern society, strong families, recommendations to manage challenges, Russian family, strengthening family relations, sociological research

INTRODUCTION

The Russian Federation (Russia) is the largest country in the world. It envelops the eastern part of Europe and the northern part of Asia and covers almost 17.1 million square km. The larger part of the Russian territory takes up the position between the 50th parallel and Arctic Circle and is situated in the middle and high latitudes with a moderate and cold climate. The maximum distance between western Russian (not counting the Kaliningrad region) and the eastern boundaries is 9,000 km. It is 4,000 km between the northern and southern boundaries. There are 11 time zones within the limits of Russia.

The population of the Russian Federation is 145,200,000 people, seventh in the world behind China, India, the USA, Indonesia, Brazil and Pakistan. Almost three-fourths of Russians are city dwellers. More than one-third of them live in the 13 largest cities with a population of more than one million people. The populations of the largest megalopolises of Russia–Moscow and St.-Petersburg–comprise 10.4 million and 4.7 million people (Statistical Bureau of Russia, 2003). The capital of the Russian Federation is Moscow.

The Russian Federation is one of the most multinational countries in the world–people of more than 160 nationalities live in the country (Statistical Bureau of Russia, 2003). Russians, the largest group, account for 116 million people (80% of the country's residents). The second largest population group is the Tartars, at 5.56 million people (almost 4% of the country's population). Of the total population, 142.6 million people (98%) have a command of the Russian language. Females outnumbered males by 10 million (77.6 million to 67.6 million). The difference results from men having a shorter lifespan. In rural areas it is 63.4 years (for men 57.1, for women 71.3) and in the urban areas 65.3 years (for men 59.0, for women 72.3).

THE RUSSIAN FAMILY THROUGH HISTORY: THE INFLUENCE OF THE CHURCH AND THE RISE OF THE COMMUNIST STATE

The historical development of the Russian family is connected, first of all, with Russian Orthodoxy. Certainly, there are other Christian religions along with Islam, Buddhism and Judaism that have existed and continue to exist in Russia. However, 80% of the Russians follow Orthodox traditions. Yet, modern research demonstrates an absence of dependence on marriage and family conditions and behavior related to national and religious traditions (Êartseva, 2003).

According to the value system of Orthodoxy, an alternative to marriage and family practically does not exist. A choice of bride by groom and groom by bride precedes marriage. Happiness in family life depends on the reasonableness of this choice and consequently, it should be originated and realized with the direct participation of parents. Premarital and extramarital sexual contacts are prohibited, at least for women.

The Christian orthodox marriage is a blending of two persons in human love. By means of the Holy Spirit, this love transforms into eternal bonds, which are not broken even by death. The marriage agreement contract was especially sacred among all human agreements. A husband is the head of an orthodox family. A husband must love his wife as he loves himself and a wife must fear her husband. One without the other cannot be. A wife's fear is not simple fear, because there is love between them. It is the same fear that is present when a person is afraid to insult God by sinning. A husband and a wife, being one flesh, have also one soul and equally provoke in each other a diligence to piety through mutual love. Children must sincerely respect parents, serve them patiently, and without complaint endure parental exhortations and *corrections*. At the same time, a child will see his parents as the real defenders of his interests. Traditionally in Russia the core or root families prevailed: the parental family and the family of the youngest son. Inheritance is divided into equal parts among all children.

Most rules of family relationships, including ones between generations, and principles of childrearing were expounded in *Domostroy*–a literary monument of the Ancient Rus (1547). In this book just as in the Christian commandments, common moral standards were advanced for both marital partners (mutual love, faithfulness and responsibility), and different family roles were recognized. A husband had the right to instruct his wife and children and even to punish them physically. A wife had to be a good, hard-working mistress and to ask her husband's advice in all things. Spheres of family activity were divided: the husband is a getter and the wife is a keeper of the home hearth. These spheres were coordinated with the necessary division of labor in the peasant economy. With development of capitalism in Russia, standards of family life, especially in big cities, have undergone some changes. More and more expressive functions (mutual understanding, mutual aid, tolerance of defects, and so forth) were entrusted with a husband and not only with a wife. For the first time in pre-Revolutionary Russia, the civil rights of women were conceded by the reform of 1864 and the Manifest of October 17, 1905. However, as a whole, patriarchal relations traditionally predominated and remained up to 1917.

After the October revolt of 1917, socialism began. The religious, economic and cultural bases of the traditional family were abolished. The new communist *family projects* appeared with the concept of family life transformation into public life and the public upbringing of children.

Under the Soviet regime, it became impossible to maintain religious practices because of antireligious propaganda and limited rights for believers. The majority of temples and churches were destroyed. The institutions of family and marriage were secularized. Industrialization and equal rights for women in all spheres of economic, cultural and socio-political life led to the elimination of the housewife. During the years of Soviet power, Russia had the highest rate of female employment (up to almost 90%) and in many respects determined a transfer of power regarding the upbringing of children. After the revolution the traditional family was declared a relic of the past and up to 1944 a so-called factual (nonregistered) marriage was equated with a registered marriage. The family was still formally recognized as *a primary cell* of Soviet society; however, interests of the family were subordinated to interests of the state.

As a whole, it is difficult to view Soviet family policy as pro-family. Elevated to the highest rank, a model socialist family—a family of communist-conscious marital partners—was a myth cultivated in the spirit of *The Moral Code of Communism Builder*. From 1936 to 1955 government orders entitled *Mother-Heroine* and *Mother's Glory* made abortion and other birth control measures illegal. Beginning in 1944 the honorary title of *Mother-Heroine of the USSR* was given to mothers who bred and brought up ten or more children. The Mother-Heroine enjoyed special privileges including a pension and public housing utilities. There were also some positive moments in Soviet family policy, especially in the second half of the 20th century. Mothers were granted four months of paid holiday on the birth of children, the preservation of their job for one and a half years, free home-visiting services for the babies and a network of free medical services, preschool and school establishments. These and some other modest free services, privileges and benefits only helped the family to stay afloat.

Communist ideology, in order to justify itself, was solicitous about achieving economic superiority over capitalism. Therefore, women, *a very uncomfortable component* of the Soviet manufacturing system, which by virtue of their gender function were sometimes switched off from building communism. On the other hand, the government decided that economic growth was the primary goal and therefore had the right to decide on all family issues, including reproduction. In the final analysis, efforts to strengthen the family were influenced by opposing social systems: absolutely everything must be better under socialism rather than capitalism.

THE CONTEMPORARY RUSSIAN FAMILY

Today there are 34 million married couples in Russia. Of every 1,000 persons age 16 and over, 572 are married; 114 are widowed; 94 are divorced; and 210 were never married. Of the total number of married couples, 3 million (10%) are in common-law relationships. Of the 4.2 thousand people under age 16 who say they are married, 2.3 thousand are in common-law relationships. The declining number of registered marriage unions has been followed since the beginning of the 1980s. Between 1989-1995 there was a period of relative stability. Nevertheless, in 1989 there were 1.4 million marriages registered, and by 2002 the number had dropped to slightly more than one million marriages (Statistical Bureau of Russia, 2003). A higher marriage level remains in rural areas. In the city 22% are unmarried and in the country 15% are unmarried (Êartseva, 2003).

The number of persons who have never been married increased at the same rate as the number of divorced. Approximately 800,000 marriages are dissolved annually. As a result, about 400,000 under-age children remain without one parent. More than one third of divorces are young married couples who have been married less than five years. This leads to an increase in divorced persons within the marriage structure of the population, especially among women, for which entry into a repeated marriage is more difficult because of a disproportion in the population based on gender and age. Repeated marriages represent only 25% to 28% of failed marriages (the grand totals of all the all-Russian populations of 2002, 2003).

From 1989-2002, the birth rate dropped considerably. Now the average number of children per woman is 1.3 (1.5 in the country; 1.25 in urban areas) in contrast to 2.0 in 1989. However, having smaller families is typical in the majority of European countries. The tendency toward increased age for parents at the birth of their first child is also studied. In 1989, the average age of the mother at birth was 25.5 years while in 2002 it rose to 26.2. The increase in non-registered marriage unions led to an increase in the number of children born outside of registered marriage. From 1989-2002 this number doubled and amounts to about 30% of the total number of annual births. The abrupt reduction of the birth rate began at the end of the 1980s has increased the age of the Russian population, similar to the process seen in other European countries. The average age of the country's population is 37.7 years (35.2 years for males and 40.0 years for females) (Statistical Bureau of Russia, 2003).

As we see, the demographic data show a decrease in the number of concluded marriages, an increase in divorces, one-child and childless families. There are two basic points of view about the explanation for these processes, which in one way or another are inherent in all Western countries. The first view may be called a paradigm of modernization and the second a paradigm of the crisis of the family as an institution (Antonov & Medkov, 1996). In the modernization paradigm, all changes in the functioning of the family are perceived as particular elements of the general, positive and progressive development of society. From the viewpoint of the modernization paradigm, times of upheaval and stress in a society are seen as temporary difficulties as the transformation progresses from traditional to modern, from autocratic to democratic relationships and to a time in which a wide variety of family structures have developed to meet changing demands on the family. The second paradigm sees a crisis in the traditional family–an increase of incomplete and ersatz families, divorces, and a continuous decrease in childbearing. In this paradigm the changes are seen as a destructive process, which in the absence of purposeful family policy will lead to the de-socialization of people and depopulation in all countries. For the most part, the author agrees with the second point of view and considers the strengthening of the family to be a global problem requiring the constant attention of national governments and international organizations.

Family functioning in many respects depends on the place the family has in the public hierarchy of values. According to public opinion polls (*Poll of population Russian citizenry about family and children*, 2004), family values do rank high in Russia. In answer to a question about values and the nature of happiness, family stability takes the first place. Researches show that the most acceptable form of family relations is the official registered marriage (72% of the population). The answers to the question, "In your opinion, how many children should be in a family, if there are sufficient material conditions for it?" were as follows: one child, 7%; two, 43%; three, 35%; four and more, 13%, no child at all, 1%; no reply, 1% of the respondents.

Data of sociological polls shows Russians place a high value on family relations, especially for those with registered marriages, and a high value on children. If you do not take into account that respondents see *family* in different configurations and have different understandings of general family activity, the picture looks safe enough. The real situation, however, as the above-cited social-demographic data show, is rather problematic. Why have pro-family values and attitudes proclaimed by respondents not been fully realized? We believe that the paradoxical situation for the family in a transforming Russian society is understood by the fact that, on the one hand for the majority of people, family may be the only island of stability in a boundless ocean of uncertainty generated by the dysfunctionality of social institutions. On the other hand, the crises in institutional systems undermine the fundamentals of the institution of the family and causes family challenges that are hard to manage. At the same time, there are families who have sufficient internal resources for their own preservation, stability and development and can successfully resist the challenges of modernity. Such families are called strong families.

THE PROBLEMS RUSSIAN FAMILIES FACE TODAY

What modern problems worry members of strong families the most and how do they manage these problems? To answer these questions, we have undertaken qualitative sociological research. In the first stage, short semi-structured interviews to select strong families were conducted. To guide the interview, questions were formulated using the following criteria for the strength of family relations: a total subjective appraisal, the perceived value of the family based on other life values, and satisfaction with family relations (warmth, mutual respect, support, and understanding,). In the second stage, brainstorming procedures were used to uncover the challenges for the modern family (For respondents who were unsure, the term *challenge* was replaced by the term *problem*). Using generalizations from the information, we formulated fourteen basic challenges or problems. In the third stage, the respondents ranked these problems in order of importance for all Russian families and for the respondent's own family. In the fourth stage, focus-group methodology was used and a discussion of problems was conducted. Possible and practical ways of overcoming these problems were revealed by the respondents.

After selecting the strong families in the first stage of the research, fifteen strong Moscow married couples were identified. Demographics of these couples show that they range in age from 26 to 60, family experience of 7 to 30 years, one to three children, average or higher education and diverse professions and income levels. However, all these characteristics influence the problems identified by the respondents in parvo. We did not study childless families in accordance with well-founded opinion formed by Russian sociology that a family is characterized by the triad of matrimony-parenthood-consanguinity (Antonov & Medkov, 1996). In the opinion of our respondents, the following modern problems are the most difficult for families (see Tables 1 and 2).

The data of our qualitative research does not contradict the data of representative research in Russia. The monitoring of family problems being conducted by the *Fund Public Opinion* (2004) demonstrates that despite different questions, financial, material and housing-domestic problems are the main problems for 80% of Russian respondents. Fears concerning violence in society (wars, terrorism, criminality, power actions of the government) are voiced by a third of those surveyed. In other research, problems of criminality and personal safety represent the views of more than 95% of the citizens (Lapin, 2004). Comparing the data in Tables 1 and 2 as a whole, we note that the problems of all Russian families are ranked higher the problems of our strong families. We conclude that our strong families have fewer problems and/or know how to manage them more effectively. In addition, the estimations of Russian family problems are more coordinated by husbands and wives than the estimations of the concrete family problems, inasmuch as the first ones (estimations) reflect a public opinion and the second, originality and variety of the concrete family biographies. Let us consider the most important problems from the point of view of our respondents.

TABLE 1. Problems from the point of view of their importance for all Russian families.

Problems threatening to modern family*	Husband		Wife		General Estimation	
	Mean*	Rank	Mean*	Rank	Mean*	Rank
Financial problems, poverty in families, including unemployment	4.7	1-2	4.5	2-3	4.6	1
Absence of effective social policy to protect families, motherhood and childhood	4.7	1-2	4.3	4-5	4.5	2
Growth of violence (criminality, terrorism, armed conflicts)	4.5	3	4.3	4-5	4.4	3
Housing limiting capabilities of creation and planning of family	4.0	4	4.7	1	4.3	4
Alcoholism and drug abuse of the population	3.8	5-6	4.5	2-3	4.2	5
Decreased family time and personal contacts resulting from paid employment	3.7	7-8	3.8	6	3.7	6
Neglecting children, increase in time children spend outside the family	3.7	7-8	3.6	7	3.6	7
Effects of mass media on the consciousness of people and the decreasing face-to-face interrelations	3.8	5-6	3.2	10-12	3.5	8
Sexual depravity in society, and a culture of promiscuity among youth	3.2	9	3.3	8-9	3.3	9
Global (technological, ecological, biological, and other) disasters	2.8	10-11	3.3	8-9	3.1	10
Increase in utilitarianism, pragmatism, and lack of spirituality in society	2.8	10-11	3.2	10-12	3.0	11
Ethnic, religious, political, and other intolerance between people	2.7	12-13	3.2	10-12	2.9	12
Elimination of the traditional socio-cultural family roles of men and women	2.5	14	3.0	13	2.8	13
Acceptance of divorce and remarriage, suggesting a decrease in the value of family life	2.7	12-13	2.8	14	2.7	14

*Items were scored 1 = Unimportant to 5 = Very Important

TABLE 2. Problems from the point of view of their importance for the polled families.

Problems threatening to modern family*	Husband		Wife		General Estimation	
	Mean*	Rank	Mean*	Rank	Mean*	Rank
Financial problems, poverty in families including unemployment	4.2	1	4.0	4-5	4.1	1-2
Absence of effective social policy to protect families, motherhood and childhood	3.5	5	4.0	4-5	3.8	4
Growth of violence (criminality, terrorism, armed conflicts)	3.7	2-4	4.3	2	4.0	3
Housing limiting capabilities of creation and planning of family	3.7	2-4	4.5	1	4.1	1-2
Alcoholism and drug abuse of the population	3.2	6-7	3.7	6	3.4	6
Decreased family time and personal contacts resulting from paid employment	3.2	6-7	4.2	3	3.7	5
Neglecting children, increase in time children spend outside the family	2.8	8	3.2	7	3.0	8
Effects of mass media on the consciousness of people and the decreasing face-to-face interrelations	2.3	9-11	2.2	12-14	2.2	12
Sexual depravity in society, and a culture of promiscuity among youth	3.7	2-4	2.6	10	3.1	7
Global (technological, ecological, biological and other) disasters	2.3	9-11	3.0	8	2.7	9
Increase in utilitarianism, pragmatism, and lack of spirituality in society	2.3	9-11	2.5	11	2.4	10-11
Ethnic, religious, political, and other intolerance between people	1.5	14	2.2	12-14	1.8	14
Elimination of the traditional socio-cultural family roles of men and women	2.0	12	2.8	9	2.4	10-11
Acceptance of divorce and remarriage, suggesting a decrease in the value of family life	1.8	13	2.2	12-14	2.0	13

*Items were scored 1 = Unimportant to 5 = Very Important

Financial Problems and Poverty in Families Including Unemployment

With the fall of communism, the years of transformation in the 1990s from a planned and centralized economic system were characterized by a decreased standard of living caused by reduction of incomes, narrowing of resources, unemployment and the absence of a constant income even at full employment. The situation led to a moral crisis in society, first expressed in a sharp growth in alcoholism, drug addiction, criminality and the death rate.

According to official data today, the income of a quarter of Russians is below the living wage (*Criminality and law in Russia. Statistical aspect*, 2003). Only one-seventh of the respondents consider themselves quite well-to-do (11%) or rich (2%) (Levashov, 2004). The spending structure of the majority of Russian families is disproportional: expenditures for food, rent and public utilities predominate. Many family members have relatively low life satisfaction due to many housing-domestic, physiological, socio-cultural and spiritual needs.

Official data indicate the unemployed number more than 6 million people or over 8% of the economically-active population (*Criminality and law in Russia. Statistical aspect*, 2003). Some social scientists believe that up to 9 million people are unemployed (Hrushev, 2006).

During financial difficulty, the main strategies of survival for strong families include: a decrease of the necessities of life, economy in everything; intensification of efforts for self-service, home repairs; a search for basic and supplementary work; individual labor and commercial activity, including activity of *shuttles* (buying goods abroad to sell), children's labor, re-sale of goods, personal, educational, cultural and other services; cottage-handicraft industry and also work on subsidiary garden plots; credit-financial operations, including opening deposits, buying shares, obtaining credit, etc.; and renting property–housing, garages, motor vehicles, different means of production.

In addition to a large variety of strategies for survival, strong families have a more realistic understanding of material problems. During the transformation of the 1990s, prosperity decreased and conditions of maintenance, upbringing and education of children became worse for the majority of families. At the same time, with the development of a market economy, the income gap between the richest and the poorest increased. The income of the top 10% of the population now exceeds the income of the lowest 10% by 14 times (*Criminality and law in Russia. Statistical aspect*, 2003). Also during the 1990s, welfare claims from the state increased. The gap between actual and desired prosperity widens when comparing groups with low incomes to groups with higher incomes. For example, the people with lower incomes wish to double their incomes, the people with average incomes wish to triple their incomes and so on (Antonov & Sorokin, 2000). In the current study, the variation in these wishes is less dramatic. The members of strong families are more satisfied with their income as a whole. In our opinion, it shows a more realistic view of material issues and the fact that they put family values above material ones. During the interviews, especially for families of modest means, they said they believed that an increase in economic well-being would strengthen their family relationships to some degree.

One of the myths advanced both by some governments and some families is that people have fewer children than they want only because of financial difficulties. The crisis of the modern family clearly shows the error in this way of thinking. According to Smith and Ricardo (Avtonomov, 1998), economic advances stimulate large families. The data above speaks only about the converse. The growth of material needs and desires along with an increase in income is one reason for the diminution of the number of children in rich families and rich countries.

The Absence of Effective Social Policy with the Aim of Protecting the Family, Motherhood and Childhood

In Russia there is no effective pro-family social policy. The government is busy rendering social help in the form of benefits and privileges to families who need it. This help is very modest and only compensates for the inflationary fall of the living standards to a minor degree. However, it is impossible to call such a policy family oriented. A family policy should attend to a whole complex of economic, legal, socio-engineering, social-pedagogical, social-psychological and other measures trended on strengthening the family institution.

In the message to the Federal Assembly of May 10, 2006, Russian President Vladimir V. Putin proclaimed a solution to the depopulation problem by the priority national project. The main purposes of this project are the decrease of death rates and the increase of birth rates. To increase birth rates, this project provides funds to women who give birth to a child. It is the so-called *mother capital* that is used by mothers for education, treatments, and other similar needs. Money is transfered for each child and increase greatly at birth of the second and the third child. The project stipulates improvement of children's health in the country.

As we see, these measures are again mainly material support but it is better than generally nothing.

Russian family policy is based mostly on its economic component. Yes, there are benefits and privileges for mothers, children, the aged, and invalids with disabilities. Free medical and educational benefits are partly preserved. Women who have the possibility of pregnancy are forced to work, and are at serious disadvantage and undergo discrimination in the labor market. The tax system equalizes families regardless of size or configuration; similarly, salaries are not supportive of families. As a result, married couples having two children are less satisfied with their economic situation than married couples with one child (Êartseva, 2003). From the strong families we learned that the absence of a pro-family policy is not so topical because, as the respondents indicate, they are used to relying on their own resources. The members of strong families believe that all problems can and should be solved using their own psychological and material resources and the help of their friends. Help from outside the family can be necessary in major circumstances such as natural calamity, military actions, technological disasters, and so forth. In general, however, it is impossible to call the relationship between families and the state a warm relationship. Today few Russians trust the power structures.

The Growth of Violence: Criminality, Terrorism and Armed Conflicts

These problems became worse during the first phase of the social transformation, when there was both a value and a legal vacuum in Russia. Criminal activity during the first five years of social reforms doubled. Half of the hard-core criminals did not have a constant source of income or employment. Today in Russia, statistics on the majority of each of the different types of criminal behavior are not out of line with crime statistics in other countries. Official statistics indicate that the number of registered crimes in 1999, following the economic crisis of 1998, was quite high: 3 million crimes. In subsequent years, the crime situation in Russia began to improve. By 2002 registered crimes had decreased to 2.5 million. However, during the same period, the number of murders and attempted murders and the number of robberies continued to grow. Repeat offenses, which are 7 or 8 times more prevalent in Russia than in central Europe, remained high (*Criminality and law in Russia. Statistical aspect*, 2003).

Terrorism merits special consideration here. The first widely-known act of terrorism occurred in a Moscow subway in 1977. Since the end of the 1990s, acts of terrorism have caused more and more alarm among Russians. Here, it is enough just to remember cynical and cruel acts of terrorism such as taking hostages in the hospital of Budennovsk in the Stavropol region (1995), the theatrical center on Dubrovka Street in Moscow (2002), and School No. 1 of Beslan in Northern Osetia (2004) that have cost several hundred lives after the fall of the communist state. The vacuum in power left by the collapse of the state gave way to the rise of armed opposition from the early Chechen separatists and to criminal acts by bandits and international terrorists today. The members of strong families we interviewed understand the seriousness of these problems. However, to a great degree, they don't regard combat operations and terrorism as a daily risk. Hazards of violence in daily life such as physical and sexual violence, kidnapping, political violence, criminal behavior, seem more likely.

Nevertheless, these kinds of violence are not so common that it forces people to change their way of life or to take extraordinary measures, for example, to arm themselves. The most widespread measures taken in opposition to possible violence involve only walking on populated streets and not late at night; an analysis of children's friends and acquaintances; establishing children's daily routine, escorting children to places; maintenance of phone contact; installation of metal doors in entrances and flats; and installation of a security systems in flats and cars. A few of those interviewed or their acquaintances (men) have gas pistols; somewhat more individuals (mainly woman) carry spray cans with tear gas. To fight against political violence and lawlessness, the respondents did not eliminate the idea of making an appeal to the courts. However, few were confident such an appeal would be effective as the protest potential of Russians is rather low, especially as it concerns non-sanctioned measures of protest (Sokolov, 2003). Finally, the members of strong families said that violence within others families, though it can be a serious problem, is unlikely to influence the strength of their relationships.

Housing Difficulties Limiting the Capability to Create and Plan for the Family's Growth

The housing problem in Russia is especially acute in the cities. Right up to the middle of the past century, city-dwellers mainly lived in communal flats constructed during the mass migration of people from the village to the city. During the Great Patriotic War, many cities and other settlements in the European part of the country were destroyed. Difficulties with housing availability spawned multigenerational families, which Russian society had abandoned. In 1989, only 12% of conjugal couples lived with one or two relatives (Êartseva, 2003). The housing problem was aggravated during the transition to a market economy. Data collected by the Russian government at the beginning of 2005 indicate that 31 million households need improvement. Insufficient financial resources and difficulties in finding rental property have caused a quarter of Russians to live with relatives (Êartseva, 2003). There are also other housing problems such as decaying housing services and an absence of sufficient financial resources to pay the rent. Certainly, all these problems complicate family life.

In Moscow, a huge megalopolis, it can be said that housing problems are traditional. Therefore, the members of strong families we interviewed consider these problems coupled with financial difficulties quite standard. In a traditional family, joint living with different generations was the standard pattern. However, today in connection with the increase of individualism in society, married couples rush to live separately. Our respondents indicate that enforced living with parents of a husband or wife often leads to conflicts and aggravation of the generation gap. The respondents prefer not to live together with their parents, but near to them so it was possible to communicate, celebrate family holidays and help parents or receive help from them. Commonly, when parents are very aged or ill and need constant help, they live with one of their children. In Russia the old men tend not to live in nursing homes or similar establishments.

Alcoholization and Narcotization of the Population

Researchers at the World Health Organization confirm that the consumption of alcohol above eight liters per capita of the population leads to the degeneration of a nation. Russian data indicate the consumption of alcohol averages 12-15 litres per capita of the population, which is much more than in such traditionally alcohol-imbibing countries as France, Italy and Germany. Although Russia ranks tenth in the world in alcohol consumption, in some areas of the country up to 90% of absolute alcohol is consumed in the condition of strong drinks. In Europe, this parameter usually does not exceed 30%. Alcohol use causes financial problems for many individuals and families, and because there is little state control over alcohol production, alcohol-related problems are increasing. Between 1995 and 2002, the number of reported health-related problems associated with the diagnosis of alcoholism and alcoholic psychoses declined slightly from 2.4 million to 2.2 million (from 1630.4 to 1543.8 health-related problems per 100,000 people). Alcohol-related problems among children and adolescents continue to grow, though they are under-reported (*Criminality and law in Russia. Statistical aspect*, 2003). It has been estimated that the total number of people dependent on alcohol now exceeds 20 million. Drunkenness is usually intimately connected with criminality. In Russia, 70-90% of the cases of hooliganism, rape, murder, robbery and assault are committed under the influence of alcohol. Other data indicate that drunkenness is the cause of more than half of all divorces.

There is also a problem with narcotics. In Russia, very few narcotics are produced, but the absence of secure borders with the former south republics of the USSR, the growth of crime and number of unemployed have all contributed to the emerging drug business. Since the mid-1990s, the number of ills associated with drug addiction has increased five times and those registered on the preventive books in connection drug use has increased three times. Both of these groups officially include almost 450,000 people (*Criminality and law in Russia. Statistical aspect*, 2003). However, data indicate that more than 12% of Russians abuse narcotics (Pozdnyakova, 2004). The overwhelming majority of people using narcotics are in very productive ages (13 to 30 years). At the same time, since 2000 the group at greatest risk (children and adolescents under 17) has decreased more than 2.5 times. Naturally, drug addiction and toxicomania are also connected with criminality, but more critical is the spreading of HIV infection. Today in Russia, about 300,000 of the HIV-positive individuals are registered and the probability of that problem continuing remains very high. We have not found data regarding the collapse of drug addicts' families, but it should be assumed that using narcotics, especially powerful ones and maintaining a family way of life are not compatible.

The problems of alcoholism and drug addiction for Russian families are severe enough to be serious. Moreover, consumption of large quantities of alcohol by Russians is traditional. In Russia, not one holiday including those celebrated with family (perhaps with the exception of children's birthdays) occurs without spirits. Strong families face these problems also, but they are resolved basically through the mutual help and support of family members and their faith in each other. In a number of cases, these problems are decided in an ultimatum-like form. The family member must choose between her/his harmful habits or the family.

Certainly, this way is applicable when the harmful habits of children are involved. As the respondents indicate, first of all it is necessary to interest children in productive activity and also to attempt to harmonize a circle of their friends and supportive older people in their lives. This last idea is especially true because about 80% of children and adolescents are regularly included and/or periodically active in different groups outside school. And practically all Russian children (98.4%) study at school.

Lack of Time Together and Personal Contact Related to Outside Employment

The research on time management in pre-reform and post-reform Russia indicates some interesting trends (Patrushev, Artemov & Novohatskaya, 2001). For working city-dwellers there was an essential decrease in the hours of general labor and an increase in free time for women. Considerable change in the content of time management for both men and women included an increase of time watching television, a reduction in visits to cultural and relaxation establishments and an increase in education and participation in training activities. For the rural population there was an increase in labor; a re-distribution of labor, especially for females, to the sphere of family economic management; and a growing dissatisfaction with less free time.

Since the economic reforms, the majority of these trends have become stronger. The actual amount of paid work for a working day has decreased, the time spent on work at home has decreased, work in the subsidiary job outside the formal job essentially has increased, but at the same time incomes have decreased. For a part of the population, especially urban dwellers, diametrically opposing tendencies are characteristic. Many members of families are forced to work very hard, at times on several jobs, to maintain a decent financial position and standard of living for the rest of the family. Often, the children carry a heavy educational burden.

Employment patterns for Russians have changed. Except for the period during the 1990s, the labor load for women decreased considerably and increased somewhat for the men (Patrushev, 2003). However, how a family spends time together depends not so much on the degree of employment but how well many family members' schedules are synchronized. It is important for them not simply to spend time together, but to spend it with interest, joy and fascination. As a rule husbands and wives work in different places and at different times and the children have their own daily routine. Spending family time, in many respects depends on the season. For winter time, the most widespread occupation is television viewing. In the summer outings are spent in nature such as on a visit to a dacha, a reservoir, lake or river, or a forest. On days off, going out to visit or receive visitors is popular. Half of the family members with free time spend it for their own entertainment. Because of the high prices of tickets, Russians seldom go to cinemas, theatres and concert halls. Few attend sporting events (Shuraleva, 2004). As a whole, spending free time in Russia means watching television. The greatest amount of the working city-dweller's free time includes viewing of telecasts, followed by reading and dialogue for the men, and dialogue and active kinds of leisure for the women (Patrushev, 2003).

Our research confirms these tendencies, though the members of strong families have a rich repertoire of joint occupations and personal interests. At the same time, because of the fast pace of life in the city, they have less free time than the inhabitants of the periphery. Strong family members have different possibilities for spending time together and follow certain rules. First, regularity in family activities is important as well as creating family traditions (rituals, symbols). Family traditions can include a joint celebration of holidays, a visit to cultural establishments, involvement in sports, games, trips into nature, walks in the city and so forth. Second, not all members of the family can participate in family activities and may have different interests, particularly between men and women. Also, it may be difficult to coordinate family activities when some of the members are working long hours or their leisure hours do not coincide.

An Increase in the Time Children Spend Outside the Family and the Neglect of Children

Data from representative research samples indicate the following problems. Parents practice child rearing passively. Slightly more than half of officially married couples have a sufficient quantity of time to raise children. Almost one-third of parents are engaged with their children only occasionally. Parents in a civil marriage are engaged with their children less than those in an official marriage. The causes of such situations are highly pragmatic, including financial difficulties and to a lesser extent workload, such as a large volume of work at home or the absence of necessary knowledge and experience (Éartseva, 2003).

At the same time, the family policy of the Soviet state usurped the function of parenting hat has led to the majority of parents who neglect traditional interaction with their children, delegating authority to professionals and state establishments. Parents frequently consider that the main function in raising children is satisfying the child's material and biological needs (clothing, food and medical care). Inconsistency and the lack of co-ordination of upbringing influences are displayed which leads to a neurotization of children and other negative consequences (Shabas, 2003). Thus, the belief that fewer children in a family provide the best conditions for the upbringing of children is without foundation.

Our strong families, to a greater degree, gravitate towards an independent realization of the childrearing function. Home schooling in Russia practically does not exist, therefore children spend a lot of time in kindergartens and schools. Parents in strong families, depending on their financial capabilities, prefer to develop the abilities of their children themselves with supplementary formal education. As the basic method of upbringing, members of strong families consider persuasion by word but first of all by deed. Parents believe their behavior should set an example for children in everything, including organization of family life and family relationships. It is quite natural and has been demonstrated in research setting a bad example by saying one thing and doing another, leads to children's deviations. Parents' divorce increases the probability of divorce for their children. Certainly the parents in our study encourage and punish their children and believe forceful approaches to childrearing may seem tough at times but are necessary. More important though, the parents think it is necessary to love their children and find a reasonable compromise between encouraging their independence and limiting their freedom.

During conversations with the strong families, the problem of coordinating upbringing influences was discussed. This includes two basic aspects. The first aspect, which may be called explicit, is the development of common strategies and tactics between parents and also between parents and other family members living with them. Often this process is very emotional at times and uncompromising. Here strong families more or less successfully attempt to reach a consensus. In this sense, it is easier to find a consensus between a smaller number of people, that is, between parents and for this purpose they should live separately from grandparents. The second aspect may be called implicit. If parents are working long hours outside the home or need time for themselves without the children around, the young are sometimes sent to the grandparents for care. In this case, grandfathers and grandmothers educate the children in their way of understanding life, but most often spoil them.

Then, when the children return to the parents, it is first necessary to re-adapt to the parents' way of thinking and this can be problematic.

The Technology of the Mass Media Mesmerizes People, Turning Them into Unconscious Zombies, Substituting Entertainment for Direct Human Interrelations

The mass media are called *the fourth authority* in Russia. It is difficult to overestimate the influence they have on people's behavior. By virtue of an integrated perception, the greatest influence on social behavior is probably television. Laboratory research by Albert Bandura and his colleagues in the 1960s gathered a significant quantity of data on the influence of television violence on social behavior, and demonstrated a connection between the frequency of viewing telecasts with violence in childhood and the quantity and severity of criminal actions at maturity. For Russians, television plays a significant role in life. For example, television viewing by the urban working population consumes 57% of free time (Patrushev, 2003). Knowing this, it is not difficult to imagine how behavior can be influenced, especially when youth are viewing programs and movies where the main characters are thieves, crooks and swindlers.

The Internet has a special place among the mass media. In Russia, *Runet*, as it is called, provides basic information, but also can form a syndrome of Internet-dependence (Voiskunski, 2000). The danger of Internet-dependence in Russian society as a whole is not great now, but the number of Internet users in the country is only about five million people. It is necessary to consider that this problem will increase because the volume of Internet use increases on the average 10-12% a year (Aimaletdinov, 2003).

As a whole, the social irresponsibility demonstrated by the press, radio, television and the Internet seriously disturbs both the average Russian and social scientists today (Zubkov, 2003). The experience of the transformation has shown that public morality as a regulator of information and entertainment plays a confined role. *Arbitrary information* flourishes and we see a situation where it is difficult to separate objectivity from estimation, facts from commentaries, opinion of experts from opinion of journalists and the personal mercenary outburst of mass-media talking heads from the genuine needs of society.

Members of strong families are tested by the influence of the mass media. This problem especially disturbs them in the context of raising children. Parents point out that children most often become admirers of actors and stars of show business and not scientists, artists or political leaders. Many children are carried away by computer games, which, to put it mildly, do not contribute to healthy development. Parents in strong families see the negative influences of the mass media. They believe it is important, instead, to introduce children to high culture, to train them in reading the best pieces of fiction, and also to plan carefully and expose the children to theatres, museums and exhibitions. The parents also believe children need enough rich experiences during the day that there will not be time to sit in front of the TV or computer. However, this is also a concern for adults, especially men who are not busy.

Sexual Dissoluteness in Society and the Low Sexual Culture of Youth

Individual freedom does not mean freedom from moral standards. But in the 20th century, moral standards in the area of sexual behavior have undergone considerable changes. These changes in many respects are connected with the democratization of society and tolerant attitudes toward sexual deviations, the appearance of pornography, and the development and widespread use of contraceptives that assisted in the division and isolation of sexual and genesial behavior. In the context of our research, sexual problem can be divided into two parts. The first part is the problem of sexual behavior before marriage and the second part is extramarital sexual behavior.

Research shows that more than half of both adolescents and their parents have not formed a strong opinion about the issue of virginity before marriage. This demonstrates that the transformation of social standards has touched not only youth who are the most receptive to change, but all society (Zhuravleva, 2003). One-third of adolescents consider it acceptable to lead a sexual life at age 15 (Orlova, 2003). Among the young, the belief in the expediency of a sexual life before marriage to check for partner compatibility is widespread.

With the steady growth of pre-marital sexual behavior and a rising teenage birth rate, the genesial health of adolescents becomes worse. During the last decade inflammatory diseases and sexually transmitted diseases as well as complications of pregnancy and childbirth for teenagers has increased five-to-seven times. Sexual education in schools is absent, and is conducted poorly in the family. Only somewhat more than one-third of adolescents indicate that their parents regularly talk with them about sexual behavior. Mothers discuss these problems with girls 1.5 to 2 times more often than with boys, which puts the traditional responsibility for the consequences of sexual relations primarily on women (Zhuravleva, 2004).

The second aspect of the problem is extramarital sexual relations. Research shows about 60% of men and about 30% of women have had extramarital sexual experiences (Gurko & Boss, 1995). Men more often hold a principle of the double standard and to a greater degree accept extramarital sexual relations for men than women. Naturally, such freedom in sexual relations does not add strength to a marriage and is one of the causes of divorce, though as numerous studies show, not the most important cause.

During our interviews, for obvious reasons we could not directly ask about their conjugal infidelities and so we asked them about the problems of sexual dissoluteness and sexual culture in general. These problems, to a great degree, disturbed the respondents in regard to raising children in an amoral society in which freedom of sexual behavior and sexuality in the mass culture are practically the norm and sexual crimes are ordinary events. Parents in strong families have concerns about further legal rights for homosexuals, which in modern Russia already have their own organizations and their own printed publications. In the opinion of strong family members, it is possible to resist these negative tendencies in society by cultivating in families the values of conjugal sexual behavior. Parents talk to their children about sexual subjects–fathers talk with sons and mothers with daughters. The parents consider regular conversations and maintain constant and close spiritual (psychological) contact with their children, believing this is important and time needs to be devoted to help the children with solutions for their new life, including sexual problems. Also, it was mentioned that a normalization of sexual behavior would probably return through Christian values. The *Christian renaissance* in Russia today, however, is to a greater degree only superficial, observing only religious holidays and rites, instead of a genuine change in one's deep world-outlook and toward a religious way of life.

Global Disasters:
Technological, Ecological, Biological and Other Types

The transition of Russian society, characterized by a large degree of uncertainty and risk, plus the natural and technogenic catastrophes shown in the mass media, have created a sharp increase in risk consciousness and uneasiness (Shlyapentoh, Shubkin, & Yadov, 1999). The greatest anxiety and fear for them is the possibility of ecological catastrophe. Two thirds of Russians believe the chemical and radiation pollution of water, air, and other resources to be more threatening than a possible accident. The monstrous consequences of the explosions of Chelyabinsk nuclear combine *Mayak* (Lighthouse) in 1957 and Chernobylskaya atomic power station in 1986, the explosion of two passenger trains in Bashkiria from a natural gas leak in 1989, numerous tests of nuclear and hydrogen bombs and the *normal* functioning of many chemical enterprises without proper safety measures have been deeply imprinted in public consciousness and in memory of many Russians.

What can strong families do to prevent global disasters? Research shows that the more there is a possibility of an individual or group to gain control of a threatening situation, the more likely there will be opposition to such dangers; the less such a possibility, the less there will be a readiness to act (Shlyapentoh, Shubkin, & Yadov, 1999). For global catastrophes there is less control. Therefore, the main reaction of strong family members to global disasters is their discussion with friends, acquaintances and colleagues. At the same time, depending on the situation, the members of strong families are ready to do everything they can to secure their own environment in the face of disaster.

Increasing Utilitarianism, Pragmatism and Decreasing Spirituality in Society

The Russian-American sociologist Pitirim A. Sorokin has created the concept of social and cultural dynamics (Sorokin, 1962). According to this concept, there are three fundamental types of culture in history. The sensate culture is oriented on material valuable and the ideational culture on spiritual ones. The integral culture is intermediate and takes on values of the first two cultures. The contrary types of cultures historically alternate one another through intermediate culture, and alternate gradually. Using the terminology of Sorokin's theory, it is possible to assert that many cataclysms going on in modern Russia are a consequence of a fast transition from an ideational (burdened with communist ideology) to a sensate type of culture, passing an integral one. During the current process of the rational, materialistic type of culture, a targeted, goal-driven type of social activity and a philosophy of consumption have begun to prevail. At this time, the spiritual component of Russian society remains rather diminished. Meanwhile, the combination of weak faith and lack of morals based on a self-centered drive for wealth is rather dangerous for society. Luckily, the spiritual culture of Russia is gradually reviving.

The growth of utilitarianism and pragmatism in society are evident in various ways. For example, among the factors indicative of social status and prestige, material possessions rank highest. Almost half of respondents put it in the first place, whereas personal achievements in education and professional activity are considered important by less than a quarter of Russians (Boikov, 2004). The narrow pragmatic (mainly connected with cash income) orientations of youth cause special concern. The position of these motives in the structure of labor motivation for young people in 1997 reached 58% and has stayed at this level until now (Zubok, 2003).

Together with the growth of utilitarianism and pragmatism such antipodes of morality as dodgerness, unscrupulousness, and corruption in ordinary consciousness are often not accepted as anomalies, but as a justifiable version of behavior in daily life, in political activity and in business. Two thirds of respondents do not consider tax evasion as shameful and even see it as morally justified. More than half of those interviewed prefer to give bribes to bureaucrats as a solution to arising problems. However, as the society becomes more and more habituated to these negative phenomena, an increase in amoral and legal nihilism has caused more and more agitation among the majority of the population (Boikov, 2004).

It is necessary to note that these problems exist more often outside the family institution than inside, functioning in the wider sphere of public activity and business. Mercantilism and formalism are not inherent in the vast majority of Russian families. Marrying Russians, as a rule, do not conclude marriage contracts. There are no books on home budgeting for Russian families as there are in many European countries. A wife more often controls the money, as she conducts housekeeping. Marriage partners put their incomes together in a *common copper* and if necessary take money from it for daily expenses. If wages are deposited a bank account and the money is spent jointly. The possibility of undertaking large purchases is discussed by the couple. Therefore, members of our strong families clash with problems of *pragmatism, unburdened by morals* basically in their relation to other people and note that as a whole, the degree of confidence in people in general has considerably decreased in recent years.

Under these conditions the members of strong families, at first, rush to protect themselves against negative displays of *wild capitalism*. Second, and especially important, strong families create a mini-environment of activity and circle of relations, optimal from their point of view of moral principles and spiritual interests. This means not only friendship and collaboration with other families, but also social connections with family members. Our research shows the special necessity of these personal connections for husbands. They underline the fact that both the man and the woman should understand and be aware of the interests of their partner and that dialogue with friends is one of the very important things in family life.

Ethnic, Religious, Political and Other Intolerant Attitudes Among People

Intolerance and tolerance are social attitudes that in the end characterize the degree of society's integration. The research of recent years demonstrates that tolerance for the religious sphere of life and intolerance in relation to the ideas of a weak state and cosmopolitanism are traditional characteristics of Russians. Despite total propagation in the mass media, Russians do not accept Western tolerance in relation to sexual minorities, sexual permissiveness, or public use of foul language. In comparison with the Soviet period, tolerance for different worldviews and political dissidence has increased. At the same time, intolerance for social injustice, such as the state, political parties, individual political leaders, reformers and businessmen has increased (Sokolov, 2003). A traditionally tolerant attitude to other nationalities was replaced by intolerant relations with some of them, especially to *persons of Caucasian nationalities* (most notably, the Chechens), which explains the infamous Chechen events. Today, 66% of Russians show hostility to Caucasian people (Sokolov, 2003).

An aggravation of interethnic relations in Russia is connected with a parade of national sovereignties that appeared after the collapse of the Soviet Union. In the majority of the post-Soviet countries the Russians and other minority groups were exposed by discrimination explicitly and gave rise to Russian-language migration to Russian territory and antipathy of the Russians, e.g., to the Estonians. There is an economic context to interethnic relations. So, the cause of antipathy of Russians toward Azerbaijanis is that in many localities the latter control the important economic sector of small-sized business trade in foodstuffs (Shefel, 2002).

Members of strong families tend to think differently about policy, public behavior and ethnic questions. There are, so to speak, *the irreconcilables* among them. The participants in our research tended to speak rather quietly when discussing problems of creed, with the exception of the Chechen problem, which is bound up with Islam. But it is likely that strong families are generally tolerant to different world-outlooks and we think that this is not accidental. Family relations necessitate the ability to understand others and to see their point of view. In daily life, members of strong families simply try not to clash with people with whom they disagree.

We already addressed the low level of protest activities by Russians. More than half of Muscovites interviewed in one study did not accept any form of protest, even legal. Only one in five respondents would participate in acts of civil insubordination or movements to take power, including the use of weapons (Sokolov, 2003). As a whole, members of strong families are not disposed to protest actions. The majority of them are tired from the shock therapy administed by the government in the 1990s and want stability and opportunity to solve their own problems.

The Decline of Traditional Socio-Cultural Family Roles for Men and Women

On Russian talk shows, rather often (especially from the lips of feminist-disposed women) one can hear that modern men are losing traditional, strong masculine traits and that women have become more firm, business-like, independent and that all this reduces the value of family life. According to available data in the 1980s wives started to dominate practically all spheres in a considerable segment of Russian families. For example, in approximately one third of families, women control the money, manage economic problems and determine the upbringing and education of the children (Gurko & Boss, 1995). Let us explore some causes of this tendency.

First, the phenomenon of female leadership in the family started during the post-war period at the end of the 1940s when there was a shortage of men and the number of working women increased sharply. Second, women's activity as governesses in preschool establishments, teachers, judges, and so forth, demands authoritative psychological capacities and is a model of professional behavior involuntarily transferred to the family. Third, as we already noted, in the Russian patriarchal family, elderly parents lived with the youngest son and now more often live with a daughter, which has some advantages for her in relation to her husband. Fourth, the young married couple, as a rule, uses the material aid of parents, which does not help establish a husband's authority in the wife's eyes (Gurko & Boss, 1995). Add to this the growth rate of the educational level of women that is now higher than men and a woman frequently becomes equivalent, if not the main *breadwinner*, while a man can end up unemployed.

In the case of female leadership, lower marital satisfaction for both wives and husbands is likely. Quite often women complain that they should be able to make decisions and they argue there is an absence of initiative in their husbands. Thus, the situation resembles a *vicious circle*. A woman becomes tired of having to lead and at the same time is constantly in a struggle for her own independence (Gurko & Boss, 1995). Another study found that in the majority of Russian families, from 40% up to 70% of couples support the idea of equal influence in decision making, depending on the family problem. There is no exception to this finding even among eastern Russian peoples. Therefore, it is reasonable to postulate that the future of the family is linked to egalitarianism. However, rural residents are more likely to hold traditional views of family roles (Êartseva, 2003; Gurko & Boss, 1995).

In the majority of strong families in our study, partner relations and attitudes on the universalization of gender roles predominate. Even so, daily housework to a greater degree remains the prerogative of the women. Problems with the upbringing of children exhibit much more parity. The family income is distributed to both marriage partners. At the same time, partners in strong families emphasize that, in spite of an eccentricity in distribution of family responsibilities, a man should be manly and a woman–womanly. Echoes of traditional family roles can be seen in the differences between the husbands and wives in their ranking of problems that all families face and the problems that their particular faces (see Tables 1 and 2). In our sample, the man is responsible for the material well-being and is inclined to give financial problems greater significance. The problems of social protection and violence for all Russian families are addressed by the men as protectors with a ranking that is slightly higher than the women. The women focus their attention on housing problems and are traditionally responsible for emotional problems and ensuring the family spends enough time together. It is understandable that the men, more inclined to the use of alcohol, are less concerned with this problem and the women as a whole give less importance to the negative effects of the mass media. It is the most difficult to interpret that problems of sexual dissoluteness and low sexual culture of youth, where men are much more concerned and they worry for the women, and especially the daughters. At the same time the mothers, much more than the fathers, are engaged with the children in sexual education and reasonably confident in its effectiveness.

Acceptance of Divorces and Repeated Marriages, Linked with a Decreased Value of the Family Way of Life

The phenomenon of divorce in modern society as indicated in public opinion polls has a dual status. On one hand under democracy, divorce is a right of personal freedom and liberation from oppressive family relations. On the other hand, a family's pain hurts both the family members and society as a whole. Divorce affects the institution of the family, the health of the people, decreases the quality of youth socialization, increases deviant behavior and a number of others.

From the end of the 1980s to the middle of the 1990s, the divorce rate in Russia increased from 40% to 50%. Now it is beginning to fall and has almost reached its former level. However, a reduction in the number of divorces should be regarded in the context of a decrease in marriage registrations and an increase in cohabitation. Approximately two thirds of the men and about half of the women enter into repeated marriages (Antonov & Sorokin, 2000). The reasons for the high divorce rate of Russians are varied, and must be regarded both on a macrolevel (societal) and on a microlevel (family). It is necessary to distinguish objective prerequisites of divorces (differences in age, creed, educational levels; their upbringing in unfavorable families; a short acquaintance time before marriage, etc.), subjective causes of divorces (social, psychological and/or sexual unpreparedness for marriage), motives for divorces and also their concrete causes. But as a whole, it is possible to speak about one more *vicious circle*, which is a significant decrease in stable, valuable family relations that leads to divorce and that divorce is slowly becoming a social standard which depreciates the value of family.

In strong families, the combination of social-demographic and psychological characteristics of marriage partners, as a rule, are optimal. However, according to the respondents when their families began, they did not understand or think about scientific recommendations. For the majority of Russians in the study, the motivation was a love attachment. As to the problem of divorces, members of strong families see a divorce as a possible way out of an unsuccessful marriage. For them, the main reason for a divorce is an absence of common views or a lack of interests and mutual understanding. At the same time, they believe that if this problem does not lead to conflicts and other problems, it is necessary if only on a formal basis to keep a marriage together for the sake of the children. Even if a divorce occurs, former marital partners should support their relationship with each other for the joint upbringing of the children. However, with so many things happening in life, these good intentions are not always possible.

THE STRENGTHS OF RUSSIAN FAMILIES

To neutralize the challenges of modern society, strong families: find their own psychological and material resources; decide problems through mutual help and support of family members and through their faith in each other; discuss problems with others and are prepared to resolve them; create their own mini-environment of activity and their own circle of interaction who share their moral principles and spiritual interests; treat material problems realistically and apply a variety of survival strategies; prefer to live near parents or with them if they need help; gravitate toward partner relationships and universalization of gender roles; hold meaningful family gatherings regularly and create family traditions; strive for independent childrearing to coordinate upbringing influences and maintain contact with children; stand for the preservation of marriage or, at least, a preservation of relations for the joint upbringing of the children; prefer not to clash with people to which they are intolerant; and in general, do not join political protests or activities, desire stability and the ability to decide problems on their own.

The respondents have offered other recommendations that in their opinion serve to strengthen family relations. Apart from mutual trust and mutual support, the just distribution of family responsibilities, spending free time together and a discussion of problems, they also recommended the following: broadening of the sphere of family members' interaction to improve mutual understanding and display their attachment to each other; participation of all family members in solving family problems, respecting the opinions of each; preserving sufficient autonomy for each family member, recognizing their uniqueness and encouraging their capacities; tolerance of unessential deviations in behavior of family members; showing positive and negative emotions (making it possible *to let out steam*); refusing to take advantage of individual weaknesses or put pressure on them or force them to do something; encouraging family members to develop a high level of self-esteem and not be overly self-critical; maintenance of spirituality in sexual relations for the married couple; introducing family relations game elements, attaching regular family roles with novelty elements; flexibility in connection with changes; and understanding the inevitability of family conflicts and the ability to move them in a structured, positive direction.

CONCLUSION

It should be noted that the subject of our research itself has predetermined that negative social processes influence the functioning of the modern Russian family. However, given the data we do not want the reader to conclude that the crisis in Russian society will intensify. As a whole, official statistics and scientific research speak about a reverse in important trends. For the period since 2000 until the present time, the gross domestic product of the country is growing; the labour motivation is increasing; the period when living conditions of more than half of the population were constantly becoming worse has been turned around as living conditions are improving; contradictions between the state and civil society are being smoothed; and although not as significant as it should be, the number of people who are optimists about the future of the country is growing (Lapin, 2003; Lapin, 2004; Levashov, 2004; *Criminality and law in Russia. Statistical aspect,* 2003). It should be assumed that these positive changes will assist to strengthen the Russian family.

REFERENCES

Aimaletdinov, T. A. (2003). High technologies and problems of information disparity in Russia. *Sociological studies, 8,* 121-126.

Antonov, A. I. & Sorokin, S. A. (2000). *The fate of the family in Russia in the XXI century.* Moscow.

Antonov, A. I. & Medkov, V. M. (1996). *Sociology of the family.* Moscow: MGU Publishing; International University of Business and Control (Karich Brothers).

Avtonomov, V. S. (1998). *Model of man in economic science.* St Petersburg: School of Economics.

Boikov, V. E. (2004). Values and orientation of Russian public consciousness. *Sociological studies, 7,* 46-52.

Fund Public Opinion (2004, Dec 23). Polls of population family problems. Database of FOM. Fund *Public Opinion*: http://bd.fom.ru/report/cat/humdrum/home_family/family

Gurko, T. A. & Boss, P. (1995). Attitudes of men and women in marriage. In *A family on the threshold of the third millennium.* Moscow: Center of General Human Values, 35-66.

Hrushev, A. T. (Ed.). (2002). *Economic and social geography of Russia: Textbook for institutions of higher education.* Moscow: Bustard.

Êartseva, L. V. (2003). The model of family in Russian society transformation. *Sociological studies, 7,* 92-100.

Kozhinov, V. V. (1999). *Russia. 20th century (1901-1939). History of the country from year 1901 up to mysterious year 1937* (The experience of impartial research). Moscow: Algorithm.

Lapin, N. I. (2003). How do the citizens of Russia feel about what they aspire? *Sociological studies, 6,* 78-87.

Lapin, N. I. (2004). Values and knowledge. The monitoring of our values and interests. *Sociology, 1,* 38-41.

Levashov, V. Ê. (2004). The moral-political consolidation of the Russian society in conditions of neoliberal transformations. *Sociological studies, 7,* 27-46.

Mozgovaya, A. V. (1999). Technological risk and ecological component of life's quality of the population. Capabilities of the sociological analysis. Moscow: Dialogue–MGU Publishing.

Orlova, N. H. (2003). Installations of the democratic behavior in the youth culture (Theses of reports and appearances at the second All-Russian sociological congress, Russian society and sociology in the 21st century: Social challenges and alternatives) Moscow: Alpha-M, 2, 124-126.

Patrushev, V. D. (2003). The time budget of the urban working population of the USA and Russia (1980-1990 years). *Sociological studies, 12,* 32-39.

Patrushev, V. D., Artemov, V. A. & Novohatskaya, O.V. (2001). The analysis of time budgets in Russia in the 21st century. *Sociological studies, 6,* 112-120.

Pozdnyakova, M. E. (2004). The drug situation in Russia on the boundary of the 20th and 21st centuries: The sociological analysis (Theses and appearances of the second All-Russian sociological congress, The Russian society and sociology in the 21st century: Social challenges and alternatives). Moscow: Alpha-M, 2, 123-128.

Criminality and law in Russia. Statistical aspect. 2003: Stat. coll. Moscow: Statistical Bureau of Russia, pp. 9-21.

Poll of population Russian citizenry about family and children. (13-18.05.2004). Database of Research Holding POMIR (Russian Public Opinion and Market Research) http://www.romir@romir.ru

Shabas, S. G. (2003). The upbringing function of a family having a child of preschool age in conditions of a socio-cultural transformation (Theses of reports and appearances of the second All-Russian sociological congress, Russian society and sociology in the 21st century: Social challenges and alternatives). Moscow: Alpha-M , 2, 109-111.

Shefel, S. V. (2002). *The personality of the post-industrial epoch as a phenomenon of the socio-cultural synthesis (A social-philosophical research).* Moscow.

Shlyapentoh, V. E., Shubkin, V. N. & Yadov, V. A. (Eds.) (1999). Disaster consciousness in modern society at the end of the 20th century (based on materials of the international research). *Series scientific reports, 9.* Moscow: Moscow Public Scientific Fund; University of Michigan.

Shuraleva, F. (2004). Free time in provincial Russia (Theses of reports and appearances of the second All-Russian sociological congress, The Russian society and sociology in the 21st century: Social challenges and alternatives). Moscow: Alpha-M, 2, 653-659.

Sokolov, V. M. (2003). Tolerance: A condition and tendencies. *Sociological studies, 8,* 54-63.

Sorokin, P. A. (1962). *Social and Cultural Dynamics*. New York: Bedminster Press.

Statistical Bureau of Russia (2003) Basic sums of the All-Russian population census of 2002, Moscow.

Voiskunski, A. E. (Ed.). (2000). *Humanitarian studies on the Internet*. Moscow.

Zhuravleva, I.V. (2003). Behavior and reproductive status of adolescents (These and appearances of the second All-Russian sociological congress, The Russian society and sociology in the 21st century: Social challenges and alternatives). Moscow: Alpha-M, 3, 48-50.

Zhuravleva, I. V. (2004). Reproductive health of adolescents and problems of sexual education. *Sociological studies, 7*, 133-142.

Zubkov, V. I. (2003). *The sociological theory of risk: Monograph*. Moscow: KUDN Publishing House.

Zubok, Y. A. (2003). *A problem of risk in sociology of young people*. Moscow: Moscow Humanitarian Social Academy.

doi:10.1300/J002v41n03_07

The Family Strengths in Greece
Then and Now

Theodora Kaldi-Koulikidou

SUMMARY. Family has a long historical course in Greece. The turbulent periods of Hellenic history and the fluctuations of the political, social and economic life have influenced Hellenic family strengths. Nevertheless, there have been some basic elements on which the family has been based and acquired a continuous stability and homogeneity. These features are: religion, language, a rich cultural heritage, tradition and customs. Roles in the family are strongly influenced by the above, though they have been readjusted and redefined in contemporary society. doi:10.1300/J002v41n03_08 *[Article copies available for a fee from The Haworth Document Delivery Service: 1-800-HAWORTH. E-mail address: <docdelivery@haworthpress.com> Website: <http://www.HaworthPress. com> © 2007 by The Haworth Press, Inc. All rights reserved.]*

KEYWORDS. Greek family strengths, Greek families, Greek family and orthodoxy, Greek family values, Hellenic family

---

Theodora Kaldi-Koulikidou is Administrator, Aristotle University of Thessaloniki, School of Modern Greek Language, 54 124 Thessaloniki, Hellas (E-mail: thkaldi@phil.auth.gr).

[Haworth co-indexing entry note]: "The Family Strengths in Greece Then and Now." Kaldi-Koulikidou, Theodora. Co-published simultaneously in *Marriage & Family Review* (The Haworth Press, Inc.) Vol. 41, No. 3/4, 2007, pp. 393-417; and: *Strong Families Around the World: Strengths-Based Research and Perspectives* (ed: John DeFrain, and Sylvia M. Asay) The Haworth Press, Inc., 2007, pp. 393-417. Single or multiple copies of this article are available for a fee from The Haworth Document Delivery Service [1-800-HAWORTH, 9:00 a.m. - 5:00 p.m. (EST). E-mail address: docdelivery@haworthpress.com].

Available online at http://mfr.haworthpress.com
© 2007 by The Haworth Press, Inc. All rights reserved.
doi:10.1300/J002v41n03_08

THE COURSE OF THE HELLENIC FAMILY THROUGH TIME

"God! How much blue you wasted so that we won't see you?" (Elytis, 1978). This land, a blue spot in the world, has ever been a blessing and curse for its people, at the same time. At the crossroads of three continents, the East meets the West and the West meets the East, so that they mix in a unique way and influence each other and are reformed.

The Hellenic People

The rough and mountainous mainland, surrounded by the infinite blue of the sea and hundreds of islands, has so deeply and strongly acted on the nature of the Hellenes that we can not say where nature has influenced the people and where people have conquered nature. The immense, unknown sea has always challenged the Hellenes to explore it and acquire knowledge. They have traveled, searched, communicated, made relations and commerce, and created new ideas. It is not by chance that even today this small country holds the fourth position worldwide in terms of commercial ships under the Hellenic flag (Ministry of Commercial Fleet of Hellas, 2001). And it is also not by chance that this country has given birth to one of the most important civilizations of the world, which has positively affected the course of the modern world.

The constant changes in historical background, the enemies who have never stopped coveting this land, and the continuous struggle to survive, have provided the Hellenic people with special talents, a fighting spirit, and a unique cultural identity. There are not many societies in the world that could be characterized by so much instability at all levels for more than three thousand years. This impermanence has become part of our race, and it has been this element which has constituted the basic characteristic of our cultural stability. The continual adjustments and adaptations we have made in response to altered circumstances, and the subsequent transformation of our society have become one of the most positive elements for our people. Immigration, navigation, and Diaspora have ever been the fundamental sources for gathering our strength and knowledge. (Kataki, 1998). The more challenges Hellenes have faced, the more flexible, resilient, and obstinate they have become. It is hard to find a people simultaneously so much the same and yet so different through time.

The Hellenic family has never evolved apart from Hellenic society. The transformation of our society from the archaic to the Hellenistic, Byzantine, and later period of history have defined the family. Though at first sight everything has changed in the society throughout the last three millennia, there are some fundamental and essential elements which remain basically the same. These characteristics constitute the backbone of the Hellenes as a nation and they reinforce the strengths of the family.

The basic components that have determined the identity of the Hellenes are their language, religion, and a rich cultural heritage, tradition and customs. These components are resilient and timeless, and they have put their indelible stamp on the formation of the nation and the family. Hellenes are very proud of their history and culture. This is a heavy burden and a huge responsibility. The culture is the source of our essence; our history is the basis of our roots; our language is part of our substance; religion is the core of our existence; our ethics, tradition and customs are the cells of our life.

Herodotus (485 B.C.) refers to ". . . the kinship of all Greeks in blood and speech, and the shrines of gods and the sacrifices that we have in common, and the likeness of our way of life. . . ." (Godley, 1925).

The Hellenic Family

The family *(oikos,* pronounced ecos) was a central and important institution in ancient times. The state did not supersede or suppress the *oikos* and there was no clear public/private split because one's civic identity derived largely from one's *oikos.* The family played a key role in the political changes that marked the history of ancient Hellas. Early Hellenic society was rooted in individual households, and a man's or woman's place in the larger community was determined by relationships within those households (Patterson, 1998).

The protection of the family was an important element of public law. The ancient Hellenes protected their families by protecting their homeland: "On, ye sons of Hellas! Free your native land, free your children, your wives, the fanes of your father's gods, and the tombs of your ancestors. Now you battle for your all." By singing this paea, the Hellenes defeated the Persians in the naval battle of Salamina near Athens in 480 B.C., as it is mentioned by Aeschylus in his work "Persians" (Weir Smyth, 1956).

The woman's role in Hellenic life was important, and the amount of influence women wielded in antiquity would surprise even today's feminists. Literature and drama accurately reflect women's importance, both in the family and in the society. Great female figures have marked Hellenic history in an unprecedented way. They were personalities of distinguished grandeur, such as Penelope (Odysseus' wife), Electra, Iphigenia and others. In order to distinguish a woman in a Hellenic tragedy, she had to be tested to the final limits of her own capacity for action and tenacity. If a woman broke the rules of society and the family in Hellenic tragedy, she was not a true Hellene (e.g., Medea). If a fratricide occurred, the punishment to the woman was horrible, because the rules of the family had been violated (e.g., Clytemnestra)

The Role of Religion

The Hellenes have a unique understanding of religion. From very early on, religion was connected with the struggle for the clarification of existence. The ancient temple summarized not only the religious sense but the ultimate substance of the people. Religion and Hellenic life were intimately connected with each other (Giannaras, 1983).

The Role of Language

The Hellenic language was another component of Hellenic identity and has been spoken since the 2nd millennium B.C. It has changed through time but it is still a living language and one of the richest surviving languages today. The language has achieved great things, created important ideas, and developed a unique philosophy. The ancient Hellenes called people who did not speak the same language "barbarians." The Hellenes avoided systematically mixing "barbarians" in the family, which was not only a matter of communication but also an issue of culture and national identity. Isocrates (436-338 B.C.), in his work *Panegyricos*, was the first to broaden the meaning of the word *Hellenes*, by attributing the term not only to the original people, but also to those who were sharing in Hellenic culture (Sakellariou, 1976). Since Alexander's the Great time (336-323 B.C.), the term *Hellene* has proven to be remarkably resilient, referring not to one's birthplace but to one's cultural roots.

During the Hellenistic period (323-201 B.C.) and the Roman Empire (200 B.C.-284 A.D.) the term *Hellene* acquired a broader philosophical significance corresponding to the new humanistic ideals of globalization. This identity was reformed through Byzantine times, one of the most amazing and long-lasting civilizations of the Western world. Byzantium, a theocratic empire, was founded on three co-equal elements, which gave direction through its one-thousand-year course: Hellenism, Orthodoxy and Roman legislation. The faith in ancient Gods, which was so unbreakable and rooted in Hellenic culture, was transformed over time into a faith that was more human and spiritual, called Christianity. Language was the vehicle for the Hellenic contribution to Byzantium. The Byzantines were delighted by age-old Hellenic literature. Ancient philosophers, historians and poets profoundly influenced the formation of Byzantine education and language (Runciman, 1969; Kyrkos, 1976).

The Orthodox Christian church exhibited an astonishing spirituality, a dogmatic character, and a feeling of mystery. While the rest of Europe was living in the Middle Ages, a relatively unenlightened time, Byzantium flourished, giving a new dimension to Hellenism that worked on the canvas in the development of the nation. And thanks to the dynamics of the ancient gnoseology, open to combining old and new ideas, the expression of the Christian experience was possible, showing an uninterrupted continuation in the Hellenic philosophic meditation. The Holy Orthodox Fathers of the fourth, fifth and sixth centuries, motivated by their Hellenic roots, advanced orthodox spirituality and morality through their treasured writings. In his address to youth, Saint Basil the Great (329-379 A.D.), one of the Holy Fathers of the Orthodox Church, focused on how young people would be able to take profit from the ancient Hellenic manuscripts. Saint John Chrysostom's (345-407 A.D.) admonitions for parents on raising their children are a treasury of wisdom that could be easily considered as if they were written today (Quasten, 1960; Bournelis, 2004; Kalliakmanis, 2005).

The Role of History

The Byzantine Empire was not a nation with racial prejudices. Everyone could be a free citizen of the empire, provided that he or she embodied Hellenic culture, spoke the Hellenic language, was of the same religion, and had Hellenic upbringing. It is believed that there has never been such a heterogeneous society with so many common characteristics. Up to the end of the Empire, its citizens remained, arguably, the most civilized representatives of the human race. Women were educated and they remained mainstays of the family as mothers or wives of important men. Married women were entirely free and many times they ran the family. They had an equal share with their husbands in the common property and the tutelage of their children. The only wedding recognized by the state was the one according to Orthodox Christian dogma, and there were only four reasons for a divorce to be allowed: the commitment of adultery by the wife; the husband's impotence; an assassination attempt by a partner; and leprosy. Children began the study of the ancient

Hellenic language at the age of six. Homer, the ancient philosophers, and the Holy Bible were the main sources of their education (Runciman, 1969).

The Byzantine Empire was conquered by the Ottoman Turks in 1453. The society was shocked and jolted. Another culture, another historical background, a different religion and language, and strange ideas were imposed on the citizens of the empire. The centuries which followed in many ways were difficult for the nation and led to a redefinition of values. Two important elements of the culture struggled for survival during this long period: the Orthodox Christian religion and the Hellenic language. The family shrank out of fear of the enemy. It became a closed society, which trusted no one but the relatives. The strengths of the nation took new forms, readjusting to changing circumstances and priorities, which were very different from those with which the Hellenes were imbued. Consequently, the strengths of the family changed, also. In order to survive and maintain its roots, the family changed in a hostile society. The more hostile the world around them became the tighter and united the members of the family became–not only the family living in each household, but the extended family or clan. Religion and language composed the common denominator of family understanding. Awareness of precious heritage and the achievements of ancestors, passed from generation to generation, became the joining links for the preservation of the inextinguishable spirit of the nation. The men learned how to succumb to overwhelming force, while simultaneously securing the safety and the survival of the family. In contrast was the position of the woman in this retrograde society. The woman in the Hellenic family could have authority and opinion, and her role was upgraded, especially during the period of the Hellenic struggle.

The Revolution against the Ottoman Turks in 1821 led to the liberation and the formation of modern Hellas in 1826. Hellas experienced considerable culture shock as a result of the change. This shock was unavoidable. Western ideas from a "civilized," progressive world invaded the country. Displacing their traditional values and principles that had fortified Hellenes during Turkish rule, the new influences from Europe led to the development of a new identity in Hellas. It took the Hellenes almost one hundred years to recover from these waves of change, and to discover again their conjunction with the past. But cultural, political, and economic stability was still not yet within the Hellenes' reach. In the early 20th century new, violent changes began to flood their world: two Balkan wars, two world wars, a civil war, and a dictatorship all were to come.

Modern Hellas and the Influence of the Past

The personality of modern Hellenes is a combination of many characteristics derived from many sources. It is the East that attracts us and literally possesses our heart. It fascinates us and expresses our temperament. It is the European West that has become our destination from the birth of modern Hellas in 1826 to our integration in 1981 as a member of the European Community. Our Hellenic personality is also influenced by the Mediterranean area, the birthplace of unique civilizations and the crossroads of three continents. And finally, we are a product of the Balkan Peninsula, a turbulent and unstable area, which carries its own history, similarities and divergences. (Moussourou, 1984).

As the Hellenic society has been transforming, so has the family. The relationship between family and society, thus, has been necessarily reciprocal and mutual. The structure of society has influenced the institution of the family, in the context of the course of events. In addition, the hopes of the nation were founded on the institution of the family: the family supported the society, and operated as a safety valve for Hellenic identity. Rapid changes and development were related mostly to regulations and the organization of the state, and less with individual or family relations.

Hellas lived through social and economic changes in the last 50 years which most of the other countries of Europe experienced over a period of 150 years. In a country of antithesis this has not seemed to be a paradox. The changes have come one after another. In less than three generations we have passed from the traditional to the nuclear family, and then to a modern family pattern. Recently, a new model of family has been born, having elements of a progressive society with a traditional foundation. In the general confusion and controversy surrounding all the changes in Hellenic life, Hellenes have begun to understand that these cultural and social shocks are not necessarily the worst things they could expect. In a society that seemingly surged down a path with no obvious end in sight, the family stood behind, tossed about numerous times, but finally realized that it could not follow this frenzied course. The last three generations have had very different experiences as the society and the family changed so rapidly.

In one way, Hellenes have adjusted rather impetuously to the structure and function of post-modern life. In other ways, the strengths and the memories have been alive and ever-present. They still exist and they pass the torch of the past to the present. Therefore, we have built our new perspectives on a solid substructure, strengthened by our memories and our traditional experience. In disorganization we have found our formation. The three and four generations living today are a guarantee that these valuable memories will survive and be passed down to subsequent generations.

The great poet of antiquity, Homer (750-650 B.C.) in the *The Odyssey* narrates Ulysses' adventures as he returns to his homeland, the island of Ithaca and his beloved family. Ten years of war against Troy and ten more years wandering around unknown lands and seas full of temptations and allurements were not adequate to prevent him from going home. He had memories and they pulled him back. For the Hellenes, everything could be a memory. The Hellenes are restless and unforeseen, like the sea. They have an incredible adaptability and flexibility. This applies also to the family. The main characteristic of the family is its ability to adjust in various circumstances. It is not the adjustment itself that is important, but the way of adjustment and how the particular basic principles and memories are used to facilitate this adaptation (Kataki, 1998).

Since the 1960s there has been a flood of Hellenic immigrants to the USA, Canada, Germany, and Sweden. About that time internal emigration also began, which led the people of the region to find jobs and a more promising future in the urban centers, especially in the capital city of Athens. Suddenly, Hellas became a country of not only of emigration but also a country of immigration. The crisis that society encountered expanded to the family and created new problems. These population shifts and the quest of many families for a better life tested the endurance of Hellenic society. Only a few years ago, people started to realize that the situation was not so bleak, and just as the storm brought water into the ship, it did not sink. On the contrary, the ship proved to be quite strong and continued its route by making some alterations and indispensable concessions in order to become more resistant to disaster.

AT THE THRESHOLD OF THE THIRD MILLENNIUM

We have reached the threshold of the third millennium facing a multicultural challenge and growing globalization. Alexander the Great, in his soul-stirring speech in front of 9,000 officers in 324 B.C. in Opi, Asia Minor (today Turkey), gave a brilliant example of how this millennium could proceed: ". . . I do not divide men . . . into Hellenes and barbarians. . . . For me any good barbarian is a Hellene and any bad Hellene is worse than a barbarian. . . ." One thousand years ago, the Byzantine Empire proved that there were no main differences among human races. Byzantium demonstrated a kind of globalization in a multicultural empire. Today we talk of globalization which affects society first and through it the family.

Globalization

In Hellenic language there are two different words that render the word *globalization* in English. One is *pagosmiopoesi* and this has a rather new meaning. The other one, *ecumenicity*, which seems quite similar at first sight, is not a new idea for the Hellenes. The word *ecumenicity* derives from the Hellenic word *ecumeny* (world); this word has roots in the verb *oiko* (to inhabit, to live) and is a synecdoche of *oikos* (family) (Metallinos, 2003). The word *pagosmiopoesi* has a negative and undesirable meaning. The word *ecumenicity* is the faith and the destiny of our entire course through history. *Ecumenicity* is the Hellenic openness, starting with the family, to what is different and it is a precautionary inclination, which means the assent of the dissimilar and its remodeling and transformation in a coessential element of the Hellenic character. The movement of Hellenism in connecting with other peoples is affirmative and beneficial, not dominating and oppressively assimilative. Globalization is the illusion of *ecumenicity* (Metallinos, 2003). *Ecumenicity* refers to a world family.

In a worldwide study, the Hellenes appear to be the most skeptical nation regarding globalization, with 72% believing somewhat or entirely that globalization creates more problems than those that it solves (ICAP TNS, 2005). It is clear that Hellenes believe that globalization is not the model that fits them. They are likely to think that globalization undermines religion, language and family. One phenomenon that globalization brought to the country was the great number of emigrants that Hellas accepted, legally or not. That has been a part of the crisis for the family with many facets. One of the repercussions of the influx of immigrants has been the advent of many young women from the post-communist countries who wanted to stay in the country. Many of them immigrated because of divorces. Hellenic society over time came to the conclusion that the influx of young immigrant women was a threat to the unity of the family. In recent years laws have been made stricter as the state attempted to deal with the phenomenon by issuing new decrees and protecting the wife's rights to alimony.

Another consequence of the immigration has been the insecurity that Hellenes feel about their finances and job stability over the past 15 years.

Unemployment is 10.5%, the fifth highest in 25 European countries (Zirganos, 2005). One national survey indicated that unemployment is the most important issue that Hellas faces, according to 60% of the respondents (compared to the EU25 average of 44%) (Eurobarometer 64, 2005). Many Hellenes feeling this insecurity have realized that they could find financial shelter in the family. Living together in the same house, the members of the family have a common budget. This takes us back to the model of the traditional family of the 1950s. The family acts as a shield, protecting those confronted by poverty, unemployment and social discrimination. The support provided by the family in this case is not only psychological and moral but also economic. In connection with unemployment, many adult children continue to live with their families of origin. Fully 68% of younger people live with their parents (Vaggelis, 2005), with Hellas and Spain sharing the first ranking among European Union countries in this regard (Symeonidou, 2005).

"A Circle of Our Own People"

In Hellas the family has several common characteristics with other families in the area of the Mediterranean, but also some differences. The *circle of our own people*, which is different from *kinship*, is very important to the support of the family (Kataki, 1998). In Hellas a parallel human group, which does not necessarily belong to the family, can join with it in personal relationships, mutual dependence, and sentimental commitments. This group could include not only relatives, but people that the family feels are very close, people who support and help the family.

The uniqueness of the Hellenes' perceptions regarding close human relationships can be seen when comparing our views with the views our neighbors the Italians have in regard to close relatives. In Italian society, the investment is based on a code of mutual reciprocity, which punishes someone who does not contribute to the support of the family. In Hellenic society, regardless of the significance of the relationship, a betrayal entails the erasure of the betrayer from the group (Kataki, 1998).

The *circle of our own people* is usually quite large. An example of how important this group is in the support of the family is when a family loses a member. The group stands by the rest of the members, assists them, becomes part of a considerable extended family and withdraws only if and when the situation improves. This also explains the phenomenon of *koumbaria*. Being the best man or the maid of honor in a wedding, or the godfather or the godmother to a baptized child in the Orthodox Church is a very prestigious and respectable distinction. This is a way often used by the Hellenes to confirm their desire to belong in a large and supportive family. The affiliation is kept for life, and many times it passes from one generation to the other.

The Hellenes basically trust the members of their family and the circle of their own people. They are suspicious of any impersonal authority or institution. They dispute anything that comes from an impersonal source.

This untamed nature, this ability to be self-governing and flexible, has led us to recognize that the right to interfere in our lives is only granted to the people who truly care personally for us. Therefore, politicians are imputed with lack of concern for citizens and the majority express distrust in the political parties (EU25, 77%; Hellas, 76%). On the other hand, trust for the army is high (EU25, 76%; Hellas, 68%) (Eurobarometer 64, 2005). Since military service is obligatory, every man in the family and the circle of their own has served or has a child who is currently serving. The entire family focuses on the *soldier* (only young men serve) and reflects concern for everything related to his duty. This makes people feel that soldiering is not an impersonal institution, but a force that can be relied upon, an element of its own family dynamism.

Quite often Hellenes make contact with each other by criticizing or doubting almost all things. This is an admittedly odd approach to commu nication, which might lead to tense situations. It is not easy for someone to force Hellenes to do something and it would likely bring completely opposite results. This extends to all levels of Hellenic society, including the family. This trait may be common among people all over the world, but it is exaggerated in Hellas and helps to explain our rebellious and undisciplined character.

The members of the family are concerned a great deal with the opinion other people have of them as a unit in society. They do not seek to find the solution to their problems through psychoanalysts and if they do, they are likely to have difficulty in applying the advice. The care and the advice of their own people are what they ask for and apply. The family is likely to be strengthened as members look in the mirror and by listening to their own peoples' opinions.

One basic principle that Hellenes strongly believe is that they have *philotimo*. This is a key value–having broad and multiple meanings which mark the Hellenes more than other nationalities (Kataki, 1998). *Philotimo* is an intense and continuous sense of honor, of personal dignity, of self respect. The agony of insecurity in regard to the future, of disturbed relations, loss of the easy life and the inability to maintain personal pursuits all reduce this self-perception. A sense of *philotimo* helps the members of the extended family or the *circle of our own people* to give and not only to ask. It would also mean things such as: not forgetting the displaced people, spending money for someone who is in need, offering a meal to friends to please them or not getting married till the moment the older sister gets married. The old Hellenic movies of the 1960s and 1970s, which are played continuously on TV, have also contributed to the maintenance of this value.

Family seems to play a more and more important role in finding an exit from the self-centered loneliness that surrounds us and threatens to isolate one from the other. Family has a multidimensional character, which includes being an environment for bringing up children, an engine of economic enterprise and a religious community, as well. The members of the family seem to be united in the face of a hostile world (Campbell & Sherrard, 1968). Modern society lives in crisis, which is related to the course of individualism. The modern family, having deeply implanted the experience of the past, the culture and the tradition, is bound up with teamwork and support for each other. This seems to be the escape from the danger of loneliness and isolation. The impressive changes in the mentality of modern Hellenic parents seem to play a leading part in the cohesion of the family. The roles of parents have also partially changed. This has happened due to the attempts at further incorporation of the father into the family and of the mother into the world of work (Kataki, 1998). Women play an especially important role in the emotional support of family members (Symeonidou, 2005). A measure of how important the institution of marriage is that Hellas has the lowest percentage of births outside of marriage in the European Union (4%), while in Scandinavian countries this figure has reached 50% (Balourdos, 2005).

The generation of the 21st century seems to have rediscovered traditional values, which appeared to be under fire during the last 20 years. Researchers have found that family comes up as the most important value among young people, receiving a rating from 9.7 on a scale of 10 (Nassopoulos, 2003) to 9.4 (Vaggelis, 2005). There are two main reasons that the new generation is turning back to the family for support. One is the psychological support that members find among the people who care for and love them. This support lasts for a lifetime, regardless of whether the members have their own families or live in a faraway place. The other reason is the financial support that the family furnishes the members for their entire life. A high percentage of young people (87.13%) feel close to the family, counting on the emotional support which family offers to its members; 6.43% of young people count on the financial support of their family, and only 1.75% state that their family means little to them (Papadioti-Athanassiou, 1994).

THE ROLES OF THE FAMILY'S MEMBERS–
WAYS OF CONTACT

The Value of Children

The child is the basic pillar on which the structure of the family and the marriage is braced. For the Hellenes, the advent of a child redistributes the priorities of the family, changes the wishes and reassigns the goals. In this game the leading role is played by the nuclear family, the secondary role by the grandparents, and a minor role is played by the *circle of our own people*. From the moment a baby comes, the parents and grandparents live through the experience together. The progress of the child, the race for its education and finally its professional and personal maturity are the socially-recognized goal of the family. Enrolling the child in the university has always been a *must* for parents (Kataki, 1998). The publicity and the public concern for high-school graduates when they take exams every year in order to enter into the universities are probably unusual when compared to other countries. Parents consider their children's success as a personal triumph and they feel successful and recognized themselves (Kataki, 1998).

In a small country where the opportunities for a job, especially an esteemed job demanding high-level qualifications, are quite limited, the numbers of well-educated people continuously increase. Hellas has grown to be an overeducated country. The desire to find socially-esteemed positions demanding high-level qualifications has created a pool of overeducated men taking more mundane jobs with less-demanding qualifications. The support of the family through the long and arduous educational process is thus necessary. It is quite common for parents to continue to financially support their children even after the children and even their grandchildren have grown up (Moussourou, 1993; Symeonidou, 1998).

The purchase of a house or land for the children in order to start their own family is considered to be an investment in the new generation's future, apart from the financial standing of the family. The house usually is located close to the parents' house, so they will be at the disposal of the new couple, one way or another. (Georgas, 1994). The frequent visits among family members and relatives indicate the preservation of features which used to characterize the nuclear family. Furthermore, the constant financial support, especially of the young people by their parents, indicates an alignment with the structure and function of a nuclear family. Functionally, the family still conserves the features of the traditional nuclear family in what has become an intense urban environment (Kataki, 1998).

The connection between mother and son is one which is emotionally laden. It is based on memories of the past. The family has more expectations from the son; it invests more in his professional preparation; it gives him extra latitude for independent behavior and it expects that he will be the head of his own family. After she gets married, a daughter remains very close to her family, more than her husband with his family. Her relatives come closer to the family because she is the one who sets the main direction of the family's social behavior. (Kataki, 1998). As the folk wisdom goes, "The man is the head, but the woman is the neck and she turns the head where she wants."

The presence of grandparents in the life of the new family is very significant, according to contemporary data. This becomes more marked in regard to issues of the care and raising of the children. Grandparents are the integral members of the family who play an influential, pedagogical, and binding role in developing the cohesion of the family. Grandparents are devoted, and regularly offer help in raising their grandchildren (Hourdaki, 1995). The grandmothers are the ones who take care of their grandchildren when the mothers work or the couple wants to go out. The percentage is quite high in Hellas. The babysitting of the children is entrusted to grandmothers at the rate of 44% for children up to six years old. Grandmothers most often care for their grandchildren at their house (Symeonidou, 1998). Nursery schools are preferred by those couples whose parents live in another place or when the children are considered to be independent enough to go to a childcare center. The grandmother's contribution to the grandchildren's care allows the grandparents, especially the grandmother, to acquire authority in the raising of the child and through it to intervene in the family. This dependence becomes stronger the more time the mother spends on her job, or when the finances of the young couple are not thriving. The more the young couple needs their help, the more interference the grandparents can exercise. On one hand, the children grow up in a familiar and friendly environment and they feel safe and secure. On the other hand the children become spoiled and untamed, and it is not easy to adjust in the school community when the time comes. Seeing grandmothers with their grandchildren in churches every Sunday is common. "My child's child is twice my child" is an expression which is not only expressed but internalized. Despite all the disadvantages this orderly system may have, it does provide a healthy bridge which connects the past with the present and prepares for the future.

Gendered Identities

No matter how life proceeds in the family, the roles of the couple are organized according to gender. In the majority of families the man, as the head of the family is responsible for its subsistence. The woman is responsible for the household and raising the children. Though the claims of modern times and the structures of the family have become more diversified, the grounding of the roles by gender has basically not changed. The wife's authority within the family is likely to be greater the more children she has (Moussourou, 1984). Cooperation between spouses increases as the educational background of husbands grows. And the more specialized the husband profession is, the more likely his relationship with his wife will be based on collaboration rather than on his authority over her (Moussourou, 1993).

The birthrate in Hellas is one of the lowest in the European Union, but is comparable to the rest of the European Mediterranean countries. There could be several reasons for this, such as people getting used to having more comforts than in the past, having more interest in an easy life and preferring to spend money for personal pleasure and women working outside the home. In Hellas as in the other countries of Southern Europe, the public retrenchment, the decrease of the state's responsibility and the absence of the welfare state have led to the increase in the responsibilities of families. However, there is another reason, diametrically opposed to the others. Hellenes prefer fewer children in order to ensure for the children that they do have a prosperous and more secure life. Hellenes believe this will become the children's weapons against a hard life. Due to the very low public expenditures for social and family support, the family itself undertakes the role of supporting children and older people. The existence of few homes for the aged in the Hellas, in comparison with the size of the population, is partially explained by the above. Also, there is a high percentage of cohabitation of two generations in the same residence (Walker, 1998). Even if the older people live alone, they are visited by their children and grandchildren quite often. Putting an old man in an old people's home is a source of stigma for a family (Vardakas, 1994). For these reasons, the chasm between the generations does not appear so sharp.

There has been a significant increase in divorces in recent years. The numbers by themselves do not necessarily mean a crisis in the institution of the family. In the past, divorce was not made easy by the state, due to restraints and time-consuming procedures. The woman did not have her own income or job; therefore, she was dependent almost entirely on her husband. The institution of the woman's dowry granted to her husband at the wedding was a contribution to the family's burdens from very old times. The enactment of the dowry's return to the woman after the dissolution of the marriage was not a pleasing event for the husband. A divorce was also not acceptable by society in former days and the church was very strict on these matters. But the modification of conditions in Hellenic society and the conformity to the circumstances in a continuously changing world have imposed a different environment for divorce in Hellas. Though the divorce rate has increased from 0.7 in 1980 to 1.0 in 2003 per 1,000 population, Hellas still has the lowest divorce rate among the 30 countries of the European Union and Euro-zone. The marriage rate in Hellas has dropped from 6.5 in 1980 to 5.1 in 2003 per 1000 population (Symeonidou, 2005; Eurostat, 2002; Karakosta, 2005). "Support the Institution of the Family" seems to be the slogan of the Hellenes; fully 94% of the Hellenes who are married for more than ten years do not get a divorce. Marriages seem to be timeless and exceptionally stable; 96% of Hellenes age of 18-49 value the family above all else in their lives (Symeonidou, 2005).The existence of children in a family functions as a restraint to the couple considering the dissolution of their marriage. Also, most of the time a divorce leads to another marriage.

Family Customs and Traditions

The influence of customs and manners of the people affects marriage rates, also. During leap years, which popular tradition considers as unlucky, there is an apparent reduction in the number of weddings. The influence of religion and tradition is also obvious in the performance of weddings in the church. During Great Lent, which lasts for 40 days before Easter, weddings are not performed in churches. People have maintained these principles since Byzantium and they do not want to break them.

It is characteristic of Hellenic culture that almost every expression of social life, such as celebrations, feasts, or gatherings, is related to religion. This kind of family gathering is very important for the unity of the family and contributes to the creation of the family's identity. People cannot imagine celebrating family feasts, Christmas or Easter without spending time with their family and their own people.

Members of the family today are more and more likely to spend time and go out together for lunch or for having fun. They also enjoy staying at home, inviting friends into their home or going to their friends' place to spend time together. The kin and network of *its own people* support the nuclear family through life challenges and the daily routine, and also provides enjoyable leisure times together. In watching a favorite television show, especially a football game or an event of national or international importance, the entire family and also many friends will gather around the set in order to enjoy the event together. Communication works, even if there are arguments and preferences.

The need for contact has also created a love of cell phones. The Hellenes are fans of cell phones but not of the internet. When the mobile telephone first started in the country in 1993, it was expected to first cover the needs of business and other enterprises. Today, all the members of the family are likely to own a cell phone. The love of parents for their children runs from being protective to dominating. This explains the wish of the parents to buy cell phones for their children, even if they are in elementary school. Thus, they could have a kind of control and know where the children are at any moment or to see if they are well. Surveys indicate that 93% of all young people own a cell phone and 96.1% of those age 18-24 (Vaggelis, 2005). By comparison, the use of the Internet is not common for communication among family and friends. In Hellas the Internet has the lowest level of usage by individuals because 65% of the population has no basic computer skills (EU25, 37%) and 82% of the population is not regularly using computers or the Internet (Eurostat, 2006). Being with friends and spending time with the family or the clan is the biggest priority. Whatever distances one from close human relationships is not acceptable (Morihovitis, 1982).

A very good excuse for being together with family and the friends is food. Meals together constitute an important aspect of our culture. All the big events in society or with family are accompanied with food. Everything that happens in life can be a good reason for a quick or more sophisticated meal. Weddings, funerals, baptisms, and celebrations are only some of the reasons. The invitation for a lunch or dinner, even for a cup of coffee, is a pretext for gathering and communication. This has always been a *return* in our way of thinking: a remembrance of the past, a contact with the present and a quest for the future together. The word *epistrofi* (return) in the Hellenic language includes the word *strofi* (turn) which includes the word *trofi* (food) (see the 2004 film *A Touch of Spice* written and directed by Tassos Boulmetis). Young couples with their children quite often go for lunch at their parents' home. The image of being together with three generations every Sunday is not a rare occasion. Mothers cook and send home-made traditional food to their children who are students or work in another city or even abroad. This is not only an expression of the care of the mother, but also the preservation of a traditional old way of maintaining the family bond. Even though in our days fast food has invaded our quick-paced life, a woman who is a good cook is the reason to gather family and friends at home. It is not accidental that in any part of the world when the Hellenes emigrate they run a successful restaurant.

During the last two decades of the previous century, the facts were disappointing because the cultural and financial shock Hellas experienced during that period of time was unexpected and intense. In this millennium, it has been observed that there is an impressive return of the new generation to its cultural roots. Many families left their homes in the 1970s, migrating outside Hellas or migrating inside Hellas, as they attempted to improve their chances in the future. Many villages were devastated and only elderly people stayed at home to keep the past alive. The generation who left to live in another city or country tried to keep contacts with family and friends. They organized themselves together in their new communities, retaining customs and traditions from home. For important occasions, holidays and feasts they returned to the home place to reunite with their roots and the members of their family and friends who stayed behind. The distance has never been an obstacle to the maintenance of cohesion (Kataki, 1998). Today, the third generation rediscovers their roots in a more forceful way, using their memories of childhood and a conscious feeling of elation in regard to their traditional values. Many Hellenes own a house at their place of origin (Moussourou, 1985). An impressive 77% of Hellenes state they are fully connected with the village or city of their origin (EU25, 53%) (Eurobarometer 62, 2004).

Their circle of their relatives and friends grows bigger and bigger. The collective expressions bring back valuable memories, but also they invest their future in an environment which is based on timeless values. This creates a resistance to the new trends of modern life.

BASIC ELEMENTS OF MODERN FAMILY STRENGTHS

We have referred briefly to the main elements which have had a continued presence in Hellenism. These elements are still present today. They have changed of course–they have developed a new face, they have assimilated other elements, and they have adjusted to the needs of the modern society and life. All the following elements coexist, march together, help and complement each other–religion, heritage, cultural identity, tradition, customs, and language. It seems that there is a strong attitude among Hellenes, more than other Europeans, for maintaining religion, family and traditional values, to preserve the cultural and religious homogeneity of the country (Nassopoulos, 2003).

Orthodox Christianity composed one of the common elements of our identity during the last two thousand years. In spite of social, political and economic changes, Christianity continues to be the faith of 98% of the Hellenes in the homeland. Religion and family are considered as the most important values. For the people, faith is a constant and unalterable value. It is a view of life which is summed up in knowledge and experience. The Hellenes are the most religious Europeans: 63.7% state that they pray every day or several times a week and 55.5% of them go to church at least once a month (Nassopoulos, 2003); 81% of Hellenes believe in God, giving Hellas the third highest ranking on this dimension among 33 European countries surveyed. There is an affirmation of traditional religious beliefs in the country where the Church has been historically strong (Eurobarometer special, 2005). The Church still uses the language of the gospels and the texts of the holy fathers written in the language of the Hellenistic period (3rd–6th centuries A.D.). This is an important fact that speaks to the vitality and power of the faith. The Hellenic language has become the main expression-bearer of Orthodoxy. At the end of the first century, the historical future of Christianity was in the Hellenes' hands. The four gospels, written in Greek have been a work of the Hellenic communities (Zizioulas, 1976). Ion Dragoumis (1878-1920), the theoretician of modern Hellenic culture, stated: "Where ten Hellenes are found, they make a community. They collect money and they build a church. Then they bring first a priest and second their wives. Then they gather money from the masses and build a school. Hellenism is a family of Hellenic communities" (Metallinos, 2004).

The sacraments and the ecclesiastical feasts held in commemoration of the saints create a social dynamic as popular and unconstrained as meetings of the family. The social activities concerning the family are almost always performed through religion and not through the state.

Faith and worship are not just a simple religious expression, but they are part of the social dynamics within the family, as natural and unconstrained links. Families who live around and in the life of the Church are proven to be very resistant to the challenges of the present. They have developed a remarkable resilience and tenacity in opposing the degenerative phenomena of modern society. The majority of families with many children are very religious and these beliefs create very strong family ties.

Marriage in the Orthodox Church has a sacred, mystic and indestructible character. Its sanctity is the essence of man and woman living together; it is the foundation of the family. Though the state has enacted civil marriage since 1983, the overwhelming majority of Hellenes prefer to get married in the Church. During the early years after civil marriage was enacted, some couples chose a civil ceremony, but were likely to soon follow with a religious ceremony, also. Today, civil marriage is adopted mainly by couples of mixed nationality and religion, because a mixed marriage is not allowed in a church, according to Orthodox Christian rules. Youth are likely to demonstrate that they want to keep their connections with the Church and tradition, despite all the negative influences.

Giving the first names of grandparents to the children is a tradition, which has been kept alive for three thousand years. In an ancient Macedonian tomb near Thessaloniki in northern Hellas, visitors can see where several generations were buried over a 200-year period. The later generations are named after the first names of their grandparents. The same tradition exists in modern times, but the names are only given in the Church through baptism and they have to be Christian names.

The interspersed feasts of names during the entire Orthodox Christian year give a new direction and dimension in time. Namedays are a special and important part of Hellenic life. Every Orthodox Hellene is named after a saint. When the Orthodox Church is commemorating a saint, anyone with the same name celebrates the same day. Name days are considered much more important than a person's birthday. It is a tradition that when a person has a nameday, relatives and friends visit the individual without an invitation. This is a wonderful way for a family to gather and a charming aspect of the Hellenic life.

The role that the English language plays today worldwide is a role the Hellenic language played for many centuries. This is something that Hellenes do not forget. The ancient language is part of our culture and identity; it is a motivation for our survival. We are proud of our language, which has been cultivated with no interruption for 4,000 years and still lives and evolves. Consequently, it has developed rich and expressive possibilities. Our language is spoken by 98.5% of the population. The mother tongue is learned in the family and the primary teacher is the mother. Language is the tool through which virtue and traditional values pass to the next generation. It is also the first code that allows someone to get acquainted with another person, which is not only the individual's achievement but also an achievement of the culture. Language is the vehicle that helps human beings achieve a peaceful coexistence with each other (Glykatzi-Arveler, 1998).

Today, the meaning of a picture is stronger than that of language. Nevertheless, the meanings of words in the Hellenic language, which come from the philosophical skepticism of our ancient ancestors, strengthen the backbone of the family. In Hellenic language, ethics are not only morals, manners and customs, but also *ethos*–the environment in which humans organize their life, and, thus, *ethos* becomes the center of culture, security, communication. The meaning of the noble words and ideas coming from our forebears support the continuation of the culture, the ties with the past and bonds with traditional values. It is the means to preserve our heritage. Mother has always been the axon around which the family rotated. Even in ancient times, when the woman's role was downgraded, the female genus had a strong presence, hidden under its obvious weakness. The Hellenic language is characterized by genders: male, female and neutral. It is characteristic that the words which express strong feelings, high-spirited ideas or expressions of the intellectual nature of the human race are of the female gender (nature, democracy, liberty, policy, sense, love, affection, protection, power, language, religion, tradition, science, philosophy, music, poetry and so forth).

Family strengths have always played a prime role in the formation of our national identity. The old is continuously mixed with the new, it is combined or differentiated, adjusted or rejected. The cultural memories and the experience of a traditional way of living are still vivid. On the other hand, new ideas and experience of other people enrich our cultural background and expand our ability to create and synthesize. The family is steeped in tradition. Tradition survives into our contemporary reality and embraces the historic changes, which happen outside and inside the family's space, continuously adjusting to the new circumstances.

Young people contribute to the preservation of the relatively strict roles in the family. They accept and enforce traditional values, such as respect, *philotimo*, helping the members of the family, obligations to the elder or the younger members, and faith in God. The preservation of tradition and customs is also upheld by the Hellenes of the Diaspora, who, via this preservation of culture, keep their bonds with their homeland and whatever this means for each one of them personally. For example, it is characteristic that the young Hellenes who were born and live in Germany participate with passion in every event which declares their Hellenic identity in comparison with all the other nationalities (Macedonian Press Agency, 2005). The Greek immigrants in Australia brought to their new homeland a powerful sense of the family and still maintain their spiritual and traditional bonds with Hellas (Voice of Greece, 2005). Fully 80% of the Hellenes feel *very proud* of their heritage (EU25, 46%) and 16% more state that they are *fairly proud* (Eurobarometer 64, 2005).

A PERPETUAL CIRCLE

During the last decade, a return to the traditional values of the family has been observed. Traditional values are most prominent in Hellas in a comparison group of 15 European nations. However, respect for tradition does not mean that everything should go back to the way it used to be (Eurobarometer flash, 2000). The rapid transformation of society, which had disputed many of these values, tends to be slowing. The family returns to what Hellenism has always meant: movement, creation, openness to *others*. During its historical course, the Hellenic family has proven to be particularly strong, based on the same axons of stability. Upon these ideas were founded the ancient Hellenes, the holy fathers of Byzantium and popular wisdom. Family life and life in society are among the main reasons that make Hellas a popular country for people to live in (Macedonian Press Agency, 2004).

A German man, the friend of a friend, who had traveled all over the world as a manager of a large German automobile factory, came to believe that every time he visited Hellas, the country was in chaos. But when he retired, he decided to live here. When asked why he decided to do this, he replied: "Do you know what I have finally realized? Yes, Hellas is in chaos, but you the Hellenes are the best managers of chaos."

REFERENCES

Balourdos, D. (2005). Crisis of the family and demographic transformations: Theoretical quest and empirical models. In *The social portrait of Greece 2003-2004* (pp. 54-55). Athens: National Centre for Social Research, Institute of Social Policy.
Bournelis, A. (2004). *Holy father logos: St. Chrysostom upbringing of the children.*

Campbell, J., & Sherrard, P. (1968). *Modern Greece*. New York/Washington, DC: Frederick A. Praeger.

Elytis, O. (1999). *Maria Nepheli*. Athens: Publishing House IKAROS.

Eurobarometer 62 (2004, Autumn). *National analysis for Hellas*. Retrieved on August 4, 2006 from http://europa.eu.int/comm/public_opinion/index_en.htm

Eurobarometer 64 (2005, Autumn). National analysis for Hellas and national report, executive summary, Greece. Retrived on August 6, 2006 from http://europa.eu.int/comm/public_opinion/index_en.htm

Eurobarometer flash (2000). European documentation. How Europeans see themselves: Looking at the mirror with public opinion surveys. Retrieved on July 29, 2006 from http://europa.eu.int/comm/publications

Eurobarometer special. (2005, June). Social values, science and technology. Retrieved on August 3, 2006 from http://europa.eu.int/comm/public_opinion/index_en.htm

Eurostat. (2002, March 17). Statistics in focus: First results of the demographic data collection for 2001 in Europe. Retrived on August 7, 2006 from from http://epp.eurostat.ec.europa.eu

Eurostat. (2006a, June). News release, 83. The e-society in 2005. Statistics in focus 17/2006 "How skilled are Europeans in using computers and the Internet?" Retrieved August 4, 2006 from http://epp.eurostat.ec.europa.eu

Eurostat. (2006b, June). Statistics in focus, 17. How skilled are Europeans in using computers and the Internet? Retrieved August 4, 2006 from http://epp.eurostat.ec.europa.eu

Georgas, D. (1994, Dec 1-3). Structure and function of the Hellenic family, and Family and family policies in a changing world. Introductions of plenary and work groups in Pan-Hellenic Congress (pp. 17-27). Athens: Eptalophos.

Giannaras, C. (1983). Religion and religiousness. In *Hellenism and Hellenikotita* (pp. 243-248). Athens: Hellenic Society 1, HESTIA, I. D. Kollaros.

Glykatzi-Arveler, H. (1998, May). Conclusions of the Forum. European Forum for the Family, Family–Europe–21st Century: Vision and Institutions. Minutes of the European Forum for the Family (pp. 694-697). Athens: NEA SYNORA.

Godley, A.D. (1925). *Herodotus*, book VIII. London: Loeb, 143-144.

Hourdaki, M. (1995). *The psychology of the family* (3rd Ed.). Athens: Ellinika Grammata.

ICAP TNS. (2005). World Gallup in 64 countries in cooperation with Gallup International Association. Retrieved June, 19, 2005 from http://www.icap.gr/news/index_gr_7153.asp

Kalliakmanis, V. (2005). *The ecclesiastical character of pastoral theology*. Thessaloniki: Mygdonia.

Karakosta, N. (2005, Aug 14). Difficult time for married people. *Typos tis Kyriakis*, p. 56.

Kataki, H. (1998). *The three identities of the Hellenic family* (8th Ed). Athens: Ellinika Grammata.

Kyrkos, V. (1974). The ecumenicity of the Hellenic civilization and its meeting with Christianity. In *History of the Hellenic Nation*, vol. 6 (pp. 392-395). Athens: Ekdotiki Athinon.

Macedonian Press Agency. (2004). The world in 2005: *The Economist's* annual compilation of forecasts. *Economist Newspaper Limited*. Retrieved on November 11, 2004 from http://mpa.gr

Macedonian Press Agency. (2005). Germany: More than 50% of the young immigrants run the risk of not being incorporated. Retrieved January 12, 2005 from http://www.mpa.gr

Metallinos, G. (2003, July 18). Globalization and Hellenic Orthodox ecumenicity. *Orthodox Press*, issue 1513, pp. 1-2.

Metallinos, G. (2004). Orthodoxy and modern Hellenic identity. A speech at the Popular University of the Church, Athens. Retrieved March 8, 2005 from http://www.ecclesia.gr

Ministry of the Commercial Fleet of Hellas. (2001). Statistics: Commercial fleet–currency. Retrieved July 17, 2006, from http://ego.yen.gr

Morihovitis, G. (2001). *Sociology of the modern family* (2nd Ed.). Florina : I. Aristeidou.

Moussourou, L. (1984). *The Hellenic family*. Athens: Goulandri–Horn Foundation.

Moussourou, L. (1985). *Family and child in Athens: Results of an empirical study*. Athens: Hellenic Society 5, HESTIA, I.D. Kollaros & Co.

Moussourou, L. (1993). *Sociology of the modern family*. Athens: Library of Social Science and Social Policy, Gutenberg

Nassopoulos, D. (2003, Nov 6). Policy-society-citizens. *TA NEA*, p. 12.

Papadioti-Athanassiou, B. (1994, Dec 1-3). Hellenes' students position on the institution of the family. Introductions of plenary and work groups in Pan-Hellenic Congress, Athens (pp. 157-167). Athens: Eptalophos.

Patterson, C. B. (1998). The family in Greek history. Cambridge, MA: Harvard University Press.

Quasten, H. (1960). *Patrology*, vol. III. Westminster, MD: The Newman Press.

Runciman, S. (1969). *The Byzantine civilization*. Translation by D. Degiorgi. Athens: Galaxias Hermeias

Sakellariou, M. (1976). *History of the Hellenic nation*, vol. C2 (pp. 87-90). Athens: Ekdotiki Athinon.

Symeonidou, H. (1998, May). The welfare state and the families in the countries of Southern Europe. The case of Hellas. European Forum for the Family, Family–Europe–21st Century: Vision and Institutions. Minutes of the European Forum for the Family (pp. 341-345). Athens: NEA SYNORA.

Symeonidou, H. (2005). *Settlement and dissolution of the family relations in Hellas*. In *The Social Portrait of Greece 2003-2004* (pp. 59-65). Athens: Centre for Social Research, Institute of Social Policy.

Vagellis, T. (2005, Feb). The Hellenes love the cell phones. Retrieved February 2, 2005 from http://news.ert.gr.

Vagellis, T. (2005, May). Hi tech and stressed. Retrieved May 27, 2005 from http://news.ert.gr.

Varidaki, L. (1994, Dec 1-3). *Nationality and family cure*. Introductions of plenary and work groups in Pan-Hellenic Congress, Athens (pp. 579-587). Athens: Eptalophos.

Voice of Greece (2005). Australian newspaper praises the Hellenes migrants. Retrieved on July 29, 2005, from www.voiceofgreece.gr

Walker, A. (1998, May). *Old age, the generations, and the family*. European Forum for the Family, Family–Europe–21st Century: Vision and Institutions. Minutes from the European Forum for the Family, Athens (pp. 140-151). Athens: NEA SYNORA.

Weir Smyth, H. (1956). *Aeschylus.* Aeschylus with an English translation, vol. I . London: Loeb, pp. 142-145.

Zirganos, N. (2005, June 19). Raining in Brussels, catching a cold in Athens. *Kyriakatiki Eleftherotypia,* p. 6.

Zizioulas, J. (1976). *History of the Hellenic nation,* vol. 6. Athens: Ekdotiki Athinon, pp. 142-145.

doi:10.1300/J002v41n03_08

Family Strengths in Romania

Bogdan Nadolu
Ioana Delia Nadolu
Sylvia M. Asay

SUMMARY. Romania is situated in the southeast of Central Europe with more than two millennia of agitated history. The main dimensions of the Romanian cultural model are represented by Latinity and Christianity and have involved very consistent principles. This article is focused on the specific aspects of the Romanian family and its present transformation under major structural changes in the socio-cultural context. In Romanian contemporary society there are two main types of effects that were generated by communism in the middle of the 20th century and by the rediscovery of democracy in 1989. The Romanian family has supported the consequences of these events, first by the abusive insertion of state control into the domestic sphere and second by the necessity of redeveloping self-reliant capacities for family survival. Under the

Bogdan Nadolu, PhD, is Lecturer, Department of Sociology, West University of Timisoara, Bd. V. Parvan, No. 4, Timisoara 300223, Romania (E-mail: bnadolu@socio.uvt.ro). Ioana Delia Nadolu, PhD, is Lecturer, Department of Anthropology, West University of Timisoara, Bd. V. Parvan, No. 4, Timisoara 300223, Romania (E-mail: deliailie@socio.uvt.ro). Sylvia M. Asay, PhD, is Associate Professor of Family Studies, University of Nebraska, Otto Olsen Hall 205 A, Kearney, NE 68849, USA (E-mail: asays@unk.edu).

Address correspondence to: Sylvia M. Asay.

[Haworth co-indexing entry note]: "Family Strengths in Romania." Nadolu, Bogdan, Ioana Delia Nadolu, and Sylvia M. Asay. Co-published simultaneously in *Marriage & Family Review* (The Haworth Press, Inc.) Vol. 41, No. 3/4, 2007, pp. 419-446; and: *Strong Families Around the World: Strengths-Based Research and Perspectives* (ed: John DeFrain, and Sylvia M. Asay) The Haworth Press, Inc., 2007, pp. 419-446. Single or multiple copies of this article are available for a fee from The Haworth Document Delivery Service [1-800-HAWORTH, 9:00 a.m. - 5:00 p.m. (EST). E-mail address: docdelivery@haworthpress.com].

Available online at http://mfr.haworthpress.com
© 2007 by The Haworth Press, Inc. All rights reserved.
doi:10.1300/J002v41n03_09

pressure of continuous change in the social context, the contemporary family has valuable resources inherent in traditional Romanian culture and in the family's internal strengths. doi:10.1300/J002v41n03_09 *[Article copies available for a fee from The Haworth Document Delivery Service: 1-800-HAWORTH. E-mail address: <docdelivery@haworthpress.com> Website: <http://www.HaworthPress.com> © 2007 by The Haworth Press, Inc. All rights reserved.]*

KEYWORDS. Communist alterations, extended family, nuclear family, mono-parental model, marital roles, Romanian family

INTRODUCTION

To talk about family can seem, at a first glance, a common topic. Everyone is connected with this, more or less, directly or indirectly, in a classical or innovative way, sometimes favorable and other times not favorable. But this is exactly the complexity of the topic. Although the family, as a social institution, can be considered a total social fact, its manifestations and concrete forms appear at a global level to reflect overwhelming diversity with considerable implications. Cultural models, community resources, economic development, social policies, formal education, the mass media, co-aging groups, and individual personality are just a few of the factors generating this diversity and they accentuate the dynamics of transformation and adjustment for each kind of family. Based on these factors, there are also clusters of various types of manifestations into patterns that are well structured and relatively stable in time and space.

Starting with these considerations and using a sociological approach, we invite you during the following pages to an anthropological description of the Romanian family in the multiple forms of its contemporary evolution. Continuing from this introductory information we will try to describe Romania from geographical, historical, and socio-demographic perspectives. After that we will outline a general view of the structural and functional modifications in the typology of the contemporary family, under the direct influences of transformations present in Romanian society and the cultural modeling of the birth rate and its direct implications. The final section will focus on the strengths of Romanian families.

ROMANIA, A "FAMILIAR AXIS-MUNDI" (FROM LATIN, "THE AXLE OF THE WORLD")

For someone who has not visited Romania, few words can outline an approximate image about this part of the world. Using the most relevant facts, an accurate description can be structured in three distinct dimensions: spatial, temporal and social.

Under the Sign of the Carpathian Arch: The Spatial Dimension

Romania is situated in the southeast of Central Europe, at the middle distance between the *Atlantic Ocean* and Ural Mountains, on the inferior course of the Danube. With a continental-temperate climate, Romania has a surface of 91,843 square miles (238,391 S Km) with varied and proportionate relief, that includes mountains (maximum altitude on Moldoveanu Peak with 2,5400 meters), tablelands, plains, valleys, a seacoast, and a delta. These are grouped relatively concentrically, around the Carpathian Arch. With 2/3 of its boundaries on water (Danube River, Prut River, Tisa River, and the Black Sea), Romania borders the Moldavia Republic, Ukraine, Hungary, Serbia and Bulgaria. Its main relief forms–the Carpathian Mountains and the Danube–have in time become strong cultural elements in the development of national identity and mentalities.

From Myth to History: The Temporal Dimension

Center and *vatra* (at the heart), the Carpathian Arch represents the *athanor* (the alchemist melting pot) where the Romanian people have been conceived, following its historical beginnings. The spatial organization centers around Dacian's *Kogaion* (the sacred mountain of the Dacians), *Axis Mundi* (from Latin, *the axis of the world*) of Romanians, generated archaic mythologies, and modern philosophies. To concentrate a few millennia of agitated history in just a few phrases is a very restrictive approach and we assume its limits.

Stable living in this territory is attested by an extensive series of archaeological sources since the Neolithic period (6,000-5,000 B.C.). During the same time, with the arrival of the Thracian people (an Indo-European civilization which came to the Carpatho-Balkanic basin), the Geto-Dacian tribes were established north of the Danube River, on the actual territory of Romania. The conquest of Dacia by the Romans is considered the first important step in the genesis of the Romanian nation, both from ethnical and cultural perspectives including the assimilation of Christianity as the dominant religion.

Because of its geographical place, with openings both to the Asiatic Steppe and the Arabian Peninsula, the population of this land (grouped in 3 distinct forms of administrative organization: Walachia, Moldavia and Transylvania) has endured many migratory waves, including Goths, Huns, Gepidaes, Avares, Slaves, Tatars, Mongols and later Turks. The successive alterations of native language development by many battles, conquests, and invasions were reflected throughout the Middle Ages. The presence of these new and various cultural models served to consolidate the current profile of the native population, which has gradually become *a Latin island in a Slavic sea*, in essence, a country whose native tongue, Romanian, is a Romance language (derived from Latin) surrounded by countries where the predominate languages are Slavic. During the Middle Ages as in modernity, Romanian principalities have experienced constant and considerable pressures from different geopolitical poles–Austro-Hungary Empire, Ottoman Empire, and the Russian Tsarist Empire–but without a fundamental alteration of the socio-cultural structure of the population.

Full development of the Romanian nation took place only in the 19th and 20th centuries, first by the union of Moldavia with Wallachia (1859) and then by the union of Transylvania with *The Old Kingdom* (1918). In the same period, Romania acquired the profile of modern development, as it participated actively in both World Wars with significant human and economic losses. The natural orientation to a capitalist economic model was abusively interrupted by the oppression of communism in 1947.

During almost half of a century until 1989, Romania suffered through a particularly destructive period. Under this totalitarian regime a major alteration of all macro-social structures and functions, by arbitrary, unlegitimized and non-efficient constraints of inadequate social and economical politics, occurred. Thus, the movement toward massive industrialization from a primarily agrarian society directly correlated with an artificial urbanization and a reorganization of the rural areas. This generated a major alteration in the orientation, consistency and dynamic of social evolution. In this way, newly-generated systems of norms and values were insufficiently grounded and did not validate the complete functionality of new profiles and societal models (e.g., "ruralized" urban communities, or "urbanized" rural communities). The exclusive orientation of the dictatorial regime to create a *communist multi-lateral developed society* that determined social evolution, resources, and expectations by completely and totally ignoring civil society, led to the collapse of the regime and an aggressive resurrection by the *"Revolution from December, 1989"* (the fall of the communist government).

The distortions generated by the communist government are still felt today, after more than 15 years since the "Revolution," both at the economic level and mostly at the social level, including social values. The changing of contexts, principles, values, norms, and mentalities is a difficult process, but has been irreversibly accomplished at a few important levels.

A Land with Its People: The Social Dimension

The demographic perspective. Romania's population is 21.7 million (Romanian Census Year Book, 2004) with a significant declining trend reflected by a negative growth of –0.25% (continuously recorded from 1990, when the population was 23.2 million). From a structural point of view, in 2003 there were 48.8% males and 51.2% females with 53.4% living in urban areas and 46.6% in rural areas. For the same year, for every one thousand people in Romania there were 6.2 marriages (compared with 8.3 in 1990), 9.8 children born (compared with 27.4 in 1967 when the government banned any contraceptive methods and 13.6 in 1990 when the abortions were liberalized) and 1.5 divorces. Another set of population distribution data was is shown for July 1st, 2004 (National Institute of Statistics, 2006) (see Table 1).

TABLE 1. Population demographics.

	2001	2002	2003	2004
Total (millions)	22.4	21.8	21.7	21.7
Gender				
Males	10.9	10.6	10.6	10.6
Females	11.5	11.2	11.1	11.1
Age				
0-14	4	3.8	3.6	3.5
15-59	14.2	13.8	13.9	14
60+	4.2	4.2	4.2	4.2
Residence				
Urban	12.2	11.6	11.6	11.9
Rural	10.2	10.2	10.1	9.8
Middle age	37.4	37.8	38.1	38.3

Population: 21,673,328 citizens
Density: 90.9 persons/ S Km

Source: National Institute of Statistic. Retrieved May 15, 2006 from http://www.insse.ro/ publicatii/Romania_in_cifre.pdf

The socio-cultural perspective. To summarize in just a few words a national cultural model is obviously a rash, risky and subjective prospect. However, we will try to outline an introductory description of the institution of the family in Romania. The Romanian cultural model is the result of a complex evolution, historically validated by tradition of over 2 millennia, with two basic components: Latinity and Christianity. These two main dimensions for Romania involved very consistent principles, with a positive axiological orientation of pro-social trends, citizenship, altruism, transcendental sensibility, dynamism, open mindedness, and a patriarchal profile. Also, the long presence among the Romanian population of two important ethnic minorities, Hungarians and Germans, established a very complex intercultural perspective.

The natural evolution of Romanian society was dramatically altered as a result of the punitive actions of the communist regime, imposed by the geopolitical context for almost a half of century. As we mentioned before, some unjustified social policies were applied without any regard for their effects on Romanian culture and with very complex negative consequences. Thus, the imposition of the communist government along with the destruction of civil society and the trend toward quasi-total control of the state over the life of the individual (with the dramatic diminution of personal freedom), forced urbanization, and artificial industrialization, have all significantly disrupted the models of social relationship and their axiological consistency. Industrialization and urbanization did not have a natural evolution as both were politically imposed, but were implemented with a complete ignorance of Romanian society's sustaining capacities. As a consequence, their limits, non-functionalities, and structural inconsistencies are still observable even 15 years after communism lost political support. One example is the collapse of some so-called "industrial" cities because their industries were too inefficient to keep them active. Also, this artificial development generated many problems for adult generations in regard to professional re-training and accessibility to jobs.

The changing of the communist regime with the Revolution from 1989 signaled the return of individual freedom. The rapid introduction of this new normative context based on democratic principles was not followed by the social confirmation of a system of values. Significant problems still exist concerning the consistency and the coherence of mentalities, especially regarding relationships between generations. However, one can note an extraordinary sensibility toward new West-European models from the public impact of new information technologies to the trends in fashion, from profiles of business to models of marriage. These trends are perceived as adaptable to the traditional cultural model, which is not necessarily in concurrence or in contradiction with them.

The family institution has experienced pressure generated by the alteration of the social context, both in the communist and the post-communist periods, continually trying to develop efficiently-adjusted models in order to survive. Atypical manifestations in the frame of the Romanian nuclear family were elaborated in the communist period and are now suppressed and changed to complementary forms, which are more efficient and viable for a society in which the contemporary mark, *the quick changes*, are completely integrated.

What Has Remained from the Classical Typology of Families?

In order to make a pertinent analysis of the strength of the contemporary marital models, it is necessary to review the evolution during the two main waves of basic changes suffered by Romanian society; the imposition of the dictatorial regime and the re-achievement of democracy. For the first half of last century, before communism was imposed on the society, we can talk about two dominant marital models in Romanian society: the extended family and the nuclear family. Both forms have a number of common characteristics: strong feelings of kinship (ascendant and descendant), high stability in the hierarchy of marital roles with a predominant patriarchal distribution of power, an important value regarding the appropriateness of the traditions, and, implicitly, permanent and significant confirmation from the community. During this period, direct experience of two World Wars and the impact of military combat that occurred on Romanian territory exerted complex consequences at the socio-demographic and economic levels. However, in the brief time directly before the advent of the dictatorial regime, there was a visible trend of economic capitalism, a well-formed social structure and a complex process of the natural redefinition of social values.

With the aim of achieving communist goals, part of the informal norms elaborated within the traditional cultural model were formalized under a large-scale series of punitive rules which were ultra-restrictive in regard to personal freedom, including marital options. The communist party needed more followers and tried by all means to increase new cohorts and to strictly control their education. Thus, the promotion of early marriage was continued with the collection of a *celibate* tax for unmarried persons older than 25 years. In the traditional model, the *age limit* for marriage was around 20 years for girls and 25 years for boys.

Divorce procedures were very difficult with constant pressure against them.

The strong orientation towards pressure to increase the population has generated some drastic restrictions in this area. Examples include the illegality of abortions since 1967, the prohibition of any contraceptive measures and family planning, supplementary taxes for families without children, and amenities for families with more than three children. Similarly, the state assumed control of formal education, which became compulsory for the first ten years of study and there was pressure to increase household density with the standardized development of apartment buildings and the number of rooms per apartment restricted for smaller families. This is a general preview of life under the communist model, with a significant decrease in personal freedom to make decisions and with the insertion of the state into the domestic realm. Without analyzing in detail the value of these components and their positive and negative consequences, it is clear that the family institution had to adjust itself to a new reality, a less flexible communist world with a strong punitive profile and increased restrictions on personal freedom.

The second wave of changes occurred after almost half a century with the change of the dictatorial regime. The functionality and the efficiency of the marital models were once again disturbed. In 1989 there were adult generations who were completely socialized and had adapted to the Romanian communist model. The state was an active presence in the domestic sphere. The rediscovery of democracy gradually decreased this presence. One example was that abortions and all the contraceptive measures were liberalized and redefined the content of sexual education; all formal restrictions were eliminated. People had personal freedom to make choices now that were previously made by the state.

Learning to assume personal freedom appears to be a difficult and dramatic process, especially if state control was perceived as a support and not as a deficit. The assumption of equality, promoted by the communist model, is now being progressively replaced by the assumption of freedom and the social inequality that results can be very frustrating. The family institution is effected completely by all these new pressures generated by the new socio-cultural contexts (sometimes convergent, other times divergent), and the family has gradually developed functional alternative models. Already after 15 years of democracy, there are young generations of Romanians who have been socialized in non-dictatorial regimes that are now the legal age of marriage. They have the freedom to try any alternative marital model, more or less legitimated by the social context, but with very complex consequences. In the following pages we will try to describe these various various configurations as sources of social power and highlight the main marital models developed in Romania.

Around the Common Table: The Extended Traditional Family

The Romanian extended traditional family has kept a classical profile. Its main characteristics that they share a common residence, strict distribution of some predefined roles, monopoly of power, unitary administration of resources (economic, cultural and societal), consistent emotional and affective support, and utilization of the marital group as a dominant self-identity factor for the development of a significant *conscience of us.* This model was developed in traditional rural communities and has integrated specific values and principles, obtaining a strong social legitimacy. The marital group is well formed and is oriented to an autocratic profile that is strongly valued and receives continuous confirmation from the community. Even economic autonomy was for a long time uncommon, because ownership of land was very limited to only the social elite, the self-control of all available resources, which often-times were insufficient, was a mark of considerable prestige in the community. The transfer of ownership between generations, including material goods and land, was established by traditional rules. Generally, the first-born son implicitly becomes an heir, the other sons receive some *compensation* and the daughters receive dowries.

With high value given to tradition, Romanian extended families assured support for the continuity of the cultural model. A strong sense of respect was promoted for the customs and habits orally transmitted from generation to generation with some elements acquired from the pre-Christian period. This coherence in the protection and conservation of the cultural model has a main role in the continuity of the rural community profile, the lifestyle and in the configuration of the extended family offering enough resources to resist all external pressures.

From the structural point of view, various forms of extended family models have a central power pole that keeps together all other members. In conformity with the patriarchal profile of Christianity, the balance between genders concerning this position has mostly a masculine orientation. The matriarchal profile can have various causes, including the death of the older male, the significant difference between the partners' economic contributions or the growing personal power of the wife. Even if the traditional cultural model usually promotes the patriarchate, the matriarchal alternative has consistent confirmation and integration in rural communities, also.

Usually, the leader (whether male or female) was legitimated by ageing (*gerontocratic*), being represented by one of the old persons of the group (the grandpa or the grandma). This distinction was given both by their group and by the community as a result of a remarkable lifestyle and became an identity model for descendents. This fact is reflected also in the actual trend in rural areas to call a person by using the name or the nickname of such a referential ascendant (parent, grandparent or grand-grandparent) such as John of Anna (for John, the Anna's son). Complementary to the gerontocratic profile, there were situations when the central status of the group is held by the person who makes a more consistent contribution to family maintenance, usually by the adult male who is employed. Thus, the leadership of the marital group was not any more established by the age criteria, but by the person that keep one's family. These cases were accentuated especially by the economical trend that was increased into the communism period: the development of the industries.

The extended family still has a main component of Romanian society, however today its foundations are not the same and its presence is reduced by the appearance of other new models.

"We," the Center of the Universe (The Nuclear Family)

Another widespread marital model in Romanian society is represented by the nuclear family (the two-parent family). This was developed as a necessary and valuable marital alternative, especially because of urbanization and industrialization during the communist period. For some time, the Romanian nuclear marital model has been perceived as an adequate answer to some political interests of the dictatorial regime. Thus, its decreased size with only two adults and children, assured direct social control and, at the same time, prevented the risk of divergent structures. Its promotion as a desirable marital model also assured relative social uniformity, with complementary confirmation of the equalitarian principle, which was so intensely affirmed by communist propaganda.

On the basis of these so-called "advantages," an artificially-sustained system was developed that was dedicated to place the nuclear family in a favorable light at the individual level with both symbolic and material rewards. For example, supports were offered by the state for families with more than three children, including priority for various services. Formal control against marital behavior that was not in conformity with the classical nuclear family model was instituted. Taxes and public opprobrium for celibates and couples without children were instituted, a very complicated and long procedure for divorce developed, and a complete interdiction of any methods of birth control were put in place. Thus, the family with many children became a major ideal for life, continuously promoted by President Ceaușescu and the communist party: "The higher patriotic and civic duty of each family is to have and to bring up children. It can not be conceived to be a family without children" (Mitrofan 1984, p. 106).

Complementary with this axiological promotion of the nuclear family, a supportive institutional mechanism was developed that, by deep interventions in the domestic space, tried to solve some specific needs. Thus, the formal educational system was given the authority to have care of the children from the third month of life and in exchange, both parents could continue their professional activities without having to depend on other family members, especially grandparents. More than that, the system of child care (the crèche and the kindergarten) developed several options: a reduced program (just 4 hours per day), an extensive program (8 hours per day, including meals and sleeping time) and a weekly program (when children could stay from Monday to Saturday). Thus, the educational functions of the family could be substituted (more or less) by the state. Medical assistance and an extension of the sanitation system also increased support to the nuclear family by taking over these tasks. Also, if we take into account the fact that both partners were employed, not necessarily as personal options but because of an official imperative, we have a generalized picture of the nuclear marital model during the communist period.

In a brief presentation its details can be grouped as follows: The parents were employed, and each made a similar contribution to the family income. This generated a reconfiguration of the resources of power to an egalitarian profile, in dissonance with the traditional patriarchal model. The time spent in the domestic space was significantly decreased, legitimizing the taking over of some fundamental functions of the family by adjacent social institutions. In conformity with European principles concerning work, all employees benefit from a month of vacation yearly, but the opportunities to spend the free time were limited to the Romanian territory (in the health resorts on the Black Sea, in various mountain locations, with relatives, and so forth).

The children were integrated into a formal educational system that started from the first months of life, but no later than four years and was compulsory until 16 years. The state educational system generalized and homogenized at the level of the entire country, assured full compatibility among various schools and a very facile transfer from school to school for scholars. A universal, non-discriminative pattern for individual performance was also developed.

Living in urban areas was oriented mostly to the blocks, with a standard profile for the apartments (with 1 to 4 rooms) and with undifferentiated access inside the community to services, such as cold water, warm water (usually just a few hours weekly), heat (under the minimum needed), electricity (generally with a daily program of energy-saving for a few hours) and partial telephone use. The house equipments were also limited to those available on the communist market: black-and-white television (color television appeared in the second half of the 1980s, with very restrictive access), refrigerator, stove and a non-automatic washing machine. The strict limitation of options for space and inside configuration assured a relative egalitarian level among families. The personalization of the domestic space was almost integrally an aesthetic problem.

The prohibition and the interdiction of any actions of family planning, including the illegality of abortions, represented a strong insertion of the state into the marital realm. The high positive birth rate was also sustained by an inconsistent and insufficient sexual education and culture. The punitive restrictions imposed, by law, against any personal choice or wishes and independent of personal situations, resources, or family conditions was one of the most aberrant communist principles for Romanian families. This dramatic limitation of personal freedom of choice (sacrificed for an idealized equality) was also reflected in the procedure of divorce, which was very difficult and took a long period of time, coupled with strong official blame against it.

The behavioral limitations imposed by the dictatorial regime and almost complete acceptance and permanent self-censuring under the direct threat of the political police caused a legitimization in the promotion and development of a lifestyle that was ultra-positivist, actively atheistic, explicitly antireligious and focused on economic and production outcomes.

Another distinct characteristic of the Romanian nuclear family model was represented by the strong support assured by continuing a relationship with the family of origin and with the spiritual world of common traditions and rituals (not only in rural areas, but also in urban areas where some traditions were adjusted and kept). This contact with an alternative cultural universe, that was continually confirmed, in many experiences from childhood, offered the nuclear family the necessary strength and resources to exceed all the constraints, the limitations and the difficulties generated by a political regime focused on the constant control of all details.

Today, social and political changes generate the revitalization of individual freedom, diversity and alternatives. Homogeneity (more or less artificial) continues to decrease, but with axiological conflicts in all systems. The new socio-cultural contexts such as new marital roles, new marital models and new lifestyles constitute major changes from inside of the family institution.

I Bring Up Him/Her; They're Mine: The Exclusive Mono-Parental Family

The third component of marital typology established in Romanian communist society is represented by the single-parent family. Even though the frequency of this model was significantly decreased, its existence and its characteristics cannot be ignored. This family was formed by a parent (usually mother) and one or many children, born inside of a marriage (which ended by a divorce or by death) or children born outside of a formal marriage such as in cohabitation. As we mentioned before, communist policy did not permit complete freedom for personal choice concerning conjugal life. However, divorces were not completed negated by the state and some marriages were dissolved in this way. In spite of these difficulties, formal support offered by the state for the care and education of these children did exist and assured minimal social protection to the single-parent family.

From a complementary perspective, the cultural profile of Romanian society (with strong conservative tendencies) has exerted constant pressure on these single-parent families, making it very difficult, especially when the children were from a cohabitating relationship. This explicit intolerance resulted in directly generating a decrease in the social life of the single parents. The direct consequence of this frequent negative feedback exerted mostly by the community correlated with financial difficulties led to a decrease in social life and forced the single parent to live a private lifestyle. The parent focused on the children's education instead of her own interest in marriage and failed many times because of this ultra-protective approach, generally with unexpected effects. The concurrence among the agents of socialization determined significant dissonances and sometime even intergenerational conflicts that were both latent and manifest.

Beyond all these limits and dysfunctional aspects, the single-parent family shows a consistent strength, exceeding in an optimal way all the internal and external difficulties, even though they are more or less seen as an unfavorable socio-cultural medium. The capacity to accomplish in a single conjugal role all the tasks of a couple but with just a half of social resources is, undoubtedly, a remarkable success. Even with minimal support from the formal institutions especially formal education, credit belongs to single parents for keeping this model alive socially. Today, the one-parent family has become a normal presence in Romanian society. Together with decreasing discriminatory pressure from the community there is a significant reduction in the supportive elements offered by the state. The changing socio-cultural context has generated new problems and challenges, now even more complex, for this family model.

These three family models can be considered representative of the Romanian family institution prior to the revolution in 1989. The specific configurations developed into the framework of each model have assured adequate answers to the problems generated by an oppressive context, without any consideration for the manifestation of personal freedom. In the following pages we will present an anthropological analysis of the evolution of contemporary Romanian marital models.

Typological Metamorphoses

The revolution of December 1989 marked the end of a difficult period of communist dictatorship, opening for Romania a long and controversial path to democracy. From a formal point of view and at the institutional level, all the macro-structures needed for an authentic democratic system were quickly developed. But at societal levels the values content, normative systems and configuration of specific behavioral models are not yet completely formed. The substantial modification of mentalities, getting passed the implicit resistance to change and identification of optimal structures and profiles are very complex processes with full impact in the domestic space. The classical typology of the family (with the three main models presented above) is now in a deep reconfiguration, with adjustments and replacements by various innovations and attempts, verified in everyday life.

In contemporary Romanian society two antagonistic trends can be evidenced: the orientation to family and the domestic group versus an orientation against the family and recognized marital patterns. The first case is about support offered by a standard social structure, well-known as socialization. In an incoherent context with many doubts and major alterations of social rationality and desirable behaviors, along with critical economic difficulties, the person can find the *classical* marital group an accessible refuge and a very stable support.

In the second case, it is about the assumption and the application of individual freedom by denying some marital patterns that were developed in the old reality. The classical family models are perceived as coming from an obsolete socio-cultural context and thus, are insufficient and dysfunctional in the new Romanian society. Some implicit conditions are denied such as the *necessity* to make cohabitation official, the pressure for beginning a marital relationship at a young age, the expectations of procreation, the assumption of some discriminatory conjugal roles, and the subordination of personal expectations at the expense of the couple who remains married.

Some alternative marital behaviors and configurations are being tried, such as an increase in the age for first marriage and child bearing; the priority of the career and professional activities over conjugal tasks; the redefinition of the conjugal role; the introduction of the marital alternatives, especially cohabitation; and easier separation for dysfunctional conjugal couples. From these new perspectives we present the main changes that have occurred in the structure, function, and configuration of the extended, nuclear and mono-parental families.

The Extended Family:
Where There Are More, the Power Is Increasing

Economic difficulties, including the high prices of houses and rent determine in many situations the impossibility of leaving the parents' home after marriage. Sometimes, even when this departure has occurred, young families come back to parents, usually after some unhappy events such as divorce, unemployment or economical difficulties. In other cases, because of difficult situations, relatives come to live together to offer or request help in solving specific problems such as to take care of an old or ill family member or to live together during the time a they are attending college. Thus, the *intermittent extended family* is formed where several generations are cohabitating temporarily but for a significant period (Ilut, 2005). This situation is not fully desirable and is a response to insufficient resources. The family structure is extended with the addition of one or more new members and they have to adjust their rules, habits and behaviors. All these changes are temporary and create specific stresses as the family accommodates to the new situation and then re-accommodates to the previous situation.

In other cases, parents or grandparents that are too old or too poor to care for themselves live together with the younger family members. The intergenerational exchanges elaborated by this kind of extended family can be structured along four distinct dimensions: (1) money, goods and foods, (2) counseling and advice, (3) care, moral and affective support, (4) services, housekeeping, farm work and care of children (Tirhas, 2003; Ilut, 2005). These exchanges are based on offer and demand between generations, with compensatory roles, adequate for their socio-demographical profile. If inside of a traditional cultural model, the extended family represents an optimal configuration for the contemporary Romanian society it can adapt to meet some very problematic economic situations. This is done even with the discomfort of the cohabitation of several generations, usually in insufficient living space with very limited resources and significant divergences of mentality between the generations. Beyond all of these, the reconfiguration of the extended Romanian family assures the survival of its members in a very difficult and unfavorable economic context.

A direct consequence of this situation is represented by the reactivation of the parental network (the kinship system), not necessarily just as a mark of identity, but for specific material support. In the beginning of rural-urban migration, the main role of the parental network was for personal social integration, especially for educational and professional orientations. Now the parental network can sometimes offer a similar support for work and emigration to a foreign country (often to Western Europe, but also to the Near East).

The contemporary extended family of Romania represents in many cases a viable solution for sustaining its members in an economic crisis. The regrouping of several generations around a common home gives a strong confirmation of the traditional cultural model. Nevertheless, since the main reason for living together is the result of material need, it can be expected that in better economic times this contemporary extended family will be less in evidence.

The Nuclear Family: The Loneliness of Two

The nuclear marital model is the most affected by the socio-cultural and economical changes suffered at the present time in Romania. On one hand, as we mentioned before, the expansion of the extended family comes as a detriment to the nuclear couple. On the other hand, the homogenous character of the nuclear model is now under significant innovative pressures to make some structural adjustments or even a total replacement with other contemporary marital alternatives (marriage without children, cohabitation single parents, and celibacy). In Romania cohabitation is not yet a significant alternative. Just 4.6% of the population older than 15 years is cohabiting, according to the 2002 Census, which studied this issue for the first time. For the analysis of the *new* Romanian nuclear family we will focus on one particular type with major social implications, the couple without children.

Increased life expectancy and the generalization of a new trend of young adults leaving their parents have generated a new stage in the life of the family group, the return to a single conjugal couple (the empty nest). Even though this is a common stage in contemporary family evolution, because of the economic restrictions for living space in Romania, it is not yet representative (Ilut, 2005). Nevertheless, this new kind of couple living together without children is a specific pattern, with specific needs, rules and resources and can become, in a short time, a significant presence in Romanian society, also.

Making career a priority. Today, the extension of private business activities, has determined a new approach to the professional career. The personal choice concerning this domain, the multitude of occupational alternatives, the dynamic of new jobs and the real chance for success are some of the new fundamentals of employment. The abandonment of the standard pattern of work imposed by the state (a single job with 44-48 hours of work weekly, 11 months a year and a stable salary) has accentuated personal control and responsibility over career building. Spending a great deal of time at work with one or more extra part-time jobs, with an irregular schedule but with adequate benefits, is not an unusual situation anymore. In this situation, conjugal life is subordinate to the professional career and parental roles are not a priority. For these couples, becoming parents is considerably delayed, causing other problems when the distance between generations becomes too great.

Cultural and educational gaps in sex education. Another type of nuclear family without children is generated by the absence of a modern affective-sexual culture. The traditional model with its taboos and with its methods and cures is not functional any more. But there still are the hyper-authoritarian parents who try to induce their children to attitudes of guilt that have a direct impact on the personality of the future adult, who consequently adopts an anxious and inhibited erotic-sexual attitude:

The preconceived ideas concerning masculine and feminine sexual roles are reflections of normative models, which are frequently obsolete from cultural, moral and social points of view, but that continue to act from the subconscious and unconscious fields of the individual. (Mitrofan, 1991, p. 96)

In this kind of family, the sexual-affective life is based on a natural or instinctive approach, because of vague, naïve and disturbed informaïtion. Religious fanaticism and high moral precepts serve to accentuate feelings of timidity, guilt and shame rather than help counsel the couple in areas of sexuality. If the traditional social norm of timidity, guilt and shame is seen as decency, inside the conjugal couple it becomes a behavioral failure, generates unjustified inhibitions and a lack of communication (Mitrofan, 1991). In this kind of family, usually if timidity, guilt and shame can be overcome, the couple is ready to accept the most advanced procreation treatments and techniques. These difficulties are not caused by closed-mindedness, but inadequate affective-sexual education.

Adoption as a solution. When the mature conjugal couple is stable from a material point of view and cannot have children of their own, there is still the possibility of adoption. This has been an option in Europe since Roman law and in Romanian principalities it has been mentioned in all codes of law since the 17th century (Mitrofan, 1991). Through adoption, couples without children can satisfy their parental needs and develop favorable conditions for long-term family stability. Nevertheless, in contemporary Romania the number of families that choose to adopt a child is small.

According to statistics released by the Romanian National Authority for the Protection of Child Rights at the beginning of 2005, there are about five million Romanian children under 18 years of age. From these, 2.2% (110,000 children) are supported by the Directorate of Social Assistance and Child Protection and are institutionalized, in placement, or supervised in the biological family. From 2003 to 2005 there were only 2,923 permanent national adoptions(National Authority for the Protection of the Children's Rights, 2005). This situation has been created first, by the difficulties inherent in the adoption procedure, which is very complex, and makes many requests. In Romania, adoption is still defined as a favor the state grants couples. Added to this, there are also some related emotional, economic, and cultural causes, including negative perceptions which limit the number of adoptions today.

The single-parent family: The Sunday father. The contemporary one-parent family attempts to find adequate answers to the pressures of the new socio-cultural context. The official economic responsibility of the parent concerning the children is a trend that extends to other major aspects of their life, such as education, professional orientation, leisure and so forth. The European protocol in this area is more complex and Romania has tried to implement all of these advanced principles. Just the payment of monthly alimony is not enough, because both parents are responsible for the care, education, protection and education of their children. The modern parental roles are not similar to the traditional profiles:

> The model of the modern mother brings to the forefront the concern for the encouragement and affective support of the child in his/her development and growth as happy person [. . .]. For the traditional father, parenthood is an obligation that society expects him to achieve, but for the modern father parenthood is, rather, an enjoyable privilege he assumes based on personal conviction. (p. 225)

A distinct and relatively new situation for contemporary Romanian families, created in the social assistance field, is represented by the new procedure of *placement*. Institutionalized children can be placed under the care of a certified individual for a pre-determined period of time. These individuals are officially called *maternal assistants* but informally, they are called *parents by profession*, because of their special relationship with the children. Although it is the recommended that they not use the classical terms *mother* and *father*, there are very few situations where the relationship between these adults and children are not the same as the parent/child relationship. Also, if the couple has their own children close to the age of the children who are placed with them, they usually develop sibling relationships. Thus, a real family is formed, albeit a *hand-crafted* one. This is not only a workable solution for adults' needs, but also for the emotional and security needs of the children (see Table 2).

At the end of the 1990s almost all institutionalized children were in placement centers, whereas today a reorientation toward substitute families has been observed (60.48% in substitute families and only 39.52% are in specialized institutions).

Contemporary Challenges for Parents

One challenge parents face today is decision-making regarding the size of the family they desire. The ideal number of children varies according to cultural values in the different historical regions of Romania.

TABLE 2. Situation of children's protection and placement.

Children in substitute families or in institutions Distributed as:	83,059	100%
children protected in substitute families	50,238	60.48%
• with maternal assistants employed by public services	15,588	18.77%
• with maternal assistants employed by private and state-authorized organizations	332	0.40%
• with relatives until the fourth grade	27,017	32.53%
• with other families or persons	6,071	7.31%
• assured for adoption	1,230	1.48%
children protected in institutions	32,821	39.52%
• placement in public centers	27,363	32.94%
• placement in private centers	5,458	6.57%

Source: National Authority for the Protection of Children's Rights. (2005, Jan 31) from
http://www.copii.ro/Prezentare_sistem_Ianuarie_2005.xls

In Moldavia in the east, a large number of children in the family have a high social value and important communitarian functions, even when economic conditions are not always adequate for optimal support. In Banat in the southwest, financial considerations are cited as reasons for a reduced number of children, usually only one. This is thought best so that land and property will not be divided, even when economic conditions are good. The main factors that directly influence contemporary family size, instead of traditional cultural prescriptions, include: the new public policies concerning birth control and family planning; the new challenges, opportunities and risks concerning parental roles; and the major changes in the socio-economical context.

Another challenge parents face is who should educate the child. Today, children's education is influenced by two strong socialization agents with high positive and/or negative impacts: the peer group and the mass media. The efficiency of the new media in quickly spreading ideas around the globe and the complete availability for exploring new challenges with friends (as a distinctive mark of personal freedom) represents serious contemporary challenges to the educational function of Romanian families. Extensive television offerings and access to all new information and communication technology are present in the everyday lives of the young generation. These electronic media promote new ideas and principles that are usually confirmed by other agents of socialization, such as friends, but are not necessarily convergent with parental principles. Thus, some tension is developing between generations, with significant consequences for all involved. In addition to this challenge, parents have to learn new educational approaches themselves and re-negotiate their position as basic socializing agents in their children's lives.

Some children may start their first class with a private tutor that assists them with homework, exams and other school tasks. To use a private tutor is sometimes a necessity, especially when parents cannot offer enough assistance or when there are special circumstances, but it also can be just a fashion or a subjective parental desire. The private tutor was a significant trend, especially during the period when admission to formal education was based only on examinations. Now, parts of these examinations have been replaced by teacher evaluations and the demand for tutorial services has decreased. The new perspective is to use a private tutor, starting from the first classes, to assist children with homework.

In Romania, to use a special person to care for children as an occasional parental substitute (as in a *babysitter*) is at the experimental level. There are several limitations to the growth of this kind of service: the absence of institutionalized training, too few professionals employed by specialized agencies, and the availability of relatives that can care for the children on a temporary basis. Even though the benefits can be significant, especially for parents involved in professional careers, this kind of service has a lot of unexplored potential. Starting in January 2006, the Romanian state began giving formal support in the form of monthly payments to mothers who do not remain at home to care for newborns (until the age of two years) and continue their professional activity. This payment, the equivalent of a minimum salary, is dedicated to assure the employment of a babysitter during this period of time.

Family Strengths in Romania: A Case Study of Three Families

Three Romanian families provide a glimpse into the family life of Romanians. Following the case study method, each family was observed and interviewed and data were recorded. As the families felt more comfortable with the interviews and observations, they were asked to identify other family members and acquaintances who were willing to talk about their family. Many other interviews were conducted with extended family members such as parents, cousins and siblings, as well as acquaintances such as neighbors and friends to provide triangulation, or agreement among sources for internal validity.

All data collected were analyzed for common themes. These themes were helpful in identifying characteristics of a strong family as described by these Romanians. Attention was also given to the differences found between families from different locations. Finally, differences were noted between what Romanians describe as a strong family and what families from the United States and other countries have described as a strong family in previous studies.

The experience of studying three Romanian families revealed the richness of their lives as well as the similarities and differences among them. These families had endured many hardships and yet they emerged as groups that were bound together and exhibited many family strengths as a result. These Romanian families willingly and in some cases, enthusiastically, provided insights into their lives that many families might seek to hide. Most of the family members and their acquaintances were not afraid to tell the very personal and gripping stories, no matter how painful or even ugly. Although these families shared common characteristics indicative of Romanian families, they each faced particular challenges within their family that differed from the other families.

The Romanian families in this study were alike in many ways and yet uniquely individual. These families were all affected in dramatic ways by the period of communism that structured their lives for so long. Economically, they struggled in various degrees to make a living and to protect their families. Emotionally, they were affected as was evident by the passionate stories that had marked their lives until the 1989 revolution. Even today, they are struggling to emerge from those years unscathed.

All the families shared the common bond of understanding what it means to be a family member. All had children and/or parents and all had experienced the loss of loved ones. They talked about their past and present understanding about what it meant to have a family and the importance of family in their lives. Even though none of these families had ever participated in a formal family education program, they had been taught by their experiences and most of them had a good understanding about what a strong family looks like.

The differences between these three families were few. Demographic differences pointed to the contrasts in living conditions and surroundings. The family from the village of Giarmata lived in somewhat primitive conditions without many facilities. They also lacked adequate transportation. Although within a few minutes of a large city and access to the same goods as all Romanians, their resources were limited and their lack of skills prevented them from achieving their goals. The family from rural Bran was geographically isolated but only by choice.

Because of their resources, they were able to travel and have the things that they wanted if they were willing to go after them. The family from the urban city of Constanta had many goods and services available to them in the large city but lacked the time and resources to take advantage of them. Their lives were stressed as they negotiated their days with thousands of other people around them.

Focusing on the three families, it became apparent from their answers to our questions and by observing them that they shared some common experiences that shaped their lives, both individually and as family members. What emerged from the study of these families are three factors that seem to describe their lives collectively. Although these families represented differences in geography, affluence, financial status and even family life stage, all three exhibited qualities of perseverance, respect and unity.

Perseverance

Enduring years of hardship and heartache has made an impact on the lives of many Romanians. These families are no exception. Each family told stories about the tough times, the crises and the deaths of their loved ones. Some of the stories were about financial hardships. The Giarmata family told about the money they lost when they trusted a friend and the hardship that resulted when they lost an expensive horse. They also reported the failure of their *magazinul* (general store) and how their agricultural endeavors sometimes ended in no profit or income. Some stories were about relationships. The grandmother and son of the Giarmata family talked about an alcoholic father and husband and their failed marriages. Both the Bran and the Constanta family spoke about the difficulties that caused strained relationships at one time. All the families have experienced the sadness of death. Even family members that had lived long and happy lives were missed and mourned. Others, like the great-grandmother of the Giarmata family, have had to deal with the untimely death of loved ones.

Other stories centered on the hardships that the communist period created. The Constanta family recalled the time that the *economic police* turned their home upside down and questioned their integrity. The Giarmata family gave many incidents in which the government had prevented them from succeeding.

Regardless of the kinds of hardships and difficulties that these families experienced, there were common reactions to them. Many of the family members talked about getting through the tough times and moving on.

Irina from the Bran family was described by her neighbor as being determined. The idea that a problem could not be overcome was not an option for these families as they worked together. Perhaps the most amazing reaction of all was the fact that many times these families did not even have any hope that the situation would get better. Dan of the Bran family recalled the time as perpetual negativity. During the communist period, choices and options were limited and yet, they kept going.

The family members spoke about the perseverance in continuing to provide for their family. The Bran family spoke about the sacrifices that they made for each other. The commitment level for most of the family members was associated with their continuing connection to the family and its preservation.

Respect

Respect plays a large part in the families of Romania. Each of the three families studied expressed the importance of respect in the family. Several of the family members referred to respect as an important ingredient in the values and belief system of the family. Doru from the Constanta family talked about respect as a key ingredient of the sacredness of the family as outlined in the Orthodox religion. Holding on to values such as respect was essential for the family during the communist period when they did not freely receive respect elsewhere.

Respect was mentioned as important in understanding each other's differences and interests. The Giarmata family had come to understand and respect the differences in religion within the family. Even though the logistics of the two religions, Romanian Orthodox and Catholicism have caused problems, they are satisfied to accept each other's beliefs. The Bran family also expressed respect for each other's opinions and interests as a strength. This family seemed to relish the idea of difference in their ideas and interests. Several family members spoke about the idea of family members *completing each other*. Celebrating the differences in each other was a crucial part of their lives. Acceptance of the other family members was important to all the families.

Another aspect of respect for these families dealt with the appreciation of accomplishments and achievements of other family members. The Constanta family talked about the achievements of the family members as being a victory for the whole family. Doru was especially interested in the achievements of his daughter and respected her accomplishments. The Bran family respected each others' endeavors and served as encouragers to support each other as they became successful in their activities and businesses.

For these three families, showing affection was often equated with respect for each other. Many family members spoke of doing things for each other as a sign of respect. The idea that actions speak louder than words seemed to be important to many of the family members. In reverse, they also spoke of showing respect as a sign of affection. For these Romanians, the idea that their family members deserved and earned respect was a traditional part of family life. Some examples given in showing respect were doing things for each other, caring for each other or buying presents.

Unity

A united family was often mentioned as the families described themselves and as their friends and neighbors described them. Being united was regarded as an important quality for a family. Some of the family members spoke of their unity as bringing them close. Maria of the Constanta family talked about the importance of unity when she said they were "preoccupied with sticking together." There are many ways in which these families displayed unity. It seemed important in a country that struggled with unity in government, that the family had unity.

Unity of purpose was found in all the families studied. The Giarmata family spoke of themselves as a work unit, working side by side to accomplish the task. The Bran family saw themselves as a group of individuals who work together to gather resources. Unity of purpose also included the way in which these families made plans together, set goals, and made decisions for the family. The Bran family spoke of being united in their view of money and their desire to work toward a common goal and succeeding. Dorel talked about making schedules, discussing events and deciding on how to spend money. Although the families recognize mistakes and failures they have made, they also work together to solve the problems that hinder their progress.

Communication is also a sign of unity for the families in this study. Their ability to compromise with each other was important. The Bran family's friends and neighbors were impressed by the family's ability to really listen to each other. The Constanta family also was found by acquaintances to be good communicators and they themselves reported spending a lot of time talking with each other. Spending time in communication was very special to the family. Many of the family members spoke about having nothing to hide from each other.

Time spent in family rituals was also a sign of unity for the families. It was obvious that holidays and birthdays were special for the members of the families in this study. Holidays centered on family and the members looked forward to the time together. Spending time with loved ones was especially important to the older family members. Perhaps they have come to realize the importance of family and how quickly the time passes in a family's life.

These three family strengths, found to be a part of the experiences in the Romanian families of this study have some relationship to the six qualities of strong families that have been identified by researchers in previous studies around the world (see Table 3). The quality of perseverance is directly tied to their abilities as families to handle and recover from crises. Each of the families have experienced crisis, many of which have involved the most basic needs of the family and have been sustained over long periods of time. One example would be when they experienced shortages of food and energy blackouts. The commitment exhibited by these family members also showed the perseverance of the individuals within the family. Although these families have weathered some challenges, they have been committed to staying together and working together to get through the tough times. In addition, perseverance was also expressed as a component of the spiritual well-being felt by many of the family members. Those family members who have strong belief systems continued to worship at their churches even though it was difficult during the communist period, especially for those not in the state-controlled Orthodox church. Even those that did not hold a strong faith seemed to be strengthened by a sense of hope that their lives would improve.

Respect was also part of the understanding of their spiritual well-being. Respect seemed to be deeply connected to their value system and

TABLE 3. Comparing family strengths in Romania with international research.

Romanian family strengths	Qualities of strong families as indicated in previous international studies
Perseverance	Ability to manage stress and crisis effectively Commitment to the family
Respect	Spiritual well-being Appreciation and affection for each other
Unity	Spending enjoyable time together Positive communication Commitment to the family

was an integral part of their daily family lives. Respect was also attached to the way in which these families expressed their appreciation and affection for each other. It was rare to see an outward sign of affection among these family members. It was also rare to hear appreciation expressed between family members. What was evident, however, was a great respect for each other. Many family members spoke very highly of each other in a way that seemed to serve, in some way, to protect each other.

Unity for these families centered on their commitment to each other and the time that they spent together working and playing. These families show commitment by the amount of time that they are together. Even the families that had many outside commitments, made an effort to spend time together. It was evident that they enjoyed being together. Communication for these families was also a sign of unity. Being able to listen to each other and to make compromises was important for the unity of the family. Sometimes those compromises were real sacrifices for the family members.

CONCLUSION

The Romanian family today is in a complex process of adaptation to the new economic and socio-cultural dimensions of the post-transition period. The main factors that directly influence the various models of the contemporary Romanian family include: the present effects of the communist period; the uncertainty and social incoherence of the post-revolutionary period; the new foundations of a capitalist society; and the perspective of the European Union integration process.

Under the pressure of a continuously changing social context, in its adaptive effort to function under new post-modern realities, the Romanian family can find valuable resources inside of the traditional cultural inheritance. The re-discovery of the old principles for life, verified for a long time in various social contexts, represent a valuable resource. The return to some unexhausted social resources in the context of Weberian *world disenchantment* (Gerth & Mills, 1946) could seem to be an odd solution. But, following the McDonaldization thesis of Ritzer (2000), the adaptability and pro-social aspects of Romanian tradition may successfully meet the challenges of an ultra-rationalized contemporary cultural pattern.

The Gender Barometer, financed by the Open Society Foundation, appeared in 2000. This sociological survey of a nationally-representative sample of 1,839 subjects, focused on Romanian attitudes and values. The survey found that the most important things for a successful marriage are: love (23.6%), trust (20.2%) and the couple having a personal home just for them alone (16%). The classical marital models sought to find adequate answers to the many pressures imposed by more or less favorable socio-political contexts. Facing new challenges, the new Romanian marital models will finally find the needed configurations to assure the optimal style of life for its members and their strengths as a family will be used to create strong families in the future.

REFERENCES

Alua°I., & Drãgan, I. (1971). *Contemporary French sociology*. Bucure°ti: Politicã.
Center Partnership for Equality *Gender barometer*. (2000). Retrieved May 15, 2006 from ttp://www.cpe.ro/romana/index.php?option=com_content&task=view&id=27&Itemid=48
Gerth, H. H., & Mills, C. W. (1946). Max Weber: Essays in Sociology. New York: Oxford University Press.
Ilut, P. (1995). *The family–Knowledge and assistance*. Cluj-Napoca, Romania: Argonaut.
Ilut, P. (2005). *The socio-psychology and the anthropology of the family*. Iasi, Romania: Polirom.
Mitrofan, N. (1984). *Love and the marriage*. Bucuresti, Romania: Editura °tiinþificã °i Enciclopedicã.
Mitrofan, N., & Mitrofan, I. (1991). *Family from* a to z. Bucuresti: Editura Stiintifica.
National Authority for the Protection of the Children's Rights (2005) *Statistics*. Retrieved May 15, 2006 from http://www.copii.ro/protect.htm
National Authority for the Protection of Children's Rights (2005) *Presentation* Retrieved May 15, 2006 from http://www.copii.ro/Prezentare_sistem_Ianuarie_2005.xls
Ritzer, G. (2000). *The McDonaldization of society*. London: Sage Publications.
Romanian Census Year Book (2004). Retrieved May 15, 2006 from http://www.insse.ro/anuar_2004/asr2004.htm
Stahl, H. (1977). *Rural family yesterday and today*. Bucure°ti: Ceres.
Tiras, C. (2003). *The life cycle. The sociology and anthropology of the age*. Unpublished PhD thesis. Cluj-Napoca: Babes-Bolyai University.
Voinea, M. (2000). *The young family–Socio-demographic particularities in the transition period*. In E.
Zamfir, I. Badescu, & C. Zamfir (Eds.). *The condition of Romanian society after ten years of transition* (pp. 734-737). Bucuresti: Expert.
Zamfir, C., & Vlãsceanu, L. (Eds.) (1993). *Dictionary of sociology*. Bucure°ti: Babel.

doi:10.1300/J002v41n03_09

Epilogue:
A Strengths-Based Conceptual Framework for Understanding Families World-Wide

John DeFrain

Sylvia M. Asay

SUMMARY. A positive and useful approach to conceptualizing families from a global perspective links family strengths, community strengths, and cultural strengths and demonstrates how families use these valued tools to meet the many challenges they face today in a difficult world. In this epilogue, we develop conceptual models from all three levels of strength from an analysis of the 18 countries discussed in this text, and two visual models are also presented in order to help students in family studies world-wide better understand and organize their thinking on the complexities of family life today. doi:10.1300/J002v41n03_10 *[Article copies available for a fee from The Haworth Document Delivery Service: 1-800-HAWORTH. E-mail address: <docdelivery@haworthpress.com> Website:*

John DeFrain is Extension Professor of Family and Community Development, Department of Child, Youth, and Family Studies, 135 Mabel Lee Hall, City Campus, University of Nebraska, Lincoln, NE 68588-0236, USA (E-mail: jdefrain1@unl.edu). Sylvia M. Asay is Associate Professor of Family Studies, Otto Olsen 205A, University of Nebraska, Kearney, NE 68849, USA (E-mail: asays@unk.edu).

Address correspondence to: John DeFrain.

[Haworth co-indexing entry note]: "Epilogue: A Strengths-Based Conceptual Framework for Understanding Families World-Wide." DeFrain, John, and Sylvia M. Asay. Co-published simultaneously in *Marriage & Family Review* (The Haworth Press, Inc.) Vol. 41, No. 3/4, 2007, pp. 447-466; and: *Strong Families Around the World: Strengths-Based Research and Perspectives* (ed: John DeFrain, and Sylvia M. Asay) The Haworth Press, Inc., 2007, pp. 447-466. Single or multiple copies of this article are available for a fee from The Haworth Document Delivery Service [1-800-HAWORTH, 9:00 a.m. - 5:00 p.m. (EST). E-mail address: docdelivery@haworthpress.com].

Available online at http://mfr.haworthpress.com
© 2007 by The Haworth Press, Inc. All rights reserved.
doi:10.1300/J002v41n03_10

<http://www.HaworthPress.com> © 2007 by The Haworth Press, Inc. All rights reserved.]

KEYWORDS. Family strengths world-wide, community strengths world-wide, cultural strengths world-wide

INTRODUCTION

Drawing conclusions about families on a global level is a most difficult task. As a starting point, we have chosen to use the discussions of the 18 countries presented here, which represent a diverse sample of all the major regions of the world. The variety of information that the authors have provided is fascinating and each presentation is unique. Perhaps that is our greatest reason for being delighted by their work: We asked eminent professionals world-wide, representing a wide variety of countries and cultures, to write about the difficulties families face today and how families use their strengths to meet these challenges; the 43 co-authors approached the task at hand from their own unique individual and cultural perspectives, and the diversity of their responses is remarkable.

From the very beginning, we believed the creation of this volume would make two major contributions to the field of family studies: First, we thought the text would help the reader conceptualize families around the world from a strengths-based perspective. We believe this is a useful way of organizing our thinking about the multiplicity of families living in so many diverse cultures, and have found that without some way to do so it can be very easy for students of the field to become overwhelmed by the differences and not be able to see the striking similarities among families from culture to culture. It simply is too easy to get lost in the cultural trees of difference and miss the cultural forest of similarities. Family strengths–those qualities demonstrating love and care for each other that help families succeed in the difficult tasks of life–are a positive, unifying conceptual frame for understanding families.

Second, we believed from the very beginning when we started working on this research project that the act of creating the text and analyzing the contributors' work on families in 18 countries would also advance the level of theoretical understanding of family strengths globally. The fact was that many of the countries represented in the text had not had studies of family strengths conducted there before, and a discussion of strengths and challenges in their cultures would be a catalyst for new investigations. This proved to be the case for, as we have seen, the research project resulted in a good deal of new thinking from a strengths-based perspective in many countries, and in a number of countries, new research on family strengths was conducted specifically for the articles the writers were developing.

Organizing this wealth of new insights into a few broad conclusions seems in some ways to minimize the depth of understanding and meaning that our co-authors present. The synopsis of a great and moving work of literature pales in the light of the work itself; as the authors of *Cliff's Notes* themselves argue, *Cliff's* version is no substitute for the real thing. And yet, we also believe that it remains very useful to think about global family strengths broadly, and the International Family Strengths Model in our mind remains a practical way to conceptualize family emotional health and well-being. In the final analysis, generally speaking, *people are people are people and families are families are families.* There does not seem to be any way to get around this metaphorical insight.

The strengths of families from culture to culture, when compared to each other, are remarkably similar and give us common ground around the world upon which to unite and develop mutual understanding. If all cultures have families in all their remarkable diversity as the foundation for their cultures, and if family strengths from culture to culture are much more similar than different as we remain convinced, a powerful bond can be built among nations when this observation from research world-wide is broadly disseminated. But the question remains: Can we find a way to love our children and our families more than we love war?

BOTH MICRO- AND MACRO-SOCIAL PERSPECTIVES

As our co-authors in this volume make exceedingly clear, to understand family strengths dictates that one also understands the cultural contexts in which families live. The lives people live within the context of their family, their extended family, the community, and the broader national culture cannot be easily understood, labeled, or judged. Myriad external factors enmesh and influence families and sometimes prove helpful and useful to individual families, and in other cases prove harmful and demanding. Countless families from culture to culture live in a desperately confounding milieu, and to judge them without understanding the social context in which they live can be patently unfair.

Thus, our discussion here will continue to include both a look at family strengths around the world from the *micro-familial perspective*: What, precisely, are the qualities that help to make families succeed in the difficult process of loving and caring for each other and surviving in a world laden with difficulties? And, at the same time, we will examine families from a *macro-familial perspective* in the light of the community, national and cultural strengths in which they are inextricably embedded.

Upon examining the various family strengths studies conducted around the world in the past three decades, we see that the researchers generally come to the conclusion that the qualities of strong families are amazingly similar, regardless of culture. Study Table 1 below carefully and we think you will come to the same conclusion.

TABLE 1. Dimensions of family strength as delineated by prominent researchers.

Theorists and Countries	Dimensions
Beavers & Hampson (1990). U.S.A.	Centripetal/centrifugal interaction, closeness, parent coalitions, autonomy, adaptability, egalitarian power, goal-directed negotiation, ability to resolve conflict, clarity of expression, range of feelings, openness to others, empathic understanding
Billingsley (1986). U.S.A.	Strong family ties, strong religious orientation, educational aspirations/achievements
Curran (1983). U.S.A.	Togetherness, respect and trust, shared leisure, privacy valued, shared mealtime, shared responsibility, family rituals, communication, affirmation of each other, religious love, humor/play
Epstein, Bishop, Ryan, Miller, & Keitner (1993). Canada.	Affective involvement, behavior control, communication
Geggie, DeFrain, Hitchcock, & Silberberg (2000). Australia.	Communication (open, positive, honest, including humor), togetherness, sharing activities, affection, support, acceptance, commitment, resilience
Kantor & Lehr (1974). U.S.A.	Affect, power
Kryson, Moore, & Zill (1990). U.S.A.	Commitment to family, time together, encouragement of individuals, ability to adapt, clear roles, communication, religious orientation, social connectedness
Mberengwa & Johnson (2003). Botswana.	Consensus as a means of settling differences, anger management, concern for the welfare of one's kin, valuing their culture, respect toward others, *kgotla* (community development associations) for strengthening neighborhoods

Theorists and Countries	Dimensions
Olson, McCubbin, Barnes, Larsen, Muxen, & Wilson (1989); Olson & DeFrain (2006); Olson & Olson (2000). U.S.A.	Strong marriage, high family cohesion, good family flexibility, effective coping with stress and crisis, positive couple and family communication
Otto (1962, 1963). U.S.A.	Shared religious and moral values; love, consideration and understanding; common interests, goals and purposes; love and happiness of children; working and playing together; sharing specific recreational activities
Reiss (1981). U.S.A.	Coordination, closure
Sani & Buhannad (2003). United Arab Emirates.	Patriarchal family structure; family-arranged marriages; gender-based rights, responsibilities and privileges; strong emotional family bonds (*muwada*); extended family (*dhurriyah*); living with or next extended family members; frequent consultation; elders as role models and advisors; crises are tests from Allah; Islamic beliefs (*taqwa*) and practices provide optimal guildeines; collectivism over individualism; the government is supportive of individual, couple and family well-being
Stinnett, DeFrain, & colleagues (1977, 1985, 2002). U.S.A.	Appreciation and affection, commitment, positive communication, enjoyable time together, spiritual well-being, effective management of stress and crisis
Xia, Xie, & Zhou (2004); Xie, DeFrain, Meredith, & Combs (1996); Xu, & Ye (2002). China.	Togetherness and time together across three generations; love, care, and commitment; communication; family support; spirituality (at peace with nature, at peace with oneself, at peace with others, at peace with the world); family oriented and harmonious
Yoo (2004); Yoo, DeFrain, Lee, Kim, Hong, Choi, & Ahn (2004). Korea.	Respect, commitment, appreciation and affection, positive communication, sharing values and goals, role performing, physical health, connectedness with social systems, economic stability, ability to solve problems

However, family strengths are based in culture and, thus, are likely to look somewhat different as they are exhibited from place to place, country to country. Using food for an analogy, everyone around the world eats but we eat different things that are prepared and served in different ways.

Although the first studies of family strengths were done in America and, thus, began with a distinctly American flavor to them, the panoply of family strengths as exhibited in cultures world-wide appears to be universal. In the articles of this volume we have heard the authors echo this same conclusion many times.

FAMILY STRENGTHS WORLD-WIDE

Using the International Family Strengths Model as a template for our discussion, we will discuss the strengths our co-authors have delineated:

- Appreciation and affection
- Positive communication
- Commitment to the family
- Enjoyable time together
- A sense of spiritual well-being
- The ability to manage stress and crisis effectively

Families around the world show their *appreciation and affection* for each other in various ways. In war-torn Somalia, "moral support becomes the currency of love and affection, a reflex strengthening of bonds within and beyond family structures." In New Zealand, the Maori families "exude a quality known as 'aroha'–or warm love. It quickly enfolds a stranger and hospitality is generous." Koreans talk about "affection (love) and affinity, expression of positive feeling and gratitude and awareness of the family as the psychological nest."

Positive communication is another strength that is valued around the world. In Russia, strong families strive to include all family members in their problem-solving and "respect the opinions of each." In Kenya "communication is a strong bonding factor where couples and children are free with one another and with their immediate relatives in matters pertaining to family life." Studies in Mexico have shown that solidarity can be found in those families who have a strong sense of cooperation.

Having a *commitment to the family* is an important characteristic of strong families. The article about India discusses the fact that an emphasis on rituals and customs "fosters feelings of security and belongingness and convey the message that family bonds are immutable, dependable, and lifelong." Israeli families see commitment as an expectation and the authors of the article believe that it is central to their resiliency as they face the violence that permeates life in their country. Commitment is exhibited by family members in Romania in the form of perseverance. Many families had endured hardship during the transition away from communism but were committed to staying together and working together to get through the tough times.

Strong families find ways to be together and enjoy sharing time with each other. *Enjoyable time together* in Greece usually involves food and the article relates that, "the image of being together with three generations every Sunday is not rare." The notion of *familism* in Brazil encourages close family ties and fosters strong relationships. The authors suggest that "frequent contact with extended and nuclear family members provides ample opportunities for multiple attachment relationships to develop."

As in previous family strength studies, spirituality and religion can take many forms. There are many ways to create *a sense of spiritual well-being* within the family. Many of the countries represented within this volume opted to speak about the role of religion in family life as a way of achieving spiritual well-being. The article about families in Mexico points to a set of values that includes happiness, optimism, hope, and faith that are established by Catholicism, the primary religion in that country. The author of the article on Botswana speaks about the concept of *botho*. The Setswana saying, "Let not our children be without soul," points to the desire and responsibility to address the moral development of children in the family. In Russia, where organized religion was severely limited under communism, the article points out that strong families "create their own mini-environment of activity" that conveys moral and spiritual beliefs. The author emphasizes that faith in each other is important and necessary for the Russian family.

Many of the countries represented in this effort have experienced tremendous upheaval as a result of political crisis or natural disaster. Examples of this include Somalia's civil war, Romania and Russia's difficult transition from communism, and the HIV/AIDS crisis in South Africa, Kenya and Botswana. Others pointed out the internal struggles of changing gender roles, structures and values within the family, such as the social challenges pointed out in the Korean article. Strong families are able to handle these stressors no matter what the circumstance. *The ability to manage stress and crisis effectively*, which demonstrates the resiliency of families around the world, is evident as you read article after article. As the author of the article on the family in Oman declares, there is confidence in the fact that traditions and heritage will "sustain the family and give it the strength it requires to survive future challenges."

COMMUNITY STRENGTHS WORLD-WIDE

Strong families contribute to the well-being of communities, and strong communities enhance the development of strong families. A number of important community strengths are described by our co-authors:

- A supportive environment that genuinely values families, and a general willingness and natural generosity infused in the culture to help when families are in need
- An effective educational delivery system
- Religious communities for families seeking this kind of support
- Family-service programs developed by government and non-governmental organizations for families who cannot find the help they need from their own extended family, friends and neighbors
- A safe, secure and healthful environment

A supportive environment. Throughout this volume it is evident that the contributions of the community to the family are undeniable. It is this connection to other individuals and families that serves as a safety net for many families. The author of the article on Canada reports that the government has suggested that families increase involvement with their community (including extended family, neighbors, and churches) to strengthen the family. Specific wording in the document suggests that "these groups must reclaim their natural functions as agents of family support."

Many societies are relatively collectivist in nature and rely on the group for support. As the Korean co-authors point out, "The concept of *We-ness* for the Korean includes homogeneity, unity, interdependence, mutual protection and acceptance as its intrinsic properties." Even those countries with a more individualistic orientation find that a supportive environment within the community is essential. As we see from the article about Botswana, it may be the community that is able to help families transition to a modern society.

Communities perform many functions that affect the family. As noted in several articles, the arranged marriage is an example of community function that impacts families. In this volume, we find discussions of arranged marriage within the context of the Indian, Omani and Chinese experience. It takes a community effort to match potential mates between families. It is also the community which will successfully support changes away from these practices to individual choice.

Another important community function for families is *an effective educational delivery system.* Several articles have mentioned the importance of education for their countries. This is an important function usually delivered by the community. During the communist period in Romania, the state controlled the education and care of children from the third month of life. Until the fall of communism in 1989, the community took full responsibility for education of its young. The authors of the article on Romania believe that this type of institutionalized form of education is difficult to change even when it may not be the best for the child or the family. Informal education is also a function of the community. The South African co-authors write about *indigenous knowledge systems* that have educated young people for centuries. These localized educational systems are based within the community and information is passed on by word of mouth. It is a precious picture of elderly community members sitting down with young boys and girls and visiting about life.

Religious communities for families seeking this kind of support. The religious community may play an important role in enhancing spiritual well-being for many families and may also play an important role in supporting families in a variety of other ways. Several articles speak about the social support that the faith community provides for families. The article on Israel describes the role of religion as that of a social regulator in terms of issues such as marriage and passing on values. The article on Botswana talks about the community prayers for marriages. In Somalia, the influence of religion is used to justify behavior and becomes the vehicle for social change within the community.

Family-service programs developed by government and non-governmental organizations for families. Social services provided by communities also play an important role in family life. In some countries such as China, family policy is well-defined and provides needed services to families within communities. The authors report that, "Parents, schools, and communities work closely together to set up programs that ensure the proper development of children today." Other articles reveal a different story and finding access to services are mentioned as challenges.

For many, the dichotomy between urban and rural, wealthy and poor becomes the dividing line between adequate and inadequate services. The article on Brazil points out that there are many regional disparities between what the communities are able to offer families. Government-sponsored welfare programs that are needed by families in the poorest areas are lacking. The article on Mexico reveals that 57% of families do not have access to social services.

A safe, secure and healthful environment. Around the world, the community usually takes on the responsibility for protecting individuals and families. A safe environment is necessary for families to carry out their functions. The article on Greece notes that the protection of the family is a component of public law. This is not the case in many countries that have been ravaged by terrorism, war and natural disaster. The civil war in Somalia has forced many to flee their country. Even though Somalis are nomadic and are accustomed to the difficulties inherent in that way of life, civil war has taken a far greater toll on the population due to starvation, maiming and killing. The authors of the article on Israel share their perspectives on the effect that relentless terrorism has on a community. "The devastating impact of this kind of violence is ubiquitous, powerful, and inescapable."

Traditional societies have elaborate and effective social security systems built into the community. Margaret Mead has said, "If we are to achieve a richer culture, rich in contrasting values, we must recognize the whole gamut of human potentialities, and so weave a less arbitrary social fabric, one in which each diverse human gift will find a fitting place" (Mead, 1935, p. 322). The difficulty arises when the community is not able to provide that safety net, as is the case with so many societies in which families have been displaced or in the case of urbanization. Rural-to-urban migration has brought about tremendous changes that have been highlighted by the authors of several articles within this volume. In the article on Somalia for example, the author writes: "Urbanization and modernization has removed the previous communal spirit of openness and sharing, with the younger generation more possessive of their privacy and less willing to share." Other changes that have occurred to weaken the community include lack of services for families, multicultural strife, urban isolation, health crises such as the HIV/AIDS pandemic, and a lack of trust.

CULTURAL STRENGTHS WORLD-WIDE

So far in this discussion we have seen how family and community strengths reinforce each other. There is a third level or dimension that we would like to include in the discussion, which could be called cultural strengths. These include:

• A rich cultural history
• Shared cultural meanings

- A stable political process
- A viable economy
- An understanding of the global society

The *rich cultural history* of these countries needs to be considered in our efforts to understand families in their social context. The heritage and historical legacy of each country contributes to the strengths of the families, giving them meaning, direction and inspiration for dealing with life's challenges. As you read through the history of each country you realize the bequest given by the people who have come before them to create a culture unlike any other, each unique in its own way. Greece is a country whose cultural heritage seems to call out to future generations, giving them a foundation and a purpose. The author talks about the instability of the area for more than three thousand years and how these constant changes and struggles have prepared the people with a fighting spirit and a sense of determination. Likewise, the article on India emphasizes how it is one of the oldest cultures in the world with a rich heritage. The author of the Russian article spends a significant amount of the beginning of the article in examination of the history and importance of understanding the heritage of a great people who have suffered throughout time. Individuals and families draw strength from knowing who they are and find comfort from a deep sense of belonging.

Shared cultural meanings. Strong families also share meanings with their culture. Many of the articles include words or maxims that are indigenous to that country. The authors sometimes struggle with translation because there is no way to explain the rich meaning or consequence of the statement in just a few words. It is so embedded in the fabric of their lives that its meaning is only something that those within the culture can really understand and appreciate. Examples of this can be found in the idea of *botho* in Botswana, the *mauri* in New Zealand, *ubuntu* in South Africa, and the *oikos* in Greece. Even the concepts of *filial piety* in China and Korea or *apartheid* South Africa are difficult for those in the western world to grasp without some explanation of the philosophical and historical background. Furthermore, the concepts may be understood at the information or knowledge level but the genuine emotional meaning will be quite different for those who have grown up in the culture and have shared personal experience.

A stable political process and *a viable economy* are beneficial for families. The political environment of a nation affects families in significant ways. A stable government provides an atmosphere in which families do not have to concern themselves with the daily responsibilities of the country, although some individuals may choose to involve them-selves in the political process. When the political process is functioning well, people may come to expect that the government will continue to provide and protect with a consistency that can be trusted. In that way, they are able to build on that stable base and have expectations that allow them to construct a bright future for themselves.

An example of this is found in the United States. Families have come to expect the stability of the government and the relative predictability of the political process. This, however, can also be a problem in that it breeds complacency and the feeling that the individual or family has no voice in the government.

The lack of a stable government has been mentioned in many of the articles in this volume. Families that live in times of political upheaval cannot rely on the political process for support, which makes family life more difficult and in some cases dangerous. In Somalia, for example, mass killings, starvation, destruction of resources, and separation of families have resulted from the political civil war that has divided the country.

A stable economy contributes to the ability of families to provide for themselves and gather resources to sustain life. In reading through the articles in this volume, almost every author has addressed issues related to economics. All families use resources to carry out their daily activities. When a country is facing economic failure, the families of that country suffer.

Just as political instability can destabilize families, economic pressures and problems often cause societies to make adjustments ultimately forcing families to change the way they carry out their functions. In some cases, families are forced to concentrate their efforts solely on survival. Although this tends to leave little time for building family strengths, the article on Russia points out that during conditions of economic hardship, there are several strategies that strong families implement while working together for solutions. The article on Mexico points out that one strategy advocates for more families members to enter the workforce, particularly women. The author suggests that although it is a viable solution to the economic crisis for families, it has also changed the basic structure of many families.

Another strategy has been migration which has also forced families to change while they are separated from each other. This is not only true for Mexico but was mentioned as a challenge for families in other countries such as Botswana.

Political instability and economic hardship are significant stressors in the lives of families and add to the difficulty of creating warm and loving family bonds. But stable politics and a vibrant economy do not guarantee that each individual family will be strong, loving and happy. And there are many families who may be caught up in a desperate political and economic environment, but who still manage somehow to create positive emotional connections with each other even as the instability of the social environment swirls around them.

An understanding of the global society. Learning from other cultures is an important tool for building strong families. Each culture develops creative ways for dealing with the many challenges that life brings. Knowledge of other cultures adds innumerable options for families as they create a meaningful, stable, and joyful life together.

Over a decade ago, Marshall McLuhan (1994) argued that a global village would eventually take the place of different cultures. When one examines the impact of the globalization of the business world, the Internet, movies, and other technologies, it would be easy to come to the conclusion that it may be possible to meld all world cultures into one. However, this idea has met with considerable criticism in terms of the importance of the vibrant differences around the world that make each culture unique. Who would want to live in such a sterile and monotonous world?

Although the world is not likely to ever become uniformly and universally the same, global influences are inevitable. Globalization has impacted countless families for better and worse, not only in the modern, developed countries but the more traditional agrarian societies as well. As we have seen in some of the articles, globalization may have contributed to the erosion of traditions such as familism and patriarchal structures by advancing the common vision that what a family should be is usually the picture of the family from the western perspective.

Fortunately, when we read carefully through the articles it becomes strikingly clear that the differences run deep and no matter how far technology advances or globalization brings people together, it cannot erase the unique history of a people and their way of life.

Globalization also has some advantages for families. Increasing information and being aware of the world outside provides a new perception of how one fits into the world and gives a sense of the human interconnectedness with all people around the globe. Increased cultural understanding erases misunderstanding and reduces fear.

In an important sense, the purpose of this volume is to help inform the global community. Knowing about strong families in other cultures helps families everywhere understand the components of what constitutes a healthy family. One key ingredient of this exercise is that it must be reciprocal. Any one culture that assumes they have all the answers has not really examined the strengths of other cultures. Although each culture may display family strengths in their own way, knowing there is a connection to strong families all around the world serves to reinforce the role and importance of the family in every society.

THE INTEGRATION OF FAMILY, COMMUNITY AND CULTURAL STRENGTHS: TWO VISUAL MODELS

From a visual perspective, how do family strengths, community strengths and cultural strengths fit together and mutually influence each other? Borrowing from the Ecological Model established by Bronfenbrenner (1977), the idea of concentric or nested circles is one way to view the three areas of strengths with family strengths in the center and moving out and away from the single family unit to the broader culture context (see Figure 1).

Ecological theory includes the microsystem, mesosystem, exosystem, and the macrosystem. The mesosystem involves the interrelationship of the near environment. This system represents the face-to-face interactions with others. The immediate family is found in this system. In some societies, this basic system would also include extended family or those that form close associations such as within a small village or a group that represents family although not blood related. For example, in the article on South Africa, the social-cultural and social-political climate has forced families to create household structures formed by the availability of resources and the ability to sustain its members rather than a group whose relationship is strictly formed through kinship.

The mesosystem and exosystem involve interaction between contexts. For families around the world, this can represent many different types of places in which people are connected and belong. In a relatively individualistic society such as the United States, this may represent very few connections–the school system for children, the workplace, and a few others. Many cultures emphasize the extended family as part of their connections. In Mexico, the extended family is the source of economic support, emotional support and personal satisfaction. In China, filial piety, which focuses on respect and obligation to the family rather than individual identity, creates a family network in which the extended family

FIGURE 1. The Relationship of Family, Community, and Cultural Strengths: Concentric Circles. In this model, the three areas of strengths move out and away from the single-family unit to the broader culture context related in a concentric fashion. The three areas not only interact from dimension to dimension but also have depth, thus, interacting on various levels.

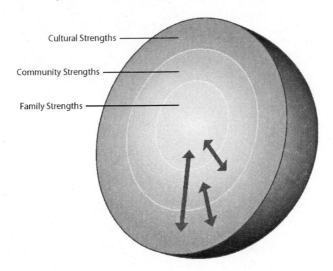

plays a critical role socially, emotionally, and economically. In other societies, there may be more connections. For example, in Kenya the *harambee* philosophy has formed communities where families work together to provide the social needs of everyone by forming connections to educational, medical and social institutions.

The macrosystem encompasses the outside influences. This system represents influences that are culturally imbedded. Deep cultural meaning is found in the macrosystem. For example, the idea of filial piety is a macrosystem within Chinese culture. Children may not be taught to honor their elders specifically by their parents (microsystem) or within the school system by their teachers (mesosystem) but it is found to permeate society as a whole (macrosystem). History is also included within the macrosystem. The historical background influences the microsystem and mesosystem of the people within those countries. This can be seen in the articles about Russian and Greek families.

As with the Ecological Model, the influence between the circles is reciprocal in that the influence of the family on the community and culture can be as significant as the influence that the community and culture have on the individual local family unit. From an examination of families around the world, families seem to take on different structures in different circumstances. An example of this is the South African households where the authors describe a family that is more "fluid" and results in more "complex family structures." Here the household is one of social organization and includes those who live together and contribute income and practical help. The common trend of all families, however, is to accomplish tasks such as childbearing, providing for the basic needs of family members, establishing social support networks, and essentially establishing family traditions. The way in which these tasks are realized ultimately influences the way society functions.

Another way to visualize how family, community, and culture strengths relate to each other is to construct a Venn diagram (see Figure 2). In this model, we might visualize the strong family as that family where the three areas of strengths intersect. A family which possesses not only internal family strengths but enjoys support from the community and a

FIGURE 2. The Relationship of Family, Community, and Cultural Strengths: A Venn Diagram. In this model, the family, community, and cultural strengths intersect. Although this intersection represents the strong family, when one or more areas are lacking, a state of equilibrium may be reached and a strong family is still possible.

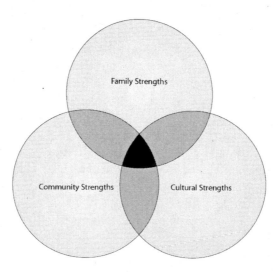

positive and empowering heritage is, indeed, in an excellent position in the world.

Unlike what may be imagined in the Venn diagram, however, those who are living in parts of the world torn apart by war, famine, or harsh political conditions can still create and maintain strong families, though the task becomes much more difficult because of external stressors impinging upon the family. In difficult circumstances such as these, families search for a new state of equilibrium within the community and/or within their culture. It could be that a family unit is preserved and thrives but the country is politically unstable. In this type of situation, the stability of the families is dependent almost solely on the strengths of the individual family and their immediate community. Even though there may be chaos in the larger environment, the family is still able to continue to nurture each other and to function as a family even though their cultural heritage is threatened. In this model, this equilibrium would be represented by the intersection of only family strengths and community strengths. When political order is re-established, cultural strengths will again have a positive influence within the family.

Another example can be found among the articles that have examined the changes that urbanization has forced among families. In South Africa, the author talks about the situation where individual families have been separated due to the need for one or more of the members to find jobs in the cities leaving families vulnerable and isolated. The authors note that, "The culture of sharing provides a buffer system for the many indigent rural families who are often without any form of social support or safety." In this case, the community and culture have intersected to meet the needs of the family in the absence of the family unit.

Other articles talk about the absence of community support. The article about Russia talks about the lack of family services. The author states that the family "may be the only island of stability in a boundless ocean of uncertainty generated by the dysfunction of social institutions." In addition, families are more divided and spend much more time in individual actions leaving little time for community activities. Here the family strengths and the cultural strengths are the two categories that carry the family through during this time in history.

In some cases where the entire culture is in a state of transition, the absence of community and cultural strengths leaves the family unit alone to survive only on their our internal strengths. One example of this is Somalia. The authors have shown that significant changes in circumstances have taken place for the predominantly nomadic population. This group of people, who for centuries have known the ways of independence and pride in caring for their own, are suddenly faced with the necessity of living in urban areas to survive. They become overwhelmed by the transition and are forced to give up their traditions and communal ways of living while at the same time often do not have the community support and the basics they need.

Both of these visual models illustrate the truly amazing ways that families all over the world are able to use their strengths to triumph over even the most horrendous conditions and insecure situations. It is also strengths that help families who live in relative prosperity and freedom to rise above complacency and the subtle erosion of the family. Certainly communities and cultural heritage contribute to the stability and support of families in all types of circumstances but ultimately it seems that the individual internal strengths of families provide the basic foundation for what keeps the family from gradually disappearing.

In conclusion, it is our belief that this study of the strengths of families, communities, and cultures around the world is still in its infancy. We know that we have only scratched the surface in our examination of global families. What we understand today may change tomorrow as we learn more about the diverse ways that families express themselves within the contexts of their local communities and cultural heritage. Over time, we hope to uncover new truths about how families live, and change, and grow in the environments where they live. We look forward to the journey.

REFERENCES

Beavers, W. R., & Hampson, R. B. (1990). *Successful families.* New York: Norton.

Billingsley, A. (1986). *Black families in White America.* Englewood Cliffs, NJ: Prentice Hall.

Bronfenbrenner, U. (1977). Toward an experimental ecology of human development. *American Psychologist, 32,* 582-590.

Curran, D. (1983). *Traits of a healthy family.* Minneapolis: Winston Press.

DeFrain, J., DeFrain, N., & Lepard, J. (1994). Family strengths and challenges in the South Pacific: An exploratory study. *International Journal of the Sociology of the Family, 24*(2), 25-47.

DeFrain, J., & Stinnett, N. (2002). Family strengths. In J. J. Ponzetti et al. (Eds.), International encyclopedia of marriage and family (2nd ed.). New York: Macmillan Reference Group, pps. 637-642.

Epstein, N. B., Bishop, D. S., Ryan, C., Miller, L., & Keitner, G. (1993). The McMaster model of family functioning. In F. Walsh (Ed.), *Normal family processes* (pp. 138-160). New York: Guilford Press.

Geggie, J., DeFrain, J., Hitchcock, S., & Silberberg, S. (2000, June). Family strengths research project. Newcastle, N.S.W., Australia: Family Action Centre, University of Newcastle.

Kantor, D., & Lehr, W. (1974). *Inside the family*. San Francisco: Jossey-Bass.

Krysan, M., Moore, K. A., & Zill, N. (1990). *Identifying successful families: An overview of constructs and selected measures*. Washington, DC: Child Trends, Inc. [2100 M St., NW, Suite 610] and the U.S. Department of Health & Human Services, Office of the Assistant Secretary for Planning and Evaluation.

Mberengwa, L. R., & Johnson, J. M. (2003). Strengths of Southern African families and their cultural context. *Journal of Family and Consumer Sciences, 95*(1), 20-25.

McLuhan, M. (1994). *Understanding media: The extensions of man*. Cambridge, MA: The MIT Press.

Mead, M. (1935). Sex and temperament in three primitive societies. New York: Morrow.

Moore, K. A., Chalk, R., Scarpa, J., & Vandivere, S. (2002, August). Family strengths: Often overlooked, but real. Child Trends Research Brief [4301 Connecticut Avenue, NW, Suite 100, Washington, DC 20008]. Website: www.childtrends.org

Olson, D. H., & DeFrain, J. (2006). *Marriages and families: Intimacy, strengths, and diversity* (5th ed.). New York: McGraw-Hill Higher Education.

Olson, D. H., McCubbin, H. I., Barnes, H., Larsen, A., Muxen, M., & Wilson, M. (1989). *Families: What makes them work* (2nd ed.). Los Angeles, CA: Sage.

Otto, H. A. (1962). What is a strong family? *Marriage and Family Living, 24*, 77-81.

Otto, H. A. (1963). Criteria for assessing family strength. *Family Process, 2*, 329-339.

Reiss, D. (1981). *The family's construction of reality*. Cambridge, MA: Harvard University Press.

Sani, A., & Buhannad, N. (2003). Family strengths in Islam: Perceptions of women in the United Arab Emirates. *National Council on Family Relations Report, 48*(4), F12-F15.

Stinnett, N., & O'Donnell, M. (1996). *Good kids*. New York: Doubleday.

Stinnett, N., & DeFrain, J. (1985). *Secrets of strong families*. Boston: Little, Brown.

Stinnett, N., & Sauer, K. (1977). Relationship characteristics of strong families. *Family Perspective, 11*(3), 3-11.

Xia, Y., Xie, X., & Zhou, Z. (2004). Case study: Resiliency in immigrant families. In V. L. Bengtson, A. Acock, K. Allen, P. Dilworth-Anderson, & D. Klein (Eds.). *Sourcebook of family theory and research* (pp. 108-111). Thousand Oaks, CA: Sage.

Xie, X., DeFrain, J., Meredith, W., & Combs, R. (1996). Family strengths in the People's Republic of China. *International Journal of the Sociology of the Family, 26*(2), 17-27.

Xu, A., & Ye, W. (2002). Quality of marriage: Major predictors of stability. *Shanghai Research Quarterly, 4*, 103-112.

Yoo, J. J. (2004). A study of the development of the Korean Family Strengths Scale for strengthening the family. *Journal of the Korean Association of Family Relations, 9*(2), 119-151.

Yoo, Y. J., DeFrain, J., Lee, I., Kim, S., Hong, S., Choi, H., & Ahn, J. (2004, June). Korean family strengths research project: A national project funded by the Korea Research Foundation. Seoul, Korea: Institute of Korean Family Strengths and Kyunghee University.

doi:10.1300/J002v41n03_10

Index

© 2007 by The Haworth Press, Inc. All rights reserved.

467